Pediatric Rheumatology Comes of Age: Part I

Editors

YUKIKO KIMURA
LAURA E. SCHANBERG

RHEUMATIC DISEASE CLINICS OF NORTH AMERICA

www.rheumatic.theclinics.com

Consulting Editor
MICHAEL H. WEISMAN

November 2021 • Volume 47 • Number 4

ELSEVIER

1600 John F. Kennedy Boulevard • Suite 1800 • Philadelphia, Pennsylvania, 19103-2899
http://www.theclinics.com

RHEUMATIC DISEASE CLINICS OF NORTH AMERICA Volume 47, Number 4
November 2021 ISSN 0889-857X, ISBN 13: 978-0-323-89680-1

Editor: Lauren Boyle
Developmental Editor: Karen Solomon

Rheumatic Disease Clinics of North America (ISSN 0889-857X) is published quarterly by Elsevier Inc., 360 Park Avenue South, New York, NY 10010-1710. Months of issue are February, May, August, and November. Business and editorial offices: 1600 John F. Kennedy Boulevard, Suite 1800, Philadelphia, PA 19103-2899. Periodicals postage paid at New York, NY and additional mailing offices. Subscription prices are USD 362.00 per year for US individuals, USD 1000.00 per year for US institutions, USD 100.00 per year for US students and residents, USD 427.00 per year for Canadian individuals, USD 1045.00 per year for Canadian institutions, USD 100.00 per year for Canadian students/residents, USD 465.00 per year for international individuals, USD 1045.00 per year for international institutions, and USD 230.00 per year for foreign students/residents. To receive student/ resident rate, orders must be accompanied by name of affiliated institution, date of term, and the *signature* of program/residency coordinator on institution letterhead. Orders will be billed at individual rate until proof of status received. Foreign air speed delivery is included in all *Clinics* subscription prices. All prices are subject to change without notice. **POSTMASTER:** Send address changes to *Rheumatic Disease Clinics of North America*, Elsevier Health Sciences Division, Subscription Customer Service, 3251 Riverport Lane, Maryland Heights, MO 63043. **Customer Service: 1-800-654-2452 (US and Canada). From outside of the US and Canada: 314-447- 8871. Fax: 314-447-8029. For print support, e-mail: JournalsCustomerService-usa@elsevier.com. For on- line support, e-mail: JournalsOnlineSupport-usa@elsevier.com.**

Reprints. For copies of 100 or more of articles in this publication, please contact the Commercial Reprints Department, Elsevier Inc., 360 Park Avenue South, New York, New York, 10010-1710; Tel.: +1-212-633- 3874, Fax: +1-212-633-3820, and E-mail: reprints@elsevier.com.

Rheumatic Disease Clinics of North America is covered in *MEDLINE/PubMed (Index Medicus), Current Contents/Clinical Medicine, Science Citation Index, ISI/BIOMED,* and *EMBASE/Excerpta Medica.*

Contributors

CONSULTING EDITOR

MICHAEL H. WEISMAN, MD
Adjunct Professor of Medicine, Stanford University, Distinguished Professor of Medicine Emeritus, David Geffen School of Medicine at UCLA, Professor of Medicine Emeritus, Cedars-Sinai Medical Center, Los Angeles, California, USA

EDITORS

YUKIKO KIMURA, MD
Professor of Pediatrics, Hackensack University Medical Center, Hackensack Meridian School of Medicine, Pediatric Rheumatology Division Chief, Joseph M. Sanzari Children's Hospital, Co-Chair, CARRA Registry and Research Oversight Committee, Co-PI, CARRA Registry, Hackensack, New Jersey, USA

LAURA E. SCHANBERG, MD
Professor of Pediatrics, Duke University School of Medicine, Duke Clinical Research Institute, Co-Chair, CARRA Registry and Research Oversight Committee, Co-PI, CARRA Registry, Durham, North Carolina, USA

AUTHORS

SHEILA T. ANGELES-HAN, MD, MSc
Associate Professor of Pediatrics, Division of Rheumatology, Department of Pediatrics, Assistant Professor of Ophthalmology, Division of Ophthalmology, Cincinnati Children's Hospital Medical Center, Department of Ophthalmology, University of Cincinnati, Cincinnati, Ohio, USA

STACY P. ARDOIN, MD, MS
Department of Pediatrics, Nationwide Children's Hospital, Ohio State University, Columbus, Ohio, USA

TIMOTHY BEUKELMAN, MD, MSCE
Associate Professor, Department of Pediatrics, Division of Rheumatology, The University of Alabama at Birmingham, Birmingham, Alabama, USA

LAURA CANNON, MD
Assistant Professor, Division of Pediatric Rheumatology, Department of Pediatrics, The University of North Carolina at Chapel Hill, Chapel Hill, North Carolina, USA

SIOBHAN MARY CASE, MD, MHS
Med-Peds Rheumatology Fellow, Division of Immunology, Boston Children's Hospital, Division of Rheumatology, Inflammation and Immunity, Brigham and Women's Hospital, Boston, Massachusetts, USA

MARGARET H. CHANG, MD, PhD
Division of Immunology, Boston Children's Hospital, Instructor of Pediatrics, Harvard Medical School, Boston, Massachusetts, USA

ROBERT A. COLBERT, MD, PhD
Senior Investigator, National Institute of Arthritis, Musculoskeletal and Skin Diseases, National Institutes of Health, Bethesda, Maryland, USA

ALESSANDRO CONSOLARO, MD, PhD
Rheumatology Unit, Istituto Giannina Gaslini, University of Genoa, Genoa, Italy

REMCO ERKENS, MD
Doctoral Candidate, Division of Pediatric Rheumatology and Immunology, Wilhelmina Children's Hospital, Center for Translational Immunology, University Medical Center Utrecht, University of Utrecht, the Netherlands

YSABELLA ESTEBAN, MD
Clinical Fellow, Division of Rheumatology, Cincinnati Children's Hospital Medical Center, Cincinnati, Ohio, USA

POLLY J. FERGUSON, MD
Professor of Pediatrics, Pediatrics - Rheumatology, Allergy and Immunology, University of Iowa Carver College of Medicine, Iowa City, Iowa, USA

JACOB J. FONDRIEST, MD
Resident Physician, Department of Internal Medicine, Summa Health System, Internal Medicine Center, Akron, Ohio, USA; Resident Physician, Department of Ophthalmology, Rush University, Chicago, Illinois, USA

ROBERT C. FUHLBRIGGE, MD, PhD
Professor of Pediatrics, Children's Hospital Colorado, University of Colorado School of Medicine, Aurora, Colorado, USA

ADAM M. HUBER, MSc, MD
Clinical Professor of Pediatrics, IWK Health Centre and Dalhousie University, Division of Pediatric Rheumatology, Halifax, Nova Scotia, Canada

SUSMITA KASHIKAR-ZUCK, PhD
Professor of Pediatrics, Division of Behavioral Medicine and Clinical Psychology, University of Cincinnati College of Medicine, Cincinnati Children's Hospital Medical Center, Cincinnati, Ohio, USA

HANNA KIM, MS, MD
Assistant Clinical Investigator, Juvenile Myositis Pathogenesis and Therapeutics Unit, National Institute of Arthritis Musculoskeletal and Skin Diseases, National Institutes of Health, Bethesda, Maryland, USA

SUSAN KIM, MD, MMSc
Associate Professor of Pediatrics, University of California, San Francisco, San Francisco, California, USA

YUKIKO KIMURA, MD
Professor of Pediatrics, Hackensack University Medical Center, Hackensack Meridian School of Medicine, Pediatric Rheumatology Division Chief, Joseph M. Sanzari Children's Hospital, Co-Chair, CARRA Registry and Research Oversight Committee, Co-PI, CARRA Registry, Hackensack, New Jersey, USA

MELISSA A. LERMAN, MD, PhD, MSCE
Department of Pediatrics, Division of Rheumatology, Perelman School of Medicine, University of Pennsylvania, Children's Hospital of Philadelphia, Philadelphia, Pennsylvania, USA

SUZANNE C. LI, MD, PhD
Professor, Department of Pediatrics, Division of Pediatric Rheumatology, Joseph M. Sanzari Children's Hospital, Hackensack University Medical Center, Hackensack Meridian School of Medicine, Hackensack, New Jersey, USA

SCOTT M. LIEBERMAN, MD, PhD
Associate Professor of Pediatrics, Division of Rheumatology, Allergy, and Immunology, Stead Family Department of Pediatrics, University of Iowa Carver College of Medicine, Iowa City, Iowa, USA

MINDY S. LO, MD, PhD
Division of Immunology, Boston Children's Hospital, Assistant Professor of Pediatrics, Harvard Medical School, Boston, Massachusetts, USA

FARZANA NURUZZAMAN, MD
Assistant Professor of Clinical Pediatrics, Pediatric Rheumatology, Stony Brook Children's Hospital, Renaissance School of Medicine at Stony Brook University, Stony Brook, New York, USA

KAREN ONEL, MD
Professor, Division of Pediatric Rheumatology, Hospital for Special Surgery, Weill Cornell Medicine, New York, New York, USA

RACHEL L. RANDELL, MD
Fellow, Pediatric Rheumatology, Department of Pediatrics, Duke University School of Medicine, Durham, North Carolina, USA

SARAH RINGOLD, MD, MS
Seattle Children's, Seattle, Washington, USA

DAX G. RUMSEY, MD, MSc, FRCP(C)
Associate Professor, Department of Pediatrics, Division of Rheumatology, University of Alberta, Edmonton, Alberta, Canada

LAURA E. SCHANBERG, MD
Professor of Pediatrics, Duke University School of Medicine, Duke Clinical Research Institute, Co-Chair, CARRA Registry and Research Oversight Committee, Co-PI, CARRA Registry, Durham, North Carolina, USA

GRANT SCHULERT, MD, PhD
Assistant Professor of Pediatrics, Division of Rheumatology, Cincinnati Children's Hospital Medical Center, Department of Pediatrics, University of Cincinnati College of Medicine, Cincinnati, Ohio, USA

JESSICA G. SHANTHA, MD
Department of Ophthalmology, Assistant Professor, Emory University, Emory Eye Center, Atlanta, Georgia, USA

SUSAN SHENOI, MBBS, MS, RhMSUS
Associate Professor, Division of Pediatric Rheumatology, Seattle Children's Hospital and Research Center, University of Washington, Seattle, Washington, USA

NATALIE J. SHIFF, MD, MHSc
Adjunct, Department of Community Health and Epidemiology, College of Medicine, University of Saskatchewan, Saskatoon, Saskatchewan, Canada

KEITH A. SIKORA, MD
Assistant Clinical Investigator, National Institute of Arthritis, Musculoskeletal and Skin Diseases, National Institutes of Health, Bethesda, Maryland, USA

MARY BETH SON, MD
Program Director, Rheumatology Program, Division of Immunology, Boston Children's Hospital, Boston, Massachusetts, USA

HEMALATHA SRINIVASALU, MD
Assistant Professor of Pediatrics, Division of Rheumatology, Children's National Hospital, George Washington University School of Medicine, Washington, DC, USA

PETER STOUSTRUP, DDS, PhD
Section of Orthodontics, Department of Dentistry and Oral Health, Aarhus University, Aarhus, Denmark

KATHRYN S. TOROK, MD
Associate Professor of Pediatrics, Division of Pediatric Rheumatology, UPMC and University of Pittsburgh Scleroderma Center, Director, Pediatric Scleroderma Clinic, University of Pittsburgh, UPMC Children's Hospital of Pittsburgh, Pittsburgh, Pennsylvania, USA

CHRISTOPHER TOWE, MD
Assistant Professor of Pediatrics, Division of Pulmonary Medicine, Cincinnati Children's Hospital Medical Center, Department of Pediatrics, University of Cincinnati College of Medicine, Cincinnati, Ohio, USA

MARINKA TWILT, MD, PhD, MSCE
Department of Pediatrics, Alberta Children's Hospital, Cumming School of Medicine, University of Calgary, Calgary, Alberta, Canada

NATALIA VASQUEZ-CANIZARES, MD, MS
Assistant Professor, Department of Pediatrics, Division of Pediatric Rheumatology, Children's Hospital at Montefiore, Albert Einstein College of Medicine, Bronx, New York, USA

SEBASTIAAN VASTERT, MD, PhD
Associate Professor of Pediatrics, Division of Pediatric Rheumatology and Immunology, Wilhelmina Children's Hospital, Center for Translational Immunology, University Medical Center Utrecht, University of Utrecht, the Netherlands

JENNIFER E. WEISS, MD
Associate Professor of Pediatrics, Pediatric Rheumatology, Hackensack Meridian School of Medicine, Hackensack University Medical Center, Hackensack, New Jersey, USA

EVELINE Y. WU, MD, MSCR
Associate Professor and Chief, Division of Pediatric Rheumatology, Department of Pediatrics, Associate Professor and Co-director of the Clinical Immunology Program, Division of Allergy/Immunology, Department of Pediatrics, The University of North Carolina at Chapel Hill, Chapel Hill, North Carolina, USA

YONGDONG ZHAO, MD, PHD
Associate Professor, Pediatric Rheumatology, Seattle Children's Hospital, University of Washington, Seattle, Washington, USA

Contents

The Childhood Arthritis & Rheumatology Research Alliance (CARRA) launched in 2000 as a small network of pediatric rheumatologists and investigators dedicated to promoting collaborative research to improve the care and outcomes of childhood-onset rheumatic diseases. Over the past 2 decades, CARRA has grown to become a major driver of advances in evidence-based medicine and career development in pediatric rheumatology. Its research approach has transformed pediatric rheumatology. CARRA is a vibrant organization that will continue to facilitate impactful research in the care of children, adolescents, and young adults with rheumatic disease in the years to come.

Juvenile idiopathic arthritis is a group of heterogeneous chronic inflammatory arthropathies occurring in childhood without a known cause. This article discusses the key clinical features of juvenile idiopathic arthritis and treatment updates for oligoarthritis, polyarthritis, enthesitis-related arthritis, psoriatic arthritis, and systemic arthritis. Paradigm changes in management include the earlier use of biologic agents and the introduction of biosimilars and targeted synthetic disease modifying agents like tofacitinib. This review summarizes recent developments while considering potential areas for improvement and study.

Spondyloarthritis represents a group of disorders characterized by enthesitis and axial skeletal involvement. Juvenile spondyloarthritis begins before age 16. Joint involvement is usually asymmetric. Bone marrow edema on noncontrast MRI of the sacroiliac joints can facilitate diagnosis. The most significant risk factor for axial disease is HLA-B27. Most patients have active disease into adulthood. Enthesitis and sacroiliitis correlate with greater pain intensity and poor quality-of-life measures. Tumor necrosis factor inhibitors are the mainstay of biologic therapy. Although other biologics such as IL-17 blockers have shown benefit in adult spondyloarthritis, none are approved by the US Food and Drug Administration.

juvenile idiopathic arthritis. Foremost among these are the risks of serious infections and malignancy. This article provides an overview of methodologies for pharmacosurveillance in juvenile idiopathic arthritis, including spontaneous reporting systems and the use of diverse data sources, such as electronic health records, administrative claims, and clinical registries. The risks of infections and malignancies are then briefly reviewed.

Reliable and responsive outcome measures that accurately detect changes in disease state, activity, and damage are crucial to conducting observational and interventional trials that can directly transform care for children with rheumatic disease. A combination of consensus-based and direct measurement approaches has led to the development of several validated, composite outcome measures in juvenile idiopathic arthritis, juvenile dermatomyositis, childhood-onset systemic lupus erythematosus, and pediatric vasculitis. This review outlines clinician-reported, disease-specific outcome measures developed for these conditions.

Juvenile dermatomyositis (JDM) is a heterogeneous disease with new classification criteria and updates in myositis-specific autoantibody and myositis-associated antibody groups. There are many validated assessment tools for assessing disease activity in JDM. Future studies will optimize these tools and improve feasibility in clinical and research contexts. Genetic and environmental risk factors, mechanisms of muscle pathology, role of interferon, vascular markers, and changes in immune cells provide insights to JDM pathogenesis. Outcomes have improved, but chronic disease, damage, and mortality highlight the need for better outcome predictors and treatments. Increased collaboration of stakeholders may help overcome research barriers and improve JDM treatment.

Chronic nonbacterial osteomyelitis, or its most severe form, chronic recurrent multifocal osteomyelitis, is an autoinflammatory bone disease that causes skeletal inflammation characterized by bone pain and swelling that primarily affects children. It is a diagnosis of exclusion and its clinical presentation may mimic underlying infectious processes and malignancy. Clinical suspicion for this diagnosis and timely referral to pediatric rheumatology is crucial to achieve earlier diagnosis, appropriate treatment, and improved quality of life of affected patients and families. This article focuses on recent insights into the pathogenesis of chronic nonbacterial osteomyelitis and outlines recent advances and ongoing research.

Sjögren disease increasingly is recognized in pediatric patients. Clinical features, primarily parotitis and sicca symptoms, and results of diagnostic tests may be different from those in adult disease. Adult criteria fail to capture most pediatric patients. Pediatric-specific criteria are urgently needed to define the natural history of the disease, identify risk and prognostic factors, and evaluate the impact of therapeutics and other interventions on disease course in young patients.

Juvenile fibromyalgia is a common referral in pediatric rheumatology settings. Providing a clear diagnosis and explanation of altered pain processing offers reassurance that pain has a biologic basis and the symptoms are part of a recognized pain syndrome. Physicians should acknowledge the impact of chronic pain and associated symptoms on patient's lives and take time to understand contributing factors including stress, mood, inactivity, and lifestyle factors. The optimal treatment for juvenile fibromyalgia is multidisciplinary, focusing on education about juvenile fibromyalgia, along with physical therapy, cognitive behavioral therapy, sleep hygiene, healthy lifestyle habits, and medications for symptom management as appropriate.

Children and adolescents with localized scleroderma (LS) are at high risk for extracutaneous-related functional impairment including hemiatrophy, arthropathy, seizures, and vision impairment. Compared with adult-onset LS, pediatric disease has a higher likelihood for poor outcome, with extracutaneous involvement twice as prevalent in linear scleroderma, disease relapses more common, and disease duration more than double. Consensus among pediatric rheumatologists on treating patients at risk for significant morbidity with systemic immunosuppressants has led to major improvements in outcome. This review discusses recent progress in assessment and treatment strategies and in our understanding of key disease pathways.

Juvenile-onset systemic sclerosis (jSSc) is a complex multisystem inflammatory-driven disease of fibrosis, requiring multifaceted treatment including pharmacologic therapy, supportive care, and lifestyle modification. Most regimens are adapted from adult SSc treatment given the rarity of the disease. Landmark trials over the past decade in adult SSc have led to 2 Food and Drug Administration–approved therapies for SSc-associated interstitial lung disease, and several ongoing trials of other biological agents are underway. Resetting the immune system with autologous stem cell transplant to halt this disease earlier in its course, especially in pediatric onset where disease burden can accumulate, is on the horizon.

This article provides an overview of the clinical presentation and diagnosis of select pediatric primary systemic vasculitides. Important advances in understanding the pathogenesis of these rare diseases also are discussed and efforts to harmonize treatment through consensus-based guidelines and multicenter and international collaborations highlighted.

This article reviews the diagnosis and treatment of infection with severe acute respiratory syndrome coronavirus 2, which causes coronavirus disease 2019, as well as a new inflammatory syndrome after severe acute respiratory syndrome coronavirus 2 infection, called multisystem inflammatory syndrome in children.

RHEUMATIC DISEASE CLINICS OF NORTH AMERICA

FORTHCOMING ISSUES

February 2022
Pediatric Rheumatology Comes of Age: Part II
Yukiko Kimura and Laura E. Schanberg, Editors

May 2022
Cardiovascular Complications of Chronic Rheumatic Diseases
M. Elaine Husni and George A. Karpouzas, Editors

November 2022
Environmental Triggers for Rheumatic Diseases
Bryant R. England, *Editor*

RECENT ISSUES

August 2021
Lupus
Alfred H.J. Kim and Zahi Touma, *Editors*

May 2021
Pain in Rheumatic Diseases
Maripat Corr, *Editor*

February 2021
Health Disparities in Rheumatic Diseases: Part II
Candace H. Feldman, *Editor*

SERIES OF RELATED INTEREST

Medical Clinics of North America
https://www.medical.theclinics.com/
Neurologic Clinics
https://www.neurologic.theclinics.com/
Dermatologic Clinics
https://www.derm.theclinics.com/
Physical Medicine and Rehabilitation Clinics of North America
https://www.pmr.theclinics.com/

THE CLINICS ARE AVAILABLE ONLINE!
Access your subscription at:
www.theclinics.com

Foreword

Pediatric Rheumatology Comes of Age: Part I

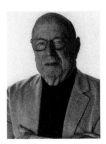

Michael H. Weisman, MD
Consulting Editor

Dr Yukiko Kimura and Dr Laura E. Schanberg have assembled two issues that reflect the remarkable changes taking place in the pediatric rheumatology community over the past 10 years. Much of this success, as reflected in the issues, is due to the strides forward in collaborative research efforts made by the various organizational care and research structures of which Laura and Yuki have played such a pivotal role and continue to do so. It is not true, however, that there has only been success, since our editors tell us that clinical remission for childhood arthritis is not achieved in a substantial number of cases. Thus, we have these two issues that point us on the journey just past and just ahead. The first focuses on the traditional roles of rheumatology to identify, measure, and achieve outcomes for pediatric rheumatic diseases, essentially addressing disease control as the item of primary interest. The second issue addresses our concerns for the impact of the diseases on the patient and the family, as well as the community at large. In this issue, the editors introduce us to the emerging technologies for patient-focused care and the impact of our diseases on comorbidities and other issues of personal health. They did an outstanding job and deserve much credit for the results.

Michael H. Weisman, MD
10800 Wilshire Blvd. #404
Los Angeles, CA 90024, USA

E-mail address:
michael.weisman@cshs.org

Rheum Dis Clin N Am 47 (2021) xv
https://doi.org/10.1016/j.rdc.2021.08.002
0889-857X/21/© 2021 Published by Elsevier Inc.

rheumatic.theclinics.com

Preface

Pediatric Rheumatology Comes of Age: Part I

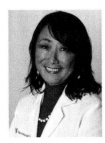 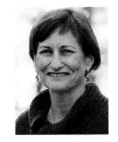

Yukiko Kimura, MD   Laura E. Schanberg, MD
Editors

The twenty-first century has been a time of enormous growth for pediatric rheumatology worldwide, spurred by the growing availability of multiple effective treatments and recognition that collaborative research is necessary to study successfully even the most common of pediatric rheumatic diseases. In North America, the incorporation and maturation of the Childhood Arthritis and Rheumatology Research Alliance (CARRA) coincides with critical progress in approaches to treatment, disease pathogenesis, and ever-expanding medication options. As treatment options expand, our understanding of autoimmunity and the recognition of the inflammatory underpinnings of disease have grown, resulting in a broadening of the definition of pediatric rheumatic diseases to include new conditions, such as autoimmune brain disease, autoinflammatory diseases, and COVID-19–related multisystem inflammatory syndrome in children (MIS-C). In addition to CARRA, the Pediatric Rheumatology Collaborative Study Group, Pediatric Rheumatology Care and Outcomes Improvement Network, Understanding Childhood Arthritis Network, the Paediatric Rheumatology European Society, and Paediatric Rheumatology INternational Trials Organisation have all greatly contributed to the growth of knowledge and understanding of pediatric rheumatic diseases over the last 20 years.

With the introduction of methotrexate for juvenile rheumatoid arthritis (JRA) in 1992, treatment expectations began to change; however, it was not until the wide use of tumor necrosis factor inhibitors that JIA outcomes drastically improved. New drugs, including other biologic disease-modifying antirheumatic drugs (DMARDs) and targeted synthetic (ts) DMARDs, are so efficacious that both families and health care providers contemplate the tantalizing possibility of cure. Despite the availability of numerous effective drugs, serious questions remain, including long-term safety, optimal use for individual patients, and which are most appropriate for JIA subtypes and other pediatric rheumatic diseases. In addition, there are significant issues

Rheum Dis Clin N Am 47 (2021) xvii–xviii
https://doi.org/10.1016/j.rdc.2021.08.001
0889-857X/21/© 2021 Published by Elsevier Inc.

concerning equity, as globally children do not have equal access to these life-altering medications. Of note, even with access to the complete menu of biologic and ts DMARDs in the United States, 30% to 50% of children in the CARRA Registry are not in clinical remission. Future research needs to focus on long-term outcomes as well as optimal, targeted use and sequence of drugs, rather than simply whether drugs are efficacious. Addressing these concerns requires the evolution of international collaborations to facilitate investigator-initiated government-sponsored, large multicenter comparative effectiveness trials that incorporate translational components in order to further the understanding of disease pathogenesis and impact of treatment.

It has been almost 10 years since the last pediatric-focused issue in the *Rheumatic Disease Clinics of North America*, and we are pleased to offer two issues that underscore the maturation and scope of the interests and expertise of the pediatric rheumatology community. Most topics reflect work of the CARRA Disease Specific Research Committees and Workgroups. Part 1 (this issue) focuses on updates to traditional pediatric rheumatic diseases, but also a new condition, COVID-19–related MIS-C. We start this issue with an article about the history of CARRA, which we believe has transformed the community's approach to research and clinical care; continue with specific disease updates and the current state of outcome measures and optimal pharmacosurveillance of medications used for pediatric rheumatic diseases. Part 2 focuses on the life impact of pediatric rheumatic disease (mental health, cardiovascular disease, pain, substance abuse, transition to adulthood) and the use of new technologies to enhance care (personalized dosing of biologics and DMARDs, treatment of pain, the role of the electronic medical record, social medial and patient engagement to enhance research and patient care). We hope that these issues will be useful to enhance the current understanding of pediatric rheumatic disease and its treatment both within the pediatric rheumatology and, perhaps most importantly, outside of it.

Yukiko Kimura, MD
Joseph M. Sanzari Children's Hospital PC344
Hackensack University Medical Center
30 Prospect Ave
Hackensack, NJ 07601, USA

Laura E. Schanberg, MD
Duke Clinical Research Institute
Duke University School of Medicine
300 W Morgan St., Suite 800
Durham, NC 27701, USA

E-mail addresses:
yukiko.kimura@hmhn.org (Y. Kimura)
Laura.schanberg@duke.edu (L.E. Schanberg)

CARRA

The Childhood Arthritis and Rheumatology Research Alliance

Robert C. Fuhlbrigge, MD, PhD[a],*, Laura E. Schanberg, MD[b],
Yukiko Kimura, MD[c]

KEYWORDS

- Pediatric • Rheumatic disease • Registry • Consensus

KEY POINTS

- The Childhood Arthritis and Rheumatology Research Alliance is an international collaborative research network dedicated to improving the care of childhood-onset rheumatic diseases.
- Over the past 20 years, the Childhood Arthritis and Rheumatology Research Alliance has created research infrastructure that supports a wide variety of clinical and translational research studies.
- The Childhood Arthritis and Rheumatology Research Alliance is committed to creating a collaborative culture of research within pediatric rheumatology, providing opportunity for every patient and the means for all clinicians to be engaged in research.

Pediatric rheumatology developed in the 1970s and 1980s out of recognition of the need for subspecialists focused on inflammatory diseases in children, supported by the expansion of knowledge in immunology and the advent of modern drug therapies.[1–3] A community of pediatric rheumatologists coalesced around North American and European specialty conferences and research initiatives to support clinical trials in children with rheumatic diseases (the Pediatric Rheumatology Collaborative Study Group [1973] and the Pediatric Rheumatology International Trials Organization [1996]). The development and operation of industry sponsored randomized clinical efficacy trials in pediatric populations by these organizations addressed a critical need, allowing the use of several new and effective treatments in children with juvenile idiopathic arthritis (JIA). However, by the late 1990s the need for broader efforts to

[a] Children's Hospital Colorado, University of Colorado, 13123 E. 16th Ave., Rheumatology B-311, Aurora, CO 80045, USA; [b] Duke University Medical Center, Pediatric Rheumatology, Box 3212 Med Ctr, Durham, NC 27710, USA; [c] Division of Pediatric Rheumatology, Joseph M. Sanzari Children's Hospital PC 344, Hackensack University Medical Center, 30 Prospect Ave., Hackensack, NJ 07601, USA
* Corresponding author.
E-mail address: robert.fuhlbrigge@childrenscolorado.org

Rheum Dis Clin N Am 47 (2021) 531–543
https://doi.org/10.1016/j.rdc.2021.07.010
0889-857X/21/© 2021 Elsevier Inc. All rights reserved.

address the full spectrum of pediatric rheumatic diseases and develop evidence-based care specific to children was clear.

Inspired by the success of collaborative pediatric oncology groups at decreasing mortality in pediatric cancer, a group of pediatric rheumatology clinician investigators in the late 1990s began discussing creation of a collaborative network focused on improving the standard of care for children with rheumatic diseases. These discussions, supported by the American College of Rheumatology and grants from the Wasie Foundation, the Lucille Packard Foundation, and the Arthritis Foundation, became a grassroots initiative to create a research network. The new network would support engagement of all providers and all patients, develop standards of care, and promote the development of a culture of research within the community of pediatric rheumatology providers.

THE CHILDHOOD ARTHRITIS & RHEUMATOLOGY RESEARCH ALLIANCE: THE BEGINNING (2000–2007)

The Childhood Arthritis & Rheumatology Research Alliance (CARRA) was created in 2000 as a collaborative network of pediatric rheumatologists and investigators in the United States and Canada seeking to address the many questions of parents and providers regarding the natural history of rheumatic disorders in children and the safety and effectiveness of medications in real-world use. A statement of the mission, vision, and guiding principles of CARRA (**Box 1**), as well the initial scientific agenda, criteria for network studies, and core scientific, leadership, and operational elements emerged from organizational meetings in 2001 and 2002, culminating in the launch of the network in late 2002. From the beginning, CARRA leaders envisioned an inclusive network that would enable widespread participation in research and create a culture of investigation among clinicians within the field. Recognition that pediatric rheumatology needed a broad-based research workforce, including clinicians, investigators, and bench scientists, led to an emphasis on support of early career investigators and small sites with few providers and limited research infrastructure.[4]

Three crucial components codified at CARRA's onset have continued to strongly influence the organization:
1. A governance structure that includes leadership positions and a steering committee elected from the membership to specific limited terms;
2. Disease- and interest-based research committees led by elected committee chairs that encompass the spectrum of diseases and interests within the pediatric rheumatology community; and
3. A commitment to include all pediatric rheumatology investigators and sites to promote research accessibility and make it possible for all children with rheumatic disease to participate in research.

To foster academic career development and facilitate widespread collaboration and participation in research, all pediatric rheumatologists, regardless of scientific or

---

Box 1
CARRA mission, vision, and values

- Vision: A world free of limitations from pediatric rheumatic diseases.
- Mission: Conduct collaborative research to prevent, treat, and cure pediatric rheumatic diseases.
- Values: Inclusiveness, trust, impact, and innovation.

academic accomplishments, were invited to participate in an inaugural CARRA Annual Meeting in 2002 (**Fig. 1**). The conference established a tradition of annual face-to-face scientific working meetings that have become a crucial community event. Through its members meeting regularly and working together to advance common interests, CARRA has fostered a culture of cooperation, collaboration, and dedication to research across the entire pediatric rheumatology community.

The Arthritis Foundation shared the CARRA vision and was an early partner, providing unrestricted grants that launched CARRA organizational and research activities and promoted development of a research infrastructure. Meeting grants from the American College of Rheumatology, National Institute of Arthritis and Musculoskeletal and Skin Diseases, Arthritis Foundation, and corporate sponsors supported the early CARRA annual meetings.

THE EARLY GROWTH YEARS: 2006 TO 2012

CARRA grew rapidly in its early years, from a handful of centers to more than 110 sites in the United States and Canada, and from 20 founding members to 180 by 2006 and more than 400 by 2012. Early funding for research studies and clinical trials came from National Institute of Arthritis and Musculoskeletal and Skin Diseases, the Arthritis Foundation, the Lupus Foundation of America, Cure Juvenile Myositis, the American College of Rheumatology, and Friends of CARRA. CARRA established a relationship with the Duke Clinical Research Institute (DCRI) to serve as data coordinating center for clinical trials and the CARRA Registry. Three successful National Institutes of Health–funded clinical trials were crucial in demonstrating the value the CARRA network in these early years.

1. Atherosclerosis Prevention in Pediatric Lupus Erythematosus (APPLE) (N01-AR-2-2265). This study, the first multicenter randomized controlled trial in pediatric lupus, tested the efficacy of atorvastatin in preventing premature carotid intimal medial thickening in children with systemic lupus erythematosus (SLE).[5]

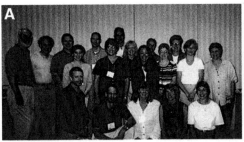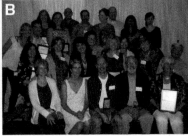

Fig. 1. (*A*) A group photo from a CARRA meeting in 2002. From left to right top row: Norman Ilowite, Lawrence Zemel, Robert Fuhlbrigge, Brian Feldman, Andrew Reiff, Marilynn Punaro, Carol Wallace, and Carol Lindsley. Middle row: Emily von Scheven, Egla Rabinovich, Yukiko Kimura, unidentified, Laura Schanberg, and Elizabeth Mellins. Bottom row: Daniel Lovell, Andrew Lasky, Christy Sandborg, Lisa Imundo, and Suzanne Bowyer. (*B*) A group photo including the CARRA Steering Committee and award winners from 2012 meeting (CARRA's 10th Anniversary). From left to right top row: Debbie Wright, Vincent DelGaizo, Susan Thompson, Justine Bushman, Kenneth Schickler, Gary Walco, Kathleen O'Neill, Robert Fuhlbrigge, Vaishali Tenkale, and Arisa Kapedani. Middle row: Nora Singer, Emily von Scheven, Yukiko Kimura, Betsy Mellins, Kathleen Haines, Laura Schanberg, Christy Sandborg, and Lawrence Jung. Bottom row: Diana Milojevic, Carol Wallace, Brian Feldman, Norman Ilowite, and Helen Emory.

2. Trial of Early Aggressive Therapy in polyarticular JIA (TREAT-JIA) (R01-AR049762), a randomized controlled trial comparing initial treatment with methotrexate versus methotrexate, steroids, and etanercept.[6]

3. Randomized Placebo Phase Trial of Rilonacept in systemic JIA (RAPPORT) (N01 AR 700015), a placebo-controlled "phased" trial comparing early versus later start of IL-1 inhibition in systemic-onset JIA.[7]

These trials created momentum for the network, operationalized a burgeoning culture of research, and established CARRA as an effective research network. Membership expanded to include nonpediatric rheumatologists engaged in research in pediatric rheumatology, including laboratory scientists, psychologists, adult rheumatologists, epidemiologists, and research coordinators.

The development and award of 2 research grants from the National Institutes of Health, funded in 2009 through the American Recovery and Reinvestment Act, provided a critical inflection point for CARRA. The first award, a Grand Opportunities Grant (RC2-AR-058934; CARRAnet: Accelerating toward an Evidence Based Culture in Pediatric Rheumatology), created an operational and informatics infrastructure for the first national scale registry for pediatric rheumatic diseases in the United States. Using the DCRI for operational support, CARRA established the basics of a research network, including central site management, standardized contracts, site training, and the development of a research coordinator network. This project, now referred to as the CARRA Legacy Registry, resulted in enrollment and data collection of more than 9500 patients representing a broad spectrum of pediatric rheumatic diseases, engagement of 250 investigators and coordinators at 60 independent sites, and creation of a US Food and Drug Administration (FDA) 21 CFR Part 11 compliant, federated open-source informatics platform. The successful implementation of CARRAnet established CARRA as an effective research organization and made real the ability to offer research participation to every provider in the field and every child affected by a rheumatic disease.

The second award, a National Institutes of Health American Recovery and Reinvestment Act Challenge Grant (CARRA-Rx, RC1-AR-058605, Comparative Effectiveness Research in Pediatric Rheumatic Diseases: Leveraging CARRA), funded the development of standardized consensus treatment plans (CTPs) in 4 pediatric rheumatic diseases: systemic JIA, pediatric lupus nephritis, juvenile dermatomyositis, and localized scleroderma. The purpose of CARRA CTPs is to facilitate comparative effectiveness research by studying the outcomes of consensus-derived, standardized treatments for pediatric rheumatic diseases in real-world observational settings and using a common data collection platform (the CARRA Legacy Registry).[8–18] The Arthritis Foundation, the Lupus Foundation of America, and the Cure Juvenile Myositis Foundation funded pilot studies testing the feasibility of using the CARRA CTPs to undertake comparative effectiveness research, which were completed successfully.[19–22] The CARRA Legacy Registry (2010–2014) continues to be a rich source of information resulting in numerous publications and presentations and supporting further development of CARRA research initiatives.

CARRA, INC., AND THE NEW CARRA (2015–PRESENT)

To better accommodate industry-sponsored research, CARRA reorganized in late 2014 and registered as a 501(c)3 tax exempt nonprofit organization (CARRA Inc.). Becoming a legal organization allowed CARRA to negotiate and execute contracts directly with pharmaceutical companies and vendors, including the DCRI data-coordinating center. A board of directors was created, along with an administrative infrastructure to move CARRA's mission forward.

A revamped CARRA Registry was launched in July 2015, creating an integrated observational registry able to fulfill global postmarketing requirements for long-term product safety monitoring.[23] The implementation of a 21CFR11-compliant electronic data capture platform for a disease-specific registry reflected a concept introduced at an FDA workshop in 2009 to improve the safety surveillance of new products brought to market to treat JIA.[24,25] The new CARRA Registry is a partnership between investigators, industry, patients, and government to rigorously follow at least 10,000 children and adolescents with JIA for 10 or more years, regardless of medication exposure and transition to adult providers. Unlike typical drug-specific safety registries, which are by nature limited in scope and participation, this inclusive registry allows a more robust estimation of the risk of rare long-term adverse events, such as malignancies and opportunistic infections in exposed and nonexposed individuals, as well as the ability to follow patients who discontinue or switch medications. The data collection platform facilitates layering of multiple types of studies, including support of data collection activities for observational studies, development of clinical outcomes measures, comparative effectiveness research, implementation science, postmarketing pharmacosurveillance, and multicenter randomized trials, as well as biosample collection to support translational studies (**Fig. 2**). Other improvements over the Legacy Registry include implementation of a reliant institutional review board model, electronic and remote consenting, enhanced patient-reported outcome measures, master agreements regulating data use and material transfer, a centralized mechanism for reporting, adjudicating and coding adverse events, and the incorporation of patient stakeholders on study teams. A DCRI call center provides remote follow-up of registry participants after transition into adult medical care, enabling improved understanding of long-term outcomes and safety events. To ensure the continued opportunity for both large and small centers to participate, CARRA has emphasized site support, providing a range of tools and training for on-site research coordinators and investigators, in addition to reimbursing sites per patient visit for data collection.

With FDA endorsement of this approach to pharmacosurveillance, CARRA has contracted with multiple drug manufacturers to satisfy their postmarketing requirements. The CARRA Registry has also become the preferred data collection vehicle for all large multicenter CARRA studies, which includes a variety of pharmacosurveillance, observational, and natural history studies, implementation science studies, comparative

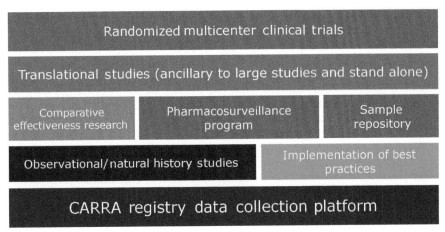

Fig. 2. CARRA research portfolio overview.

effectiveness research, and clinical trials, among other formats (see **Fig. 2**). As of spring 2021, the CARRA Registry had enrolled over 11,500 patients, including more than 10,000 patients with JIA, 950 patients with SLE (initiated in 2017), 250 with juvenile dermatomyositis (initiated in 2017), and 80 with localized and systemic forms of scleroderma (initiated in 2019).

Examples of research enabled by the CARRA Registry infrastructure include STOP-JIA (Start Time Optimization of biologics in Poly-JIA), funded by the Patient-Centered Outcomes Research Institute (PCORI), which compared the effectiveness of the polyarticular JIA CTPs to answer the pressing question of when biologics should be started in a patient with new-onset polyarticular JIA. This first large-scale study of the CARRA CTPs successfully recruited 400 patients with untreated polyarticular JIA to participate in a prospective, nonrandomized study, one of the largest cohorts of its kind. The primary results and a secondary trajectory analysis were recently published.[26,27] FROST (First-Line Options for Systemic JIA Treatment) is a similarly designed project funded by Genentech to compare the CARRA systemic JIA CTPs in children with new-onset disease. Because these are observational studies with standard of care treatments, use common data collection methods defined by the general CARRA Registry protocol, and use existing site contracts, operationalizing these studies is relatively easy and cost-efficient compared with conducting stand-alone trials. Thus, registry-based studies of comparative effectiveness in a real-world observational setting are both feasible and economical, compared with randomized active comparator or placebo-controlled trials, and provide a research model for studies in other rare diseases. Additional investigator-initiated and industry-sponsored clinical trials are being conducted that leverage the CARRA Registry infrastructure and network.

Translational studies and biospecimen collection are increasingly routine in CARRA studies, creating a robust resource of samples linked to highly curated longitudinal clinical data. The samples and linked data fuel further translational and basic science investigations. Both STOP-JIA and FROST included companion translational research studies leveraging the CARRA biospecimen collection infrastructure, focusing on sample collection before and after starting biologic or disease-modifying antirheumatic drug therapy and aiming to identify biomarkers that predict response and nonresponse, as well as potentially aiding in diagnosis. Additional studies involving biospecimen collection in other cohorts (juvenile dermatomyositis, systemic sclerosis and localized scleroderma, JIA patients initiating methotrexate, and pediatric lupus) are currently underway.

Recent initiatives to increase patient and stakeholder engagement have broadened the perspectives of research investigators. Parents and patients are a growing presence at the CARRA annual meeting, participating in workgroup activities and serving on study teams. Patient and parent study team activities include guiding study design, including developing research questions, assisting with patient recruitment issues, developing patient-facing research materials, serving on grant review committees, and participating on various stakeholder advisory panels. One inspiring example of these efforts is a video created to encourage patients and families to participate in research (Research is Hope video; available at: https://carragroup.org/patients-families/research). CARRA also participates in the PARTNERS (Patients, Advocates and Rheumatology Teams Network for Research and Service) Consortium, a patient-powered research network funded by the PCORI as part of the National Patient-Centered Clinical Research Network (PCORnet).

CARRA has expanded dramatically since reorganization as a 501(c)3, growing to include more than 575 members (see **Fig. 3**) and supporting a diverse portfolio of research. Members include more than 90% of all pediatric rheumatology providers

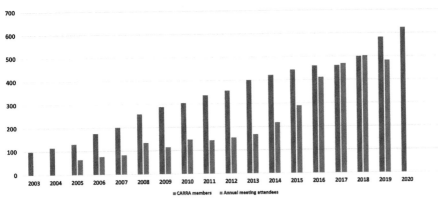

Fig. 3. CARRA membership and annual meeting attendance by year (no meeting was held in 2020).

in the United States and Canada, as well as clinicians from adult rheumatology and other pediatric subspecialties, PhD scientists, rheumatology health professionals, and research personnel engaged in pediatric rheumatology research at 175 centers in the United States, Canada, and internationally. Seventy-nine centers are CARRA Registry sites, including sites the United States, Israel, and in development in Italy. The CARRA Steering Committee has expanded to include 10 committees: 5 disease-specific research groups (JIA, Juvenile Dermatomyositis, SLE, Pain, and Rare Diseases), 3 stakeholder groups (Early Investigator, Research Coordinator Network, and Small Centers), the Translational Research and Technology Committee, and a Crosscutting Committee supporting research in areas that bridge committees. The work of the committees is distributed among more than 40 workgroups focused on specific projects and areas of research development (**Table 1**). Besides the steering committee, CARRA has organized committees that provide oversight of the registry and externally funded research (Registry and Research Oversight Committee) and intramural research (Internally-funded Research Oversight Committee). Other specific committees support development of CARRA-endorsed CTPs and scientific review of sponsored grants, as well as oversight of data and sample sharing, publications, and membership.

Through periods of intense growth, CARRA has maintained focus on its founding principles of inclusiveness and the promotion of a culture of research across all members and centers, with the goal of providing all children the opportunity to participate in research. To expand and improve the research community, CARRA has created a strong program for research workforce development. Activities include providing training in research methodology, developing peer connections within CARRA as well as with international networks, connecting early investigators with mentors who have similar interests, and providing a variety of grant mechanisms focused on early career investigators. The CARRA data warehouse makes it possible for investigators to acquire preliminary data needed to compete for external grant mechanisms. CARRA career development programs aim to increase the productivity and quality of research performed during the early faculty years, as well as the number of active clinician investigators engaged in pediatric rheumatology research. CARRA has also created a Registry Associates program, which provides promising faculty with protected time to obtain experience with CARRA Registry operations, develop registry research opportunities, and promote the career development of future CARRA Registry investigators.

Table 1
Committees and workgroups of the CARRA steering committee

Committee	JIA	JDM	SLE	PAIN	RD	TRTC	Cross-Cutting	EI	RCN	Small Centers
Workgroups	Inactive disease	JDM/SLE dermatology	Decision support in JIA	ANCA-associated vasculitis	Standard operating procedures	Mental health	Medical education research			
	Systemic JIA	Quality of care	Lupus nephritis	FIT teens (Fibromyalgia Integrative Training)	Autoimmune encephalitis/inflammatory brain diseases	Archiving	Reproductive health			
	Temporomandibular joint	Biologics	Antiphospholipid syndrome	Pain and symptom assessment tool for FM	Chronic noninfectious osteomyelitis	CARRA translational initiative	Implementation science			
	Musculoskeletal ultrasound examinations	Calcinosis	Lupus genetics		Kawasaki disease	EI outreach	Transition			
	Uveitis	Virtual care			Juvenile systemic sclerosis	Patient and family advisory council	Clinical informatics			
	Spondylo-arthropathy	JDM translational medicine			Juvenile localized scleroderma	Biosample collection and COVID-19	Vaccination			
	Outcomes	Rehabilitation and exercise			PFAPA/auto-inflammatory syndromes		Health equity Research			
		COVID-19			Sjogren syndrome					

Abbreviations: ANCA, Anti-neutrophil cytoplasmic antibody; EI, early investigators; FM, fibromyalgia; JDM, juvenile dermatomyositis; JIA, juvenile idiopathic arthritis; PFAPA, periodic fever, aphthous stomatitis, pharyngitis and adenopathy syndrome; RCN, research coordinator network; RD, rare diseases; SLE, systemic lupus erythematosus; TRTC, Translational Research & Technology Committee.

A critical factor in CARRA's recent growth is the expansion of a longstanding relationship with the Arthritis Foundation, which partners with CARRA on long-term strategic planning and the development of new programs. Examples include intramural grant programs to develop collaborative, early stage projects emerging from the workgroups, a pediatric resident scholarship program to attend the CARRA annual meeting, and the creation of CARRA early investigator development programs, among many others. Ongoing areas of codevelopment between CARRA and the Arthritis Foundation include support for translational research development, initiation of an implementation science program to explore and enhance dissemination of research results; expansion of efforts related to diversity, equity, and inclusion (addressing issues in both patient and investigator recruitment); and continued engagement of patients and parents in research development. Another focus area is advocating for rapid and expedited regulatory approval of new medications to treat children with pediatric rheumatic diseases. Together, CARRA and the Arthritis Foundation sponsored an externally led Patient Focused Drug Development program for the FDA in 2018 (available at: https://www.arthritis.org/getmedia/25118249-ea68-45b5-bfe4-c20904ddc 32c/FINAL-JIA-PFDD.pdf), as well as a CARRA-sponsored meeting to bring together investigators, patients, parents, the FDA, the EMA (European Medicines Agency), the Arthritis Foundation, and pharma companies to discuss issues related to pediatric drug development in rheumatology in late 2018.[28] This meeting led to an FDA workshop in 2019 that raised significant potential changes in regulatory approval of new medications using extrapolation from adult data accompanied by pharmacokinetic and pharmacodynamic studies in children.

EVOLUTION AND CHALLENGES

As CARRA celebrates entering its third decade of operation, the organization continues to focus on mission, addressing key research questions and challenges faced by our patients and providers. As the organization has expanded in scope and complexity, CARRA seeks to maintain transparency and a democratic governance structure, improving member and stakeholder engagement, optimizing methods for communicating with all members and the public, and ensuring leadership succession.

As of July 2021, the CARRA Registry has enrolled more than 11,000 unique patients and recorded more than 60,000 visits (**Fig. 4**). The registry is actively enrolling patients from 4 disease groups (JIA, SLE, juvenile dermatomyositis, and scleroderma), supporting the operation of 3 phase IV postmarketing studies and 7 separate cohort studies. There are 11 biosample cohorts available or in collection for investigators to study. Recent enhancements to the registry include expanded site management and data management protocols, augmented long-term follow-up and safety approaches, and the hiring of a dedicated biostatistician to support manuscript development. CARRA investigators are actively consulting on studies to test new therapeutics, including innovative pharmacokinetic and pharmacology study designs.

Increasing effective collaborations with the international pediatric rheumatology research community will be critical to making major scientific advances in rare diseases. CARRA is committed to facilitating international research efforts, which increases the complexity of the research process, but creates more opportunities. Working collaboratively with current partners and continuing to develop new funding streams is also critical to ensure the organization's financial sustainability.

Last, the current leadership of CARRA, many of whom were part of the creation of the organization, is reaching retirement age and CARRA is committed to engaging

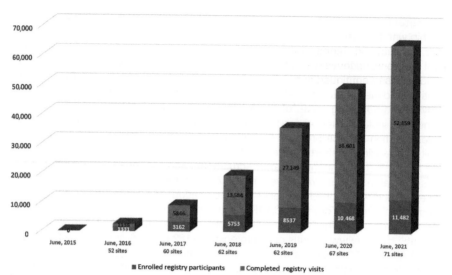

Fig. 4. Cumulative CARRA registry enrollment, completed visits and number of registry sites over time.

new leaders to ensure sustainability. As the rheumatology community has expanded, CARRA has supported and nurtured investigators to lead CARRA into the future. CARRA developed the CARRA Registry Associates program and Early Investigator Committee with the stated intention of promoting the career development of promising young investigators, encouraging participation in all levels of CARRA activities, providing experience with registry operations, and fostering engagement with international counterparts. In addition, there are formal leadership development programs for steering committee members, as well as informal mentoring of each committee chair by members of the CARRA executive team. The Registry and Research Oversight Committee is also actively engaged in enhancing research leadership skills.

THE FUTURE OF THE CHILDHOOD ARTHRITIS & RHEUMATOLOGY RESEARCH ALLIANCE

The future of academic pediatric rheumatology seems brighter than ever, with a growing clinical and research workforce and improving research infrastructure, as well as an array of effective medications to treat pediatric rheumatic diseases and prevent life-altering disability; however, there is still much to do.

The CARRA Registry will continue to be the core activity of CARRA and an engine for a wide range of research and research–workforce development activities. The infrastructure of the registry provides access to the large majority of patients with pediatric rheumatic diseases in the United States and Canada. Combined with centralized and standardized modes of data entry, communication, contracting, and regulatory compliance, as well as upcoming innovations, including platforms for remote consenting and patient-reported outcomes reporting, CARRA's research efforts will continue to expand and innovate. Through these efforts, CARRA will continue to promote the development of an evidence base for best practices in pediatric rheumatology, supporting FDA-compliant clinical trials and a range of investigator-initiated observational and translational research activities.

The culture of inclusiveness and scientific collaboration that CARRA has fostered and maintained has led directly to its current level of success. The challenge to the pediatric rheumatology community is to maintain the principles that have allowed CARRA to grow and thrive while translating the knowledge gained into changes in clinical practice and continued improvement in health outcomes.

CLINICS CARE POINTS

- CARRA is an international collaborative research network based in North America that is dedicated to improving treatment and outcomes in childhood-onset rheumatic diseases while maintaining a culture of inclusiveness and opportunity for both patients and providers.

- CARRA has demonstrated that Registry-based studies of comparative effectiveness and pharmacosurveillance are both feasible and cost-efficient compared with conducting stand-alone clinical trials and are a model for studies in other rare diseases.

- The CARRA Registry will continue to be the foundation and engine for research within CARRA and for research-workforce development in pediatric rheumatology.

DISCLOSURE

R.C. Fuhlbrigge: Salary support from CARRA, Elsevier and UpToDate royalties. L.E. Schanberg: Salary support from CARRA, research grant Bristol Myers Squibb, DSMB Sonofi, and Union Chimique Belge. Y. Kimura: Salary support from CARRA, research grant from Genentech, and UpToDate royalties.

REFERENCES

1. Cassidy JT, Athreya B. Pediatric rheumatology: status of the subspecialty in United States medical schools. Arthritis Rheum 1997;40(6):1182.
2. Schaller JG. The history of pediatric rheumatology. Pediatr Res 2005;58(5): 997–1007.
3. Athreya BH. History of Pediatric Rheumatology. In: Sawhney S., Aggarwal A. (eds) Pediatric Rheumatology. Springer, Singapore. 2017. p. 3–9, https://doi.org/10.1007/978-981-10-1750-6_1.
4. Ota S, Cron RQ, Schanberg LE, et al. Research priorities in pediatric rheumatology: the Childhood Arthritis and Rheumatology Research Alliance (CARRA) consensus. Pediatr Rheumatol Online J 2008;6:5.
5. Schanberg LE, Sandborg C, Barnhart HX, et al. Premature atherosclerosis in pediatric systemic lupus erythematosus: risk factors for increased carotid intima-media thickness in the atherosclerosis prevention in pediatric lupus erythematosus cohort. Arthritis Rheum 2009;60(5):1496–507.
6. Wallace CA, Giannini EH, Spalding SJ, et al. Trial of early aggressive therapy in polyarticular juvenile idiopathic arthritis. Arthritis Rheum 2012;64(6):2012–21.
7. Ilowite NT, Prather K, Lokhnygina Y, et al. Randomized, double-blind, placebo-controlled trial of the efficacy and safety of rilonacept in the treatment of systemic juvenile idiopathic arthritis. Arthritis Rheumatol 2014;66(9):2570–9.
8. Ringold S, Nigrovic PA, Feldman BM, et al. The childhood arthritis and rheumatology research alliance consensus treatment plans: toward comparative effectiveness in the pediatric rheumatic diseases. Arthritis Rheumatol 2018;70(5): 669–78.

9. Li SC, Torok KS, Pope E, et al. Development of consensus treatment plans for juvenile localized scleroderma: a roadmap toward comparative effectiveness studies in juvenile localized scleroderma. Arthritis Care Res (Hoboken) 2012; 64(8):1175–85.

10. Huber AM, Giannini EH, Bowyer SL, et al. Protocols for the initial treatment of moderately severe juvenile dermatomyositis: results of a Children's Arthritis and Rheumatology Research Alliance Consensus Conference. *Arthritis Care Res (Hoboken)* 2010;62(2):219–25.

11. Huber AM, Kim S, Reed AM, et al. Childhood arthritis and rheumatology research alliance consensus clinical treatment plans for juvenile dermatomyositis with persistent skin rash. J Rheumatol 2017;44(1):110–6.

12. Huber AM, Robinson AB, Reed AM, et al. Consensus treatments for moderate juvenile dermatomyositis: beyond the first two months. Results of the second Childhood Arthritis and Rheumatology Research Alliance consensus conference. Arthritis Care Res (Hoboken) 2012;64(4):546–53.

13. Amarilyo G, Rothman D, Manthiram K, et al. Consensus treatment plans for periodic fever, aphthous stomatitis, pharyngitis and adenitis syndrome (PFAPA): a framework to evaluate treatment responses from the childhood arthritis and rheumatology research alliance (CARRA) PFAPA work group. Pediatr Rheumatol Online J 2020;18(1):31.

14. Angeles-Han ST, Lo MS, Henderson LA, et al. Childhood arthritis and rheumatology research alliance consensus treatment plans for juvenile idiopathic arthritis-associated and idiopathic chronic anterior uveitis. Arthritis Care Res (Hoboken) 2019;71(4):482–91.

15. Kim S, Kahn P, Robinson AB, et al. Childhood Arthritis and Rheumatology Research Alliance consensus clinical treatment plans for juvenile dermatomyositis with skin predominant disease. Pediatr Rheumatol Online J 2017;15(1):1.

16. Mina R, von Scheven E, Ardoin SP, et al. Consensus treatment plans for induction therapy of newly diagnosed proliferative lupus nephritis in juvenile systemic lupus erythematosus. Arthritis Care Res (Hoboken) 2012;64(3):375–83.

17. Ringold S, Weiss PF, Colbert RA, et al. Childhood Arthritis and Rheumatology Research Alliance consensus treatment plans for new-onset polyarticular juvenile idiopathic arthritis. Arthritis Care Res (Hoboken) 2014;66(7):1063–72.

18. DeWitt EM, Kimura Y, Beukelman T, et al. Consensus treatment plans for new-onset systemic juvenile idiopathic arthritis. Arthritis Care Res (Hoboken) 2012; 64(7):1001–10.

19. Kimura Y, Grevich S, Beukelman T, et al. Pilot study comparing the Childhood Arthritis & Rheumatology Research Alliance (CARRA) systemic Juvenile Idiopathic Arthritis Consensus Treatment Plans. Pediatr Rheumatol Online J 2017; 15(1):23.

20. Cooper JC, Rouster-Stevens K, Wright TB, et al. Pilot study comparing the childhood arthritis and rheumatology research alliance consensus treatment plans for induction therapy of juvenile proliferative lupus nephritis. Pediatr Rheumatol Online J 2018;16(1):65.

21. Li SC, Torok KS, Rabinovich CE, et al. Initial results from a pilot comparative effectiveness study of 3 methotrexate-based consensus treatment plans for juvenile localized scleroderma. J Rheumatol 2020;47(8):1242–52.

22. Liu K, Tomlinson G, Reed AM, et al. Pilot study of the juvenile dermatomyositis consensus treatment plans: a CARRA registry study. J Rheumatol 2021;48(1): 114–22.

23. Beukelman T, Kimura Y, Ilowite NT, et al. The new Childhood Arthritis and Rheumatology Research Alliance (CARRA) registry: design, rationale, and characteristics of patients enrolled in the first 12 months. Pediatr Rheumatol Online J 2017; 15(1):30.
24. Smith MY, Sobel RE, Wallace CA. Monitoring the long-term safety of therapies for children with juvenile idiopathic arthritis: time for a consolidated patient registry. Arthritis Care Res (Hoboken) 2010;62(6):800–4.
25. Lionetti G, Kimura Y, Schanberg LE, et al. Using registries to identify adverse events in rheumatic diseases. Pediatrics 2013;132(5):e1384–94.
26. Kimura Y, Schanberg LE, Tomlinson GA, et al. The childhood arthritis & rheumatology research alliance Start Time Optimization of Biologics in Polyarticular Juvenile Idiopathic Arthritis Study (STOP-JIA): a comparative effectiveness study of CARRA consensus treatment plans for untreated polyarticular JIA. Arthritis Rheumatol 2021. https://doi.org/10.1002/art.41888.
27. Ong MS, Ringold S, Kimura Y, et al. Improved disease course associated with early initiation of biologics in untreated polyarticular juvenile idiopathic arthritis: a trajectory analysis of the STOP-JIA study. Arthritis Rheumatol 2021. https://doi.org/10.1002/art.41892.
28. Schanberg LE, Ramanan AV, De Benedetti F, et al. Toward accelerated authorization and access to new medicines for juvenile idiopathic arthritis. Arthritis Rheumatol 2019;71(12):1976–84.

Juvenile Idiopathic Arthritis Treatment Updates

Karen Onel, MD[a], Dax G. Rumsey, MD, MSc, FRCP(C)[b], Susan Shenoi, MBBS, MS, RhMSUS[c],*

KEYWORDS

- Juvenile idiopathic arthritis • Treat to target (T2T)
- Disease-modifying antirheumatic drugs (DMARDs) • Biologics • Biosimilars

KEY POINTS

- A multidisciplinary, holistic approach to treatment should be used for juvenile idiopathic arthritis.
- Although similarities in treatment approach exist across juvenile idiopathic arthritis categories, there are important differences in the approach to juvenile idiopathic arthritis – oligoarthritis/polyarthritis versus enthesitis-related arthritis/psoriatic juvenile idiopathic arthritis versus systemic juvenile idiopathic arthritis.
- There has been a recent trend toward using a treat to target approach for the treatment of juvenile idiopathic arthritis.

INTRODUCTION

This article reviews juvenile idiopathic arthritis (JIA)-related treatment updates in 3 sections: (1) JIA—oligoarticular and polyarticular, (2) JIA—enthesitis-related (ERA) arthritis and psoriatic JIA (PsJIA), and (3) systemic JIA (sJIA). Each section outlines key clinical/laboratory features (**Table 1**), recent treatment updates (**Table 2** with recommended drug doses), and future directions.

JUVENILE IDIOPATHIC ARTHRITIS: OLIGOARTHRITIS AND POLYARTHRITIS
Key Clinical and Laboratory Features

Oligoarticular JIA involves less than 5 joints at onset per International League of Associations of Rheumatologists criteria[1] and is most common in young girls presenting with arthritis of large lower extremity joints such as knees.[2] It is separated into persistent or extended disease (involvement of >5 joints, ≥6 months after onset). Of all the categories, persistent oligoarticular JIA is most likely to remit overtime.[3] Polyarticular

All 3 authors contributed equally and are listed alphabetically.
[a] Division of Pediatric Rheumatology, Hospital for Special Surgery, Weill Cornell Medicine, 535 E 70th St 5th Floor, New York, NY 10021, USA; [b] Department of Pediatrics, Division of Rheumatology, University of Alberta, 3-502 ECHA, 11405 87 Ave NW, Edmonton, AB T6G 1C9; [c] Division of Pediatric Rheumatology, Seattle Children's Hospital, University of Washington, MA.7.110, Sand Point Way NE, Seattle, WA 98105, USA
* Corresponding author.
E-mail address: susan.shenoi@seattlechildrens.org

Table 1
Comparison of various classification criteria, key systemic and laboratory features for JIA and MAS

	sJIA	AOSD	MAS (in sJIA)	OJIA	PJIA	ERA	PsA
Classification criteria and exclusions	International League of Associations of Rheumatologists	Yamaguchi Criteria	Ravelli	International League of Associations of Rheumatologists			
Criteria	Quotidian fever for 2 wks (documented for ≥3 d) with 6 wks of arthritis with onset ≤16 y and additionally (one of below): 1. Evanescent rash 2. Serositis 3. Organomegaly 4. Lymphadenopathy	PRINTO — Quotidian fever documented for 3 consecutive days and recurring over 2-wk duration and 2 major or 1 major and 2 minor criteria. A. Major criteria: 1. Evanescent rash 2. Arthritis B. Minor criteria: 1. Generalized lymphadeno-pathy or hepatomegaly or splenomegaly 2. Serositis 3. Arthralgia >2 wk (if no arthritis) 4. Elevated WBC (≥15,000/mm3) with elevated neutrophils	Presence of any 5 (≥2/5 must be major criteria): A. Major criteria 1. Fever >39 °C 2. Typical rash 3. Leukocytosis (WBC >10,000 with >80% granulocytes) 4. Arthralgias for >2 wk B. Minor criteria: 1. Sore throat 2. Splenomegaly or lymphadeno-pathy 3. Abnormal liver function tests 4. Seronegative status (negative ANA and RF)	Presence of fever, and ferritin >684 ng/mL and any 2 of the following: 1. Platelets ≤181 × 10^9/L 2. AST >48 U/L 3. Triglycerides >156 mg/dL 4. Fibrinogen ≤360 mg/dL	Arthritis in ≤4 joints in first 6 mo of onset 2 subcategories include 1. Persistent: no additional joints 2. Extended: additional joints are involved after the first 6 mo	Arthritis in ≥5 joints in first 6 mo of onset 1. RF negative 2. RF positive ×2 done 3 mo apart	Arthritis plus enthesitis or arthritis or enthesitis plus ≥2 of the following: 1. Presence of or a history of sacroiliac joint tenderness and/or inflammatory lumbosacral pain, presence of HLA-B27 antigen, onset of arthritis in a male >6 y of age, acute (symptomatic) anterior uveitis, history of AS, ERA, sacroiliitis with IBD, reactive arthritis, or acute anterior uveitis in a first-degree relative	Arthritis plus psoriasis or Arthritis plus ≥2 of the following: 1. Dactylitis 2. Nail pitting or onycholysis 3. Psoriasis in a first-degree relative

Exclusions	1. Presence or history of psoriasis in patient or first-degree relative 2. Arthritis in HLA-B27 positive male >6 y 3. Presence or history of HLAB27-associated diseases in child or first-degree relative. Example: AS, ERA, sacroiliitis with IBD, reactive arthritis, acute anterior uveitis 4. Positive rheumatoid factor test ×2 done 3 mo apart	Known malignant, autoimmune, or monogenic autoinflammatory diseases	Known infection, malignancy, or other rheumatic diseases	None	1–4 as noted in sJIA and 5) presence of sJIA	1–3 as noted in sJIA and presence of sJIA	1. Presence or history of psoriasis in patient or first-degree relative 2. Presence of IgM RF on ≥2 occasions, ≥3 mo apart 3. sJIA in the patient	1. Arthritis in an HLA-B27 positive male beginning after the sixth birthday 2. AS, ERA, sacroiliitis with IBD, reactive arthritis, or acute anterior uveitis, or a history of one of these disorders in a first-degree relative 3. Presence of IgM RF on ≥2 occasions, ≥3 mo apart 4. sJIA in the patient
Key clinical features								
Sex	No predilection			No predilection	Females > Males	Females > Males	Males > Females	Females > Males
Age	Any			Any	Peak 2–3 y	Peak 2–5 y and 10–14 y	Mean age of onset is 10–13 y	Bimodal peak at ages 2–3 then in later childhood

(continued on next page)

Table 1
(continued)

	sJIA	AOSD	MAS (in sJIA)	OJIA	PJIA	ERA	PsA
Involved joints	Any (sometimes arthritis may be delayed)		Any	Typically, large, often asymmetric (usually not hips)	Large and small joints, often symmetric bilateral small joints, c-spine involvement	Lower limb joints, hips, axial disease; enthesitis	Younger patients often start with oligoarticular presentation, but also present with dactylitis and often progress to polyarticular disease; older patients present with enthesitis and can have axial disease, (similar to adult PsA)
Extra-articular features	High quotidian fevers, evanescent macular rash, lymphadenopathy, hepatosplenomegaly, pericardial effusion, peritonitis, arthritis, sore throat, and pharyngitis		Sick appearing, persistent fevers, fixed rashes, multiorgan failure (respiratory, cardiac, renal, neurologic) and coagulopathy	Leg length discrepancy may be noted	Low-grade fever, rheumatoid nodules	Gastrointestinal inflammation, aortic insufficiency (rare)	Psoriasis, nail pitting and onycholysis, gastrointestinal inflammation

Uveitis	Rare, <1%	Not usually seen	20%–30% asymptomatic anterior	15% Asymptomatic anterior	Acute, usually unilateral, and is frequently recurrent	10%–15% Chronic (asymptomatic anterior)
Key laboratory features	Leukocytosis, anemia, elevated inflammatory markers (ESR, CRP), negative serology (ANA, RF, CCP)	Decreasing: platelets, white count, hemoglobin, ESR Increasing: CRP, AST, ALT, lactate dehydrogenase, prothrombin time/partial thromboplastin time, triglycerides, and ferritin, soluble CD25 Other: hemophagocytosis on bone marrow or tissue biopsies	Normal ESR and CRP usually Often are ANA positive (70%)	Elevated ESR and CRP and WBC, anemia of chronic inflammation, RF or CCP positive (in RF-positive disease). Can be ANA positive (30%)	HLA-B27 positive (40%–80%) mild anemia, sometimes elevated ESR/CRP; RF is characteristically absent; ANA is no more common than in the general population	ANA positive in 60% of younger patients and 30% of older patients; RF typically negative; ESR/CRP are frequently normal, but could be mildly to moderately elevated

Abbreviations: ALT, alanine aminotransferase; ANA, antinuclear antibodies; AS, ankylosing spondylitis; AST, aspartate aminotransferase; CCP, cyclic citrullinated peptide; CRP, C-reactive protein; ESR, erythrocyte sedimentation rate; IBD, inflammatory bowel disease; RF, rheumatoid factor; WBC, white blood cell.

Table 2
Medications used to treat JIA, mechanisms of action, typical dosing and route[a]

Medication	Mechanism of Action	Typical Dosing and Route
Nonsteroidal anti-inflammatory drugs		
Naproxen[b]	Reversibly inhibits cyclo-oxygenase-1 and 2 to block production of proinflammatory prostaglandins	15–20 mg/kg/d divided BID; PO Maximum: 500 mg BID
Meloxicam[b]	Reversibly inhibits cyclo-oxygenase-1 and 2 to block production of proinflammatory prostaglandins	0.2 mg/kg once daily; PO Maximum: 15 mg/day
Celecoxib[b]	Selectively inhibits cyclo-oxygenase-2 to block production of proinflammatory prostaglandins	10–25 kg: 50 mg BID; PO 25+ kg: 100 mg BID; PO Maximum 400 mg/d
Conventional Synthetic Disease Modifying Anti-Rheumatic Drugs (csDMARDs)		
Methotrexate[b]	Inhibits DNA synthesis, repair, and cellular replication.	15 mg/m^2 weekly; PO or SC 0.5–1 mg/kg weekly; PO or SC Maximum: 40 mg/week
Sulfasalazine[b]	Inhibits enzymes and transcription factors involved in production of proinflammatory cytokines	30–50 mg/kg/d divided BID; PO Maximum: 2000 mg/d
Hydroxychloroquine	Impairs complement-dependent antigen–antibody reactions	5 mg/kg/d once daily; PO Maximum: 400 mg/d
Leflunomide	Inhibits pyrimidine synthesis and, thus, interferes with lymphocyte proliferation.	<20 kg: 100 mg single dose then 10 mg EOD; PO 20–40 kg: 100 mg for 2 d then 10 mg daily; PO >40 kg: 100 mg for 3 d then 20 mg daily; PO
Biologic DMARDs		
Etanercept[b]	Soluble fusion protein composed of TNFa receptor and Fc portion of human IgG1 that binds circulating TNFa.	0.8 mg/kg/wk; SC Maximum: 50 mg weekly
Infliximab	Human-murine monoclonal antibody against circulating and membrane-bound TNFa.	6 mg/kg every 8 wk after loading doses at 0, 2, and 6 wk; IV (Often higher doses are required 6–20 mg/kg every 4 wk; IV) Maximum 1000 mg/dose
Adalimumab[b]	Human monoclonal antibody against circulating and membrane-bound TNFa.	<15 kg: 10 mg q2weeks SC 15–30 kg: 20 mg q2weeks SC >30 kg: 40 mg q2weeks SC

(continued on next page)

Table 2
(continued)

Medication	Mechanism of Action	Typical Dosing and Route
Golimumab[b]	Human monoclonal antibody against TNF-a.	80 mg/m^2 at 0, 4 then every 8 wk; IV 30 mg/m^2 q4weeks; SC Maximum: 50 mg/dose
Abatacept[b]	Selectively modulates the CD80/CD86:CD28 Costimulatory signal required for full T cell activation	<75 kg: 10 mg/kg at 0, 2, 4 then q4 weeks IV 75–100 kg: 750 mg at 0, 2, 4 then q4 weeks IV >100 kg: 1000 mg at 0, 2, 4 then q4 weeks IV OR 10–25 kg: 50 mg weekly; SC 25–50 kg: 87.5 mg weekly; SC ≥50 kg: 125 mg weekly; SC
Tocilizumab[b]	Humanized monoclonal antibody against the IL-6 receptor	For PJIA q 4 wk; IV <30 kg: 10 mg/kg ≥30 kg: 8 mg/kg Maximum: 800 mg/dose For SJIA q 2 wk; IV <30 kg: 12 mg/kg ≥30 kg: 8 mg/kg Maximum: 800 mg/dose OR <30 kg: 162 mg q 2 wk; SC ≥30 kg: 162 mg q week; SC
Anakinra	Blocks IL-1 receptor to prevent proinflammatory signaling.	1–4 mg/kg daily SC or IV (Higher doses have been used in cases complicated by MAS or in other severe presentations; up to 10 mg/kg)
Rilonacept	Blocks IL-1b signaling by acting as a decoy receptor for IL-1b.	Loading dose: 4.4 mg/kg SC Loading dose may be divided into 1 or 2 separate injections on the same day at different sites (maximum injection 160 mg/injection) Maximum loading dose: 320 mg/dose. Maintenance dose: begin 1 wk after loading; 2.2 mg/kg/dose weekly SC (Maximum maintenance dose: 160 mg/dose)
Canakinumab[b]	Human monoclonal antibody that binds to IL-1b to prevent proinflammatory signaling.	4 mg/kg/dose every 4 wk SC Maximum: 300 mg/dose
Secukinumab	Human IgG1 monoclonal antibody that selectively binds to IL-17A to inhibit the	150 mg at weeks 0,1, 2, 3, and 4 then 150 mg q 4 wk SC (adult Ankylosing Spondylitis dosing)

(continued on next page)

Table 2
(continued)

Medication	Mechanism of Action	Typical Dosing and Route
	release of proinflammatory cytokines and chemokines.	
Ustekinumab	Human monoclonal antibody that binds to and interferes with IL-12 and IL-23.	45 mg at weeks 0 and 4 then every 12 wk; SC (adult PsA dosing)
Targeted Synthetic DMARDs (tsDMARDs)		
Tofacitinib[b]	Inhibits JAK enzymes and subsequent production of select cytokines (interleukins and interferons).	Immediate release: 10–20 Kg: 3.2 mg BID; PO (oral solution) 20–40 kg: 4 mg BID; PO (oral solution) ≥40 kg: 5 mg BID; PO (tablet or oral solution) Extended release (approved for adult rheumatoid arthritis): 11 mg once daily; PO

Abbreviations: BID, 2 times per day; TNF, tumor necrosis factor; EOD, every other day; PO, oral; IV, intravenous; SC, subcutaneous.

[a] Information from LexiComp Version: 3.0.2, 2021 and A Resident's Guide to Pediatric Rheumatology, 4th Edition, 2019, SickKids Hospital and Canadian Rheumatology Association (CRA).

[b] Approved by the US Food and Drug Administration for the treatment of JIA.

JIA involves more than 5 joints at the onset and is separated by the presence or absence of rheumatoid factor. Polyarticular JIA is more common in girls and has a bimodal peak of presentation (1–3 and 9–14 years).[4] Rheumatoid factor–positive polyarticular JIA, which usually occurs in the later age peak, has a course most similar to rheumatoid arthritis.

Specific laboratory testing is not required for a JIA diagnosis. Defining categories by joint counts and other physical examination features has significant limitations; the joint examination can be insensitive owing to joint location (eg, temporomandibular joint arthritis), examiner ability, and patient cooperation.[5] Genetic studies demonstrate overlap among both forms of oligoarthritis as well as rheumatoid factor negative polyarthritis[6] and they have similar treatment approaches. For this review, the categories of oligoarticular and polyarticular JIA are viewed as being on a spectrum of the same disease.

Key Treatment Updates

Except for persistent oligoarticular JIA, which may respond to nonsteroidal anti-inflammatory drugs (NSAIDs) and/or intra-articular corticosteroid injections (IAGC) alone, most children with JIA require more intensive therapy.

Medications

CsDMARDs and intra-articular corticosteroid injections. Methotrexate remains the cornerstone of JIA treatment, irrespective of joint count, and is the most commonly used csDMARD.[7,8] Methotrexate is generally safe and effective; however, gastrointestinal intolerance remains a significant barrier to its use. Up to one-third of patients with JIA can experience an adverse drug reaction on methotrexate monotherapy.[9] Leflunomide, sulfasalazine, and hydroxychloroquine are less commonly used alternative csDMARDs.

IAGC are commonly used for oligoarthritis. Triamcinolone hexacetonide provides more complete and longer duration of clinical response than the alternative triamcinolone acetonide.[10] IAGC may require sedation and/or imaging and are not appropriate for polyarthritis or repeated injections into the same joint where escalation of systemic therapy is preferred.

Biologic disease-modifying antirheumatic drugs

Tumor necrosis factor inhibitors JIA treatment was altered and improved dramatically with the introduction of the tumor necrosis factor inhibitor (TNFi) etanercept.[11] The importance of TNFi cannot be overstated. Before the use of biologic DMARDs (bDMARDs), inactive disease and low disease activity were difficult goals to achieve and cumulative damage and disability were common. In the United States, Canada, and Germany, TNFi are the most commonly prescribed biologic treatments and efficacy has been well-documented.[12–14] There are limited head-to-head TNFi trials.

Concerns remain regarding long-term use of TNFi, including the potential risk of malignancy, increased serious infections, and provocation of new autoimmune diseases and pharmacovigilance studies are critical for this medication as well as all medications discussed to treat JIA and are discussed in a separate article in this volume.

IL-6 inhibitors Tocilizumab is approved for polyarthritis and can be given by intravenous (IV) or subcutaneous administration. The 2-year extension phase of the CHERISH trial evaluated its safety and efficacy for polyarticular course JIA and found that children experienced a more than 80% decrease in pain and improvement in well-being.[15] Neutropenia (<1500 L/10^9) was common, but no increased risk of infections was seen during periods of neutropenia.[16]

Costimulation modulators Abatacept is available in IV and subcutaneous formulations approved for use in polyarticular JIA. The results of trials have demonstrated efficacy and safety for JIA.[17,18] Abatacept is also being used in an interesting prevention trial in oligoarticular JIA. The standard approach to a patient with oligoarticular JIA is to treat with NSAIDs and/or IAGC and institute a DMARD if these fail. The Childhood Arthritis and Rheumatology Research Alliance (CARRA) LIMIT-JIA clinical trial represents a novel approach for oligoarthritis treatment (NCT03841357) and evaluates whether a short course of once-weekly abatacept injection can prevent the extension of oligoarthritis and uveitis development. If effective, this study shifts focus from treating disease to preventing disease, which is exciting.

TsDMARDs

Janus kinase inhibitors

A newer class of drug for the treatment of JIA are the Janus kinase inhibitors (see **Table 2**). The results of a tofacitinib phase III trial demonstrated improvements in disease signs and symptoms, physical functioning, and a sustained clinically meaningful improvement in disease activity for polyarticular course JIA.[19] The safety profile was similar in children receiving tofacitinib or placebo. A warning of thromboembolic events and malignancies has been added recently to the label based on adult studies.

Future Directions

The optimal sequence and timing of csDMARD and bDMARD administration in JIA remains unclear. Start Time Optimization of biologics in Polyarticular JIA (STOP-JIA) was a prospective, observational CARRA Registry study comparing the effectiveness of (1) step up treatment—initial csDMARD monotherapy, adding a biologic if needed; (2) early combination—csDMARD and bDMARD started together; and (3) biologic first—

bDMARD monotherapy.[20] Achievement of clinical inactive disease off steroids did not differ significantly between the groups at 12 months. However, there was a statistically significant greater likelihood of achieving clinical Juvenile Arthritis Disease Activity Score—10 joints (refer to Sarah Ringold and colleagues' article, "Outcome Measures in Pediatric Rheumatic Disease," in this issue), low disease activity and Pediatric ACR70 in the early combination group. These results require further exploration.[21]

In recent years, the paradigm of explicitly defining a treatment target and applying tight control with necessary therapeutic adjustments to reach the target has been incorporated into treat to target (T2T) recommendations for adult rheumatoid arthritis. A JIA task force–defined remission as the treatment target upon which to base future research studies.[22] Klein and colleagues[23] evaluated 63 children with active JIA treated using T2T methods and found that T2T greatly improved the likelihood of achieving remission and/or low disease activity. Buckley and colleagues[24] reported similar excellent results by standardizing point-of-care disease activity monitoring and implementing clinical decision support to decrease treatment variation. More work is needed to understand the feasibility of T2T methods within usual clinical management.

It is also important to note that not all children require a bDMARD. Many children in the STOP-JIA trial treated with methotrexate only never required a bDMARD.[20] However, many children do require treatment with a bDMARD and many, more than one. More than one-half of children with JIA required a switch in biologic treatment and many required more than 2 biologics.[25] An 18-year follow-up study of Nordic children showed that remission on and off medication could be achieved in a large percentage of children; however, active disease remained in almost one-half of the patients with variability between categories.[3] Once disease is controlled, medication stoppage becomes an important goal for many children and their families. However, data on TNFi withdrawal have revealed a disappointingly high relapse rate with few predictive variables of success.[26,27]

ENTHESITIS-RELATED ARTHRITIS AND JUVENILE PSORIATIC ARTHRITIS

ERA is a form of juvenile spondyloarthritis (JSpA), which is discussed at length in a separate article (see Hemalatha Srinivasalu and colleagues' article, "Recent Updates in Juvenile Spondyloarthritis," in this issue).[28] Generally, PsJIA presents in a bimodal distribution, with younger patients resembling oligoarticular JIA and older patients presenting with disease reminiscent of adult PsA.[29] In this section, we focus on the latter set of patients with PsJIA, which we group with ERA, for the purpose of discussing treatment.

Key Clinical and Laboratory Features

ERA is often associated with axial disease and enthesitis or inflammation at the insertion sites of tendons, ligaments, fascia, or capsule into bone. However, younger children more often present initially with asymmetric lower limb large joint oligoarticular disease and less commonly with axial disease.

PsJIA that presents in middle to older childhood exhibits a sex ratio of 1:1, with a tendency to enthesitis and axial disease, which results in them being classified as undifferentiated JIA.[30] The American College of Rheumatology guidelines for the treatment of nonsystemic polyarthritis, sacroiliitis, and enthesitis are relevant for ERA treatment.[7]

Key Treatment Updates

Children with ERA experience worse quality of life, function, and pain, as compared with children with other JIA categories resulting in significant morbidity over time.[31]

A multidisciplinary approach including monitoring for signs and symptoms of ocular, dermatologic, and gastrointestinal disease with the involvement of these subspecialists, is essential.

For foot and ankle enthesitis, custom foot orthotics or heel cups may be helpful. Topical anti-inflammatories, such as diclofenac gel (5% or 10%), can be an effective adjunct therapy.

Medications

Nonsteroidal anti-inflammatory drugs

NSAIDs are the initial treatment of choice for many patients with ERA and patients with PsJIA with peripheral arthritis, enthesitis, and sacroiliitis.[7,32] Cyclo-oxygenase 2 inhibitors, like celecoxib, which have fewer gastrointestinal side effects, are preferred in patients with gut disease.

CsDMARDs

Two pediatric randomized controlled trials (RCTs) demonstrate the benefit of sulfasalazine for the peripheral arthritis of JIA, including ERA.[33,34] It is also conditionally recommended for sacroiliitis treatment in children with contraindications to TNFis or who have failed more than 1 TNFi.[7] This recommendation is supported by a low level of evidence and sulfasalazine is largely ineffective for treating axial disease in adult spondyloarthritis. Methotrexate or leflunomide are sometimes used, especially in PsJIA or ERA with predominantly peripheral arthritis.

Biologic disease-modifying antirheumatic drugs

Tumor necrosis factor inhibitors. Several TNFi have been shown to be safe and effective treatments for peripheral arthritis, sacroiliitis, enthesitis, and extra-articular manifestations (including uveitis, psoriasis, and gut inflammation). Etanercept was the most commonly prescribed bDMARD for ERA and PsJIA in the CARRA Registry.[34] Its effectiveness for these children has been shown in several studies, including an RCT and several prospective, retrospective, and registry-based studies.[35–38] It is effective for arthritis (peripheral and axial) and enthesitis, but ineffective for uveitis or gut inflammation.

Infliximab is effective for arthritis, enthesitis, inflammatory markers, pain, and physical function up to 1 year after treatment initiation.[39] Although the recommended starting dose and interval for Infliximab is 5 mg/kg IV every 8 weeks after loading doses,[32] many children need higher doses and/or more frequent infusions to maintain remission. A concomitant csDMARD, such as methotrexate (even low dose) with infliximab has been shown to prevent the formation of anti-Infliximab antibodies.[40]

Adalimumab was shown to be effective in juvenile ankylosing spondylitis in an RCT.[41] It was shown to significantly reduce active joint count, enthesitis count, and pain in a phase III multicenter study of ERA out to 1 year in the extension phase.[42] Similar improvements with adalimumab have been observed in retrospective and registry studies.[32]

Future Directions

IL-12 and IL-23 inhibitors

Biologics targeting the IL-12/IL-23 pathway are effective for adult plaque psoriasis and PsA, but ineffective for axial disease. One retrospective pediatric study showed that 4 of 5 patients with refractory ERA responded to ustekinumab, with improvements in active arthritis, enthesitis, and pain.[43]

IL-17 inhibitors

Secukinumab and ixekizumab are effective for adult patients with ankylosing spondylitis and PsA.[44] A clinical trial evaluating the safety and efficacy of secukinumab in children with JPsA and ERA has now been completed with the analysis underway (NCT03031782). These drugs are not used for inflammatory bowel disease and, in fact, may flare or unmask inflammatory bowel disease in a susceptible patient.

TsDMARDs

Janus kinase inhibitor. Janus kinase inhibitors are now being used to treat adult spondyloarthritis and PsA. However, these tsDMARDs are not yet approved for pediatric ERA.[45] One advantage of these medications is that they are administered orally.

SYSTEMIC JUVENILE IDIOPATHIC ARTHRITIS

The landscape for management of sJIA has radically evolved over the last 2 decades from a heavy reliance on corticosteroids to the early introduction of bDMARDs against IL-1 and IL-6 for targeted therapy with either no or minimal use of corticosteroids. Up to 40% of cases of sJIA are associated with macrophage activation syndrome (MAS), a life-threatening complication requiring urgent recognition and treatment.[46] Complications and treatment of refractory sJIA are reviewed elsewhere in this volume.

Key Clinical and Laboratory Features

sJIA is unique owing to its associated systemic features and despite its polygenic autoinflammatory origin is currently categorized under the International League of Associations of Rheumatologists JIA umbrella.[1] sJIA is distinguished from adult-onset Stills' disease by an arbitrary age cut-off of 16 years, although the 2 diseases are essentially equivalent.[47] The recently proposed Pediatric Rheumatology INternational Trials Organization (PRINTO) criteria for sJIA are an adapted version of the adult Yamaguchi criteria, not requiring the presence of arthritis.[48] MAS can present at any time during sJIA, including when patients are on IL-1 or IL-6 inhibitor therapy. Despite advances in treatment, sJIA remains a clinical diagnosis of exclusion. Other causes of fever, including infections, malignancy, and other autoinflammatory syndromes, must be excluded before treatment. NSAIDs may be useful for symptomatic management of fevers during the initial work-up phase.

Novel biomarkers

Although the S100 proteins (S100A8, S100A9, and S100A12) are increased in sJIA and elevated S100A8/9 levels may be useful to monitor treatment response, they are not yet readily available for clinical use.[49] Elevated IL-18 levels in sJIA may distinguish a subset predisposed to MAS.[50] INFγ is elevated in MAS and surrogate markers of INFγ including chemokine (C-X-C motif) ligand 9 or (CXCL9) that belongs to the chemokine family and is induced by INFγ have been explored as biomarkers.[51]

Key Treatment Updates

Given the heterogeneity of sJIA at presentation, treatment is tailored to the severity of the systemic, arthritic, or MAS features. Early aggressive and targeted therapy is favored given a postulated window of opportunity[52]: a biphasic model of sJIA has been proposed with a preponderance of innate and systemic features in the initial phase that, if not controlled, then transitions to an adaptive phase dominated by chronic arthritis.[52] Controlled trials for anakinra, canakinumab, rilonacept, and tocilizumab provide ample proof of both the efficacy and safety of these medications, which have revolutionized sJIA management. Before the availability of these medications, many patients with sJIA had to be treated with chronic glucocorticoids, sometimes for years, which caused many side effects and growth failure. Standardized CARRA consensus treatment plans and German guidelines for sJIA have been published.[53,54] The American College of Rheumatology is in the process of publishing updated sJIA treatment guidelines.[8] A pilot study assessed the feasibility of CARRA sJIA CTPs[55] and results of the First Line Options in sJIA (FROST) CARRA registry study of these CTPs (NCT02418442) are pending.

Medications

CsDMARDs

The csDMARDs are inappropriate for use as monotherapy in sJIA, but are sometimes used in conjunction with bDMARDs for arthritic involvement. Although glucocorticoids can be used effectively for initial therapy or monotherapy in sJIA, there is a trend toward early IL-1 or IL-6 inhibition, eliminating or decreasing the use of glucocorticoids altogether.[56]

Biologic disease-modifying antirheumatic drugs

IL-1 inhibitors. Canakinumab and anakinra are used for IL-1 inhibition in sJIA. Potential predictors of anakinra response include use as initial therapy or use early in disease course, higher ferritin levels, less active arthritic joints, higher systemic features, leukocytosis or neutrophilia, and older age at disease onset.[57] Conversely, homozygous IL-1 receptor antagonist gene high expression alleles have been identified as a potential genetic marker for lack of response to anakinra thus paving the way for precision therapy in sJIA.[58] An adapted JIA–American College of Rheumatology 50 response by 15 days and glucocorticoid discontinuation was predictive of achieving clinical remission with canakinumab treatment.[59] A shorter disease duration and no prior bDMARD exposure are associated with improved long-term remission on canakinumab.[60] Canakinumab response is associated with the upregulation of neutrophil- and IL-1–associated genes,[61] higher IL-18:CXCL-9 and INFr:CXCL9 ratios at baseline,[62] whereas upregulated CD163 expression was associated with nonresponse.[61]

IL-6 inhibitors. Tocilizumab is an effective treatment for sJIA[63] and, given the lack of head-to-head trials between initial IL-1i and IL-6i therapy, physicians or patients may opt for initial treatment of sJIA with tocilizumab, depending on availability, preference, and/or other factors. In the German autoinflammatory disease registry, 46 of 200 total sJIA patients received tocilizumab, of which 46% (21/46) received this as the first biologic.[64] Among these, 67% of patients (14/21) achieved inactive disease or clinical remission on medications at 1 year.

Other biologic disease-modifying antirheumatic drugs

Although IL-1i and IL-6i are becoming the mainstay of initial sJIA management, nonresponders can be switched to a different IL-1 or IL-6 agent. For active disease refractory to IL-1i or IL-6i, other bDMARDS like TNFi, rituximab, or combination bDMARDs, can be considered, although control of systemic features may be suboptimal. Please see the article on refractory sJIA (please refer to Remco Erkens and colleagues' article, "Pathogenesis and Treatment of Refractory Disease Courses in Systemic Juvenile Idiopathic Arthritis: Refractory Arthritis, Recurrent MAS and Chronic Lung Disease," in this issue).

Macrophage activation syndrome treatment

MAS treatment involves the swift and rapid administration of pulse methylprednisolone (30 mg/kg/d for 3 continuous days, maximum 1000 mg/d) followed by lower daily doses of steroids (1–2 mg/kg/d) with or without additional cyclosporine (IV or orally 3–5 mg/kg/d) or anakinra (IV or subcutaneously at 4–15 mg/kg/d). Anakinra works rapidly in MAS and is being studied in a current trial (NCT02780583). Patients with MAS have elevated IFNγ as well as IL-18 and the ratio of high IL-18 with a relatively lower CXCL9 (surrogate for INFγ), seems to be both sensitive and specific for MAS.[65] Corollary therapeutic implications of these biomarkers include the use of IL-18–binding protein (Tadekinig alfa), which antagonizes excessive IL-18 or the anti-INF agent emapalumab (NCT03311854) as possible treatments. Other treatments tried in MAS include IV immunoglobulin, tacrolimus, rituximab, plasma exchange, or the hemophagocytic lymphohistiocytosis 2004 protocol (used in familial hemophagocytic lymphohistiocytosis).[66] Please again see the Remco Erkens and colleagues' article, "Pathogenesis and Treatment of Refractory Disease Courses in Systemic Juvenile Idiopathic Arthritis: Refractory Arthritis, Recurrent MAS and Chronic Lung Disease," in this issue on refractory sJIA.

Future Directions

Tofacitinib is being studied in a double-blind placebo controlled randomized withdrawal study for sJIA use (NCT03000439) and is used off-label for sJIA or related lung disease. Other agents on the horizon for sJIA include other Janus kinase inhibitors (eg, baricitinib) and other IL-6 inhibitors (eg, sarilimumab). Like other JIA categories, T2T approaches can be effective in sJIA. Ter Haar and colleagues[67] used a dose escalation (2 mg/kg to 4 mg/kg) strategy for anakinra for new-onset sJIA with dose taper and discontinuation at 3 months if the target of inactive disease was achieved. Seventy-six percent and 96% of patients achieved inactive disease at 1 and 5 years, respectively, with 52% and 75% being off medication, respectively. Damage (articular/extra-articular) was noted in less than 5% and the majority of patients (67%) not need corticosteroids. Quartier and colleagues[68] evaluated 2 differing tapering strategies for canakinumab withdrawal in a phase IIIb/IV open-label multicenter RCT. Patients in remission on canakinumab monotherapy were randomized to either taper by dose reduction or prolongation of interval. Seventy-one percent of those with dose reduction taper versus 84% of those on prolongation of interval taper for canakinumab maintained clinical remission for 24 weeks and 33% overall discontinued canakinumab. There was insufficient power to determine superiority between the 2 tapering strategies in this trial. Regardless, these data demonstrate that remission off medications is an achievable and feasible target for sJIA and precision medicine with the identification of the most effective therapies for heterogeneous subsets of sJIA may be a wave of the future. Novel biomarkers that could distinguish such subsets are required and new targets for those that are refractory to anti–IL-1 and anti–IL-6 therapies need to be explored. Nonetheless, the future for sJIA seems to be bright.

CLINICS CARE POINTS

- The treatment of JIA requires a multidisciplinary and holistic approach, using both pharmacologic and nonpharmacologic treatments.
- For different JIA categories (polyarticular, oligoarticular, sJIA, and ERA) rheumatologists should take into consideration nuances between differences in treatment approaches.
  - sJIA responds best to early introduction of anti–IL-1 or anti–IL-6 agents with or without additional glucocorticoids.
- Standardized disease activity measures and patient-reported outcomes whenever possible can help to guide treatment decisions, potentially using a T2T approaches with shared decision-making.

DISCLOSURE

The authors have nothing to disclose.

REFERENCES

1. Petty RE, Southwood TR, Baum J, et al. Revision of the proposed classification criteria for juvenile idiopathic arthritis: Durban, 1997. J Rheumatol 1998;25(10): 1991–4.
2. Ringold S. Oligoarticular juvenile idiopathic arthritis. In: Petty RE, Lindsley C, Wedderburn L, et al, editors. Textbook of pediatric rheumatology. 8th edition. Elsevier; 2020. p. 241–9.
3. Glerup M, Rypdal V, Arnstad ED, et al. Long-term outcomes in juvenile idiopathic arthritis: eighteen years of follow-up in the population-based Nordic juvenile idiopathic arthritis cohort. Arthritis Care Res (Hoboken) 2020;72(4):507–16.
4. Rosenberg AM, Cron RQ. Polyarticular juvenile idiopathic arthritis. In: Petty RE, Lindsley C, Wedderburn L, et al, editors. Textbook of pediatric rheumatology. 8th edition. Elsevier; 2020. p. 228–40.
5. Pawlaczyk-Kamienska T, Pawlaczyk-Wroblewska E, Borysewicz-Lewicka M. Early diagnosis of temporomandibular joint arthritis in children with juvenile idiopathic arthritis. A systematic review. Eur J Paediatr Dent 2020;21(3):219–26.
6. Nigrovic PA, Raychaudhuri S, Thompson SD. Review: genetics and the classification of arthritis in adults and children. Arthritis Rheumatol 2018;70(1):7–17.
7. Ringold S, Angeles-Han ST, Beukelman T, et al. 2019 American College of Rheumatology/Arthritis Foundation guideline for the treatment of juvenile idiopathic arthritis: therapeutic approaches for non-systemic polyarthritis, sacroiliitis, and enthesitis. Arthritis Rheumatol 2019;71(6):846–63.
8. Onel KH, Shenoi S. 2021 American College of Rheumatology guideline for the treatment of juvenile idiopathic arthritis (JIA): therapeutic approaches for oligoarthritis, temporomandibular joint arthritis (TMJ), and systemic JIA, medication monitoring, immunizations and non-pharmacologic therapies. In: Presented at: ACR Convergence; 11/08/2020. 2020.
9. Kearsley-Fleet L, Vicente Gonzalez L, Steinke D, et al. Methotrexate persistence and adverse drug reactions in patients with juvenile idiopathic arthritis. Rheumatology (Oxford) 2019;58(8):1453–8.
10. Zulian F, Martini G, Gobber D, et al. Triamcinolone acetonide and hexacetonide intra-articular treatment of symmetrical joints in juvenile idiopathic arthritis: a double-blind trial. Rheumatology (Oxford) 2004;43(10):1288–91.
11. Lovell DJ, Giannini EH, Reiff A, et al. Etanercept in children with polyarticular juvenile rheumatoid arthritis. Pediatric Rheumatology Collaborative Study Group. N Engl J Med 2000;342(11):763–9.
12. Mannion ML, Xie F, Horton DB, et al. Biologic switching among non-systemic juvenile idiopathic arthritis patients: a cohort study in the childhood arthritis and rheumatology research alliance registry. J Rheumatol 2021;48(8):1322–9.
13. Chhabra A, Oen K, Huber AM, et al. Real-world effectiveness of common treatment strategies for juvenile idiopathic arthritis: results from a Canadian cohort. Arthritis Care Res (Hoboken) 2020;72(7):897–906.
14. Klein A, Becker I, Minden K, et al. Biologic therapies in polyarticular juvenile idiopathic arthritis. comparison of long-term safety data from the German BIKER registry. ACR Open Rheumatol 2020;2(1):37–47.
15. Brunner HI, Chen C, Bovis F, et al. Functional ability and health-related quality of life in randomized controlled trials of tocilizumab in patients with juvenile

idiopathic arthritis. Arthritis Care Res (Hoboken) 2020. https://doi.org/10.1002/acr.24384.

16. Pardeo M, Wang J, Ruperto N, et al. Neutropenia during tocilizumab treatment is not associated with infection risk in systemic or polyarticular-course juvenile idiopathic arthritis. J Rheumatol 2019;46(9):1117–26.

17. Brunner HI, Tzaribachev N, Vega-Cornejo G, et al. Subcutaneous abatacept in patients with polyarticular-course juvenile idiopathic arthritis: results from a phase III open-label study. Arthritis Rheumatol 2018;70(7):1144–54.

18. Hara R, Umebayashi H, Takei S, et al. Intravenous abatacept in Japanese patients with polyarticular-course juvenile idiopathic arthritis: results from a phase III open-label study. Pediatr Rheumatol Online J 2019;17(1):17.

19. Brunner HAJ, Al-Abadi E, Bohnsack J, et al. Tofacitinib for the treatment of patients with juvenile idiopathic arthritis: an interim analysis of data up to 5.5 years from an open-label, long-term extension study [abstract]. Arthritis Rheumatol 2020;72(suppl 10).

20. Kimura YSL, Tomlinson GA, Riordan ME, et al, the CARRA STOP-JIA Investigators. The Childhood Arthritis & Rheumatology Research Alliance Start Time Optimization of Biologics in Polyarticular Juvenile Idiopathic Arthritis Study (STOP-JIA): A Comparative Effectiveness Study of CARRA Consensus Treatment Plans for Untreated Polyarticular JIA. Arthritis Rheumatol 2021. https://doi.org/10.1002/art.41888.

21. Ong MRS, Kimura Y, Schanberg LE, et al, the CARRA Registry Investigators. Improved disease course associated with early initiation of biologics in untreated polyarticular Juvenile Idiopathic Arthritis. A trajectory analysis of the STOP-JIA study 2021. https://doi.org/10.1002/art.41892.

22. Ravelli A, Consolaro A, Horneff G, et al. Treating juvenile idiopathic arthritis to target: recommendations of an international task force. Ann Rheum Dis 2018; 77(6):819–28.

23. Klein A, Minden K, Hospach A, et al. Treat-to-target study for improved outcome in polyarticular juvenile idiopathic arthritis. Ann Rheum Dis 2020;79(7):969–74.

24. Buckley L, Ware E, Kreher G, et al. Outcome monitoring and clinical decision support in polyarticular juvenile idiopathic arthritis. J Rheumatol 2020;47(2):273–81.

25. Brunner HI, Schanberg LE, Kimura Y, et al. New medications are needed for children with juvenile idiopathic arthritis. Arthritis Rheumatol 2020;72(11):1945–51.

26. Lovell DJ, Johnson AL, Huang B, et al. Risk, timing, and predictors of disease flare after discontinuation of anti-tumor necrosis factor therapy in children with polyarticular forms of juvenile idiopathic arthritis with clinically inactive disease. Arthritis Rheumatol 2018;70(9):1508–18.

27. Simonini G, Ferrara G, Pontikaki I, et al. Flares after withdrawal of biologic therapies in juvenile idiopathic arthritis: clinical and laboratory correlates of remission duration. Arthritis Care Res (Hoboken) 2018;70(7):1046–51.

28. Weiss PF, Colbert RA. Juvenile spondyloarthritis: a distinct form of juvenile arthritis. Pediatr Clin North Am 2018;65(4):675–90.

29. Stoll ML, Zurakowski D, Nigrovic LE, et al. Patients with juvenile psoriatic arthritis comprise two distinct populations. Arthritis Rheum 2006;54(11):3564–72.

30. Zisman D, Gladman DD, Stoll ML, et al. The juvenile psoriatic arthritis cohort in the CARRA registry: clinical characteristics, classification, and outcomes. J Rheumatol 2017;44(3):342–51.

31. Rumsey DG, Guzman J, Rosenberg AM, et al. Worse quality of life, function, and pain in children with enthesitis, irrespective of their juvenile arthritis category. Arthritis Care Res (Hoboken) 2020;72(3):441–6.

32. Tse SML. Enthesitis-related arthritis. In: Petty RELR, Lindsley CB, Wedderburn L, et al, editors. Textbook of pediatric rheumatology. 8th edition. Elsevier; 2020. p. 250–67.

33. Burgos-Vargas R, Vazquez-Mellado J, Pacheco-Tena C, et al. A 26 week randomised, double blind, placebo controlled exploratory study of sulfasalazine in juvenile onset spondyloarthropathies. Ann Rheum Dis 2002;61(10):941–2.

34. van Rossum MA, Fiselier TJ, Franssen MJ, et al. Sulfasalazine in the treatment of juvenile chronic arthritis: a randomized, double-blind, placebo-controlled, multicenter study. Dutch Juvenile Chronic Arthritis Study Group. Arthritis Rheum 1998;41(5):808–16.

35. Rumsey DG, Lougee A, Matsouaka R, et al. Juvenile spondyloarthritis in the CARRA registry: high biologic use, low prevalence of HLA-B27, and equal sex representation in sacroiliitis. Arthritis Care Res (Hoboken) 2021;73(7):940–6.

36. Horneff G, Foeldvari I, Minden K, et al. Efficacy and safety of etanercept in patients with the enthesitis-related arthritis category of juvenile idiopathic arthritis: results from a phase III randomized, double-blind study. Arthritis Rheumatol 2015;67(8):2240–9.

37. Constantin T, Foeldvari I, Vojinovic J, et al. Two-year efficacy and safety of etanercept in pediatric patients with extended oligoarthritis, enthesitis-related arthritis, or psoriatic arthritis. J Rheumatol 2016;43(4):816–24.

38. Windschall D, Muller T, Becker I, et al. Safety and efficacy of etanercept in children with the JIA categories extended oligoarthritis, enthesitis-related arthritis and psoriasis arthritis. Clin Rheumatol 2015;34(1):61–9.

39. Burgos-Vargas RC, Gutierrez-Suarez R. A 3-month, double-blind, placebo-controlled, randomized trial of infliximab in juvenile-onset spondyloarthritis (SpA) and a 52-week open extension. Clin Exp Rheumatol 2008;26:745.

40. Chi LY, Zitomersky NL, Liu E, et al. The impact of combination therapy on infliximab levels and antibodies in children and young adults with inflammatory bowel disease. Inflamm Bowel Dis 2018;24(6):1344–51.

41. Horneff G, Fitter S, Foeldvari I, et al. Double-blind, placebo-controlled randomized trial with adalimumab for treatment of juvenile onset ankylosing spondylitis (JoAS): significant short term improvement. Arthritis Res Ther 2012;14(5):R230.

42. Burgos-Vargas R, Tse SM, Horneff G, et al. A randomized, double-blind, placebo-controlled multicenter study of adalimumab in pediatric patients with enthesitis-related arthritis. Arthritis Care Res (Hoboken) 2015;67(11):1503–12.

43. Mannion ML, McAllister L, Cron RQ, et al. Ustekinumab as a therapeutic option for children with refractory enthesitis-related arthritis. J Clin Rheumatol 2016; 22(5):282–4.

44. McGonagle DG, McInnes IB, Kirkham BW, et al. The role of IL-17A in axial spondyloarthritis and psoriatic arthritis: recent advances and controversies. Ann Rheum Dis 2019;78(9):1167–78.

45. Wang L, Ping X, Chen W, et al. Performance of Janus kinase inhibitors in psoriatic arthritis with axial involvement in indirect comparison with ankylosing spondylitis: a retrospective analysis from pooled data. Clin Rheumatol 2021;40(5):1725–37.

46. Minoia F, Davi S, Horne A, et al. Clinical features, treatment, and outcome of macrophage activation syndrome complicating systemic juvenile idiopathic arthritis: a multinational, multicenter study of 362 patients. Arthritis Rheumatol 2014;66(11):3160–9.

47. Colafrancesco S, Manara M, Bortoluzzi A, et al. Management of adult-onset Still's disease with interleukin-1 inhibitors: evidence- and consensus-based statements by a panel of Italian experts. Arthritis Res Ther 2019;21(1):275.

48. Martini A, Ravelli A, Avcin T, et al. Toward new classification criteria for juvenile idiopathic arthritis: first steps, pediatric rheumatology international trials organization international consensus. J Rheumatol 2019;46(2):190–7.

49. Holzinger D, Frosch M, Kastrup A, et al. The Toll-like receptor 4 agonist MRP8/14 protein complex is a sensitive indicator for disease activity and predicts relapses in systemic-onset juvenile idiopathic arthritis. Ann Rheum Dis 2012;71(6):974–80.

50. Shimizu M, Nakagishi Y, Inoue N, et al. Interleukin-18 for predicting the development of macrophage activation syndrome in systemic juvenile idiopathic arthritis. Clin Immunol 2015;160(2):277–81.

51. Mizuta M, Shimizu M, Inoue N, et al. Clinical significance of serum CXCL9 levels as a biomarker for systemic juvenile idiopathic arthritis associated macrophage activation syndrome. Cytokine 2019;119:182–7.

52. Nigrovic PA. Review: is there a window of opportunity for treatment of systemic juvenile idiopathic arthritis? Arthritis Rheumatol 2014;66(6):1405–13.

53. Hinze CH, Holzinger D, Lainka E, et al. Practice and consensus-based strategies in diagnosing and managing systemic juvenile idiopathic arthritis in Germany. Pediatr Rheumatol Online J 2018;16(1):7.

54. DeWitt EM, Kimura Y, Beukelman T, et al. Consensus treatment plans for new-onset systemic juvenile idiopathic arthritis. Arthritis Care Res (Hoboken) 2012;64(7):1001–10.

55. Kimura Y, Grevich S, Beukelman T, et al. Pilot study comparing the Childhood Arthritis & Rheumatology Research Alliance (CARRA) systemic Juvenile Idiopathic Arthritis Consensus Treatment Plans. Pediatr Rheumatol Online J 2017;15(1):23.

56. Vastert SJ, de Jager W, Noordman BJ, et al. Effectiveness of first-line treatment with recombinant interleukin-1 receptor antagonist in steroid-naive patients with new-onset systemic juvenile idiopathic arthritis: results of a prospective cohort study. Arthritis Rheumatol 2014;66(4):1034–43.

57. Saccomanno B, Tibaldi J, Minoia F, et al. Predictors of effectiveness of anakinra in systemic juvenile idiopathic arthritis. J Rheumatol 2019;46(4):416–21.

58. Arthur VL, Shuldiner E, Remmers EF, et al. IL1RN variation influences both disease susceptibility and response to recombinant human interleukin-1 receptor antagonist therapy in systemic juvenile idiopathic arthritis. Arthritis Rheumatol 2018;70(8):1319–30.

59. Brunner HI, Quartier P, Alexeeva E, et al. Efficacy and safety of canakinumab in patients with systemic juvenile idiopathic arthritis with and without fever at baseline: results from an open-label, active-treatment extension study. Arthritis Rheumatol 2020;72(12):2147–58.

60. Maritsi DN, Vougiouka O, Eleftheriou D. Discontinuation of canakinumab following clinical disease remission is feasible in patients with systemic juvenile idiopathic arthritis. J Rheumatol 2020;47(4):634–5.

61. Verweyen EL, Pickering A, Grom AA, et al. Distinct gene expression signatures characterize strong clinical responders vs non-responders to Canakinumab in children with sJIA. Arthritis Rheumatol 2021;73(7):1334–40.

62. Hinze T, Kessel C, Hinze CH, et al. A dysregulated interleukin-18/interferon-gamma/CXCL9 axis impacts treatment response to canakinumab in systemic juvenile idiopathic arthritis. Rheumatology (Oxford) 2021;keab113. https://doi.org/10.1093/rheumatology/keab113.

63. De Benedetti F, Brunner HI, Ruperto N, et al. Randomized trial of tocilizumab in systemic juvenile idiopathic arthritis. N Engl J Med 2012;367(25):2385–95.

64. Bielak M, Husmann E, Weyandt N, et al. IL-6 blockade in systemic juvenile idiopathic arthritis - achievement of inactive disease and remission (data from the German AID-registry). Pediatr Rheumatol Online J 2018;16(1):22.
65. Weiss ES, Girard-Guyonvarc'h C, Holzinger D, et al. Interleukin-18 diagnostically distinguishes and pathogenically promotes human and murine macrophage activation syndrome. Blood 2018;131(13):1442–55.
66. Griffin G, Shenoi S, Hughes GC. Hemophagocytic lymphohistiocytosis: an update on pathogenesis, diagnosis, and therapy. Best Pract Res Clin Rheumatol 2020;34(4):101515.
67. Ter Haar NM, van Dijkhuizen EHP, Swart JF, et al. Treatment to target using recombinant interleukin-1 receptor antagonist as first-line monotherapy in new-onset systemic juvenile idiopathic arthritis: results from a five-year follow-up study. Arthritis Rheumatol 2019;71(7):1163–73.
68. Quartier P, Alexeeva E, Tamas C, et al. Tapering canakinumab monotherapy in patients with systemic juvenile idiopathic arthritis in clinical remission: results from an open-label, randomized phase IIIb/IV study. Arthritis Rheumatol 2021; 73(2):336–46.

Recent Updates in Juvenile Spondyloarthritis

Hemalatha Srinivasalu, MD[a], Keith A. Sikora, MD[b], Robert A. Colbert, MD, PhD[c],*

KEYWORDS

- Enthesitis-related arthritis • Juvenile psoriatic arthritis • Spondyloarthritis
- Pediatrics • Juvenile idiopathic arthritis

KEY POINTS

- Juvenile spondyloarthritis, an umbrella term that includes enthesitis-related arthritis, juvenile psoriatic arthritis, and undifferentiated juvenile idiopathic arthritis, exists on a continuum with adult onset spondyloarthritis.
- The hallmark characteristic of juvenile spondyloarthritis is enthesitis, with HLA-B27 being a risk factor for axial skeletal involvement, acute anterior uveitis, and prolonged disease course.
- Lower extremity oligoarticular disease usually occurs before the onset of axial inflammation, defined by characteristic bone marrow edema on MRI of sacroiliac joints.
- Although HLA-B27 is the most significant risk factor for axial spondyloarthritis, the majority of HLA-B27+ individuals are healthy, highlighting the role of additional genetic factors.
- Genome-wide association studies have only identified about 7% of the non-MHC heritability of ankylosing spondylitis, but genetic variants support the therapeutic benefit of targeting IL-17.

INTRODUCTION

Spondyloarthritis (SpA) encompasses a group of disorders characterized by presence of enthesitis, axial skeletal involvement and a common genetic predisposition most notably related to HLA-B27. Ankylosing spondylitis (AS) is the prototypic form of SpA. Children who develop features of SpA before their 16th birthday have juvenile SpA (JSpA). This article highlights recent advances in clinical features and pathogenesis of JSpA.

[a] Division of Rheumatology, Children's National Hospital, George Washington University School of Medicine, 111 Michigan Avenue Northwest, Washington, DC, USA; [b] National Institute of Arthritis, Musculoskeletal and Skin Diseases, National Institutes of Health, Building 10, Room 12N240, 10 Center Drive, Bethesda, MD 20892, USA; [c] National Institute of Arthritis, Musculoskeletal and Skin Diseases, National Institutes of Health, Building 10, Room 12N240E, 10 Center Drive, Bethesda, MD 20892, USA
* Corresponding author.
E-mail address: colbertr@nih.gov

Rheum Dis Clin N Am 47 (2021) 565–583
https://doi.org/10.1016/j.rdc.2021.07.001
0889-857X/21/Published by Elsevier Inc.

rheumatic.theclinics.com

CLASSIFICATION

JSpA is best understood as an umbrella term that encompasses enthesitis-related arthritis (ERA), juvenile psoriatic arthritis (JPsA) and undifferentiated arthritis categories of the International League of Associations for Rheumatology (ILAR) juvenile idiopathic arthritis (JIA) classification system. Children may also satisfy the European Spondylitis Study Group or Amor criteria for undifferentiated arthritis, the Assessment of SpondyloArthritis International Society (ASAS) criteria for axial or peripheral SpA or the modified New York criteria for AS, which are generally applied to adults over 18 years of age. Conditions such as chronic noninfectious osteomyelitis, synovitis, acne, pustulosis, hyperostosis, and osteitis (SAPHO syndrome), and hidradenitis suppurativa are sometimes clustered with SpA. For the purposes of this article, we discuss ERA, JPsA, and undifferentiated subcategories included in the ILAR classification. We also include studies in which children were classified as having JSpA based on the European Spondylitis Study Group, Amor and ASAS criteria, or the modified New York criteria for AS. The limitations of the current classification system have been extensively covered elsewhere.[1–3] Adult classification systems such as Amor, ASAS axial SpA, European Spondylitis Study Group, Garmisch–Partenkirchen, and ASAS peripheral SpA criteria have been applied to children with good sensitivity (approximately 90%) using expert opinion by pediatric rheumatologists as the gold standard.[4,5] Recently, new JIA classification criteria have been proposed that include JSpA.[4,6] However, a lack of harmony with adult arthritis classification and nomenclature continues to be an issue.[7] Considering JSpA on a continuum with adult SpA is crucial for long-term care because most of these children continue to have active disease well into adulthood. It also leverages advances made understanding pathogenesis of adult SpA and developing new treatments.

CLINICAL FEATURES
Epidemiology

The demographics and frequency of HLA-B27 in JSpA vary by geographic region. The mean age at diagnosis is 9.55 to 10.80 years for ERA,[5,8,9] and there is a male preponderance (56.0% to 82.5%).[8,10,11] HLA-B27 positivity in ERA ranges from 38% to 68%.[5,8,11] However, these demographics may be influenced by the fact that male sex, age over 6 years, and HLA-B27 status are included in the ILAR classification criteria for ERA. HLA-B27 positivity in ERA is associated with prolonged disease course, a higher incidence of acute anterior uveitis, a family history of SpA, and a higher erythrocyte sedimentation rate.[11]

Children with JPsA classically separate into 2 subgroups,[12] with those less than 4 to 5 years of age similar to children with early onset oligoarticular and polyarticular JIA with a female preponderance, dactylitis, and higher incidence of antinuclear antibody (ANA) positivity and uveitis. Children with a later age at onset are more likely to be male and have enthesitis, sacroiliitis, and psoriasis.[9,12] The mean age at diagnosis is 3.1 years for early onset JPsA and 8.2 to 11.2 years for late-onset JPsA.[8,9] Early-onset JPsA has a female preponderance of 78%. Late-onset JPsA also has a modest female preponderance of 57.7%.[9] HLA-B27 is positive in only 10.6% to 12.0% with JPsA with a similar distribution in early-onset and late-onset JPsA[8,9] and does not correlate with axial disease.

Enthesis

Tenderness at entheses where tendons and ligaments attach to bones is a characteristic feature of SpA. Enthesitis is defined as tenderness on palpation of entheseal sites.

However, patients with chronic pain may be tender on palpation in the absence of true enthesitis; the use of ultrasound examination or MRI may improve sensitivity.[13,14] Although enthesitis is classically present in JSpA, it is seen in other subtypes of JIA as well.[15] Enthesitis is reported at diagnosis in 64% to 72% of patients with ERA,[5,15] 18% of patients with undifferentiated JIA, and only 2% of patients with JPsA.[15] Over time, 78% of patients with ERA and 19% of patients with JPsA develop enthesitis.[8] Patients with late-onset JPsA tend to have enthesitis more frequently (36.8%) compared with early-onset JPsA (16.9%).[9] Classically, entheses around the patella and Achilles tendon are most commonly involved in JSpA.[10] **Table 1** summarizes the entheseal sites involved in various historical JSpA cohorts. There are several enthesitis indices for adult SpA, but no validated JSpA-specific enthesitis index for use in clinical practice or research.

Peripheral Arthritis

Patients with JSpA have peripheral arthritis more frequently than axial arthritis at disease onset. At presentation, the pattern of peripheral arthritis in ERA and JPsA is predominantly oligoarticular (approximately 75%).[10,16] However, over the disease course, patients with ERA and JPsA both tend to develop polyarticular arthritis.[8,9] In general, the lower extremity joints such as the hips, knees, ankles, and tarsal joints are more commonly involved compared with upper extremity joints. Hip joint involvement is present in 20% of patients at inception in ERA[10] and increases up to 46% over the disease course.[5] Hip joint involvement predicts development of sacroiliitis[17] and is one of the major causes of morbidity, including hip arthroplasty in adulthood for patients with juvenile onset AS.[18] Foot joint involvement is common in JSpA, with midfoot and subtalar joint involvement accounting for 58% of cases.[19] Classically, dactylitis is associated with JPsA (approximately 30%) with higher prevalence in early-onset JPsA (approximately 40%) (**Fig. 1**).[9]

Axial Arthritis

Sacroiliitis is the heralding sign of axial disease and the basis of significant disease burden in JSpA. Sacroiliitis negatively impacts physician global, parent/patient global

Table 1	
Entheseal sites studied in historical JSpA cohorts	
Entheseal Sites	**Percentage**
Insertion of infrapatellar tendon on patella	27–44
Achilles tendon	21–74
Interosseous ligaments of the sacroiliac joint	30.3
Plantar fascia insertion to calcaneus	12–39
Tibial tuberosity	23–30
Quadriceps insertion to upper poles of patella	22–46
Second MTP	21
Third MTP	16
First MTP	14
Greater trochanter	14
Iliac crest	14

Abbreviation: MTP, metatarsophalangeal.
Data from Refs.[5,10,13,15]

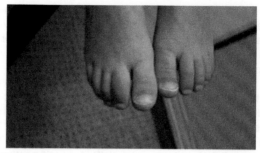

Fig. 1. Dactylitis of the second toe on the right foot in a child with JPsA. (*Courtesy of* Dr. Carlos Rose.)

and Clinical Juvenile Arthritis Disease Activity scores and predicts a high rate of biologic use (81%).[8] Clinically, sacroiliitis is defined as tenderness on palpation of the sacroiliac (SI) joint(s) and/or inflammatory lumbosacral pain by the ILAR criteria[20]; however, concordance between these findings and joint inflammation and/or bone marrow edema on imaging is unclear. In contrast with adult SpA, inflammatory back pain and clinical sacroiliitis are present in only 20% to 40% of patients with JSpA at diagnosis.[5,8,17,21] Factors associated with a higher pretest probability of finding sacroiliitis by MRI at diagnosis include HLA-B27 positivity and elevated C-reactive protein.[21] In addition, patients with a family history of SpA have a higher risk of developing both sacroiliitis and persistent active disease.[5] As noted in the study by Lin and colleagues,[17] although the majority of patients with sacroiliitis by MRI at initial diagnosis had back pain, hip pain, morning stiffness, or abnormal physical examination, 50% of patients had a normal examination and one-third were asymptomatic with a normal examination despite continued evidence of active sacroiliitis on imaging during follow-up. Thus, physical examination alone lacks sensitivity and specificity in monitoring axial disease. Children are known to have silent sacroiliitis, with evidence of inflammation on imaging in the absence of inflammatory back pain and/or clinical signs of sacroiliitis such as SI joint tenderness, pain on SI distraction maneuvers, and an abnormal Schober test.[22] Sacroiliitis at disease presentation in ERA varies from 29.0% to 55.6% based on the cohort and the definition of sacroiliitis used in the study.[5,10] Approximately 40% to 60% of patients with ERA develop sacroiliitis during their disease course.[5,8] In JPsA, sacroiliitis is more common in the late-onset subgroup with a prevalence of around 12% to 19%.[8,9] Although classically male sex is considered a risk factor for development of sacroiliitis, the CARRA registry reveals an equal sex distribution for sacroiliitis defined clinically and/or by imaging in a cohort that included patients with ERA and patients with JPsA.[8] Whether this finding is a result of increased clinical recognition of SpA in females is unknown, but this observation is similar to the equal sex distribution of nonradiographic axial SpA seen in adults.[23]

Extra-articular Manifestations

Nails

The nail bed is an entheseal organ; extensor tendons of the distal interphalangeal joints and joint collateral ligament entheses send interdigitating collagen fibers from the bone that envelop the nail root. Additionally, the nail plate is tethered to the underlying periosteum by collagen fibers.[24] Nail abnormalities classically seen in psoriatic arthritis include nail pitting and onycholysis (**Fig. 2**). Nail pitting occurs in 37% of patients with early- and late-onset JPsA.[9]

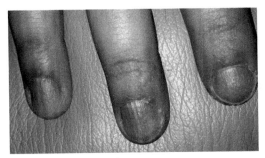

Fig. 2. Nail pitting in a 9-year old girl with JPsA.

Uveitis

Patients with JSpA can present with chronic idiopathic uveitis or acute anterior uveitis. The overall prevalence of uveitis in JSpA is approximately 7% to 11%,[25,26] and is similar in ERA (7%–13%) and JPsA (7%–10%). The prevalence of chronic idiopathic uveitis and ANA positivity in early-onset JPsA (18.8%) is similar to that of oligoarticular JIA.[9] Patients with ERA, late-onset JPsA, and undifferentiated JIA generally develop acute anterior uveitis (79%), which is typically associated with HLA-B27 positivity. Contrary to idiopathic uveitis, acute anterior uveitis classically presents with pain, photophobia, and redness. As per the recent American College of Rheumatology guidelines, ophthalmology screening should occur every 3 months for children with JPsA and undifferentiated arthritis who are ANA positive and less than 7 years of age. Patients with JPsA and undifferentiated arthritis who are older than 7 and are ANA negative and patients with ERA should be screened every 6 to 12 months.[27]

Gastrointestinal Inflammation

Gastrointestinal inflammation is strongly associated with SpA and peripheral and axial arthritis are well known extraintestinal manifestations of inflammatory bowel disease. Further, up to two-thirds of patients with SpA have subclinical gut inflammation.[28,29] Intestinal inflammation on ileocolonic biopsy has been noted in children with late-onset pauciarticular juvenile chronic arthritis,[30] which may be due to the inclusion of patients with JSpA. Fecal calprotectin, a surrogate marker for gastrointestinal inflammation, can be elevated in ERA.[31,32] The levels of calprotectin vary between children with active and inactive disease and between those with and without sacroiliitis by MRI.[32] Although in adults with axial SpA, a link between bone marrow edema in SI joints and gut inflammation has been found,[33] it is not known if such an association exists in children. New insights into changes in the gut microbiome are helping to shape understanding of the link between gut immunity and systemic inflammatory changes in patients with JSpA.[34–37]

Other Extra-articular Manifestations

Obesity and the metabolic syndrome are important comorbidities in adult psoriatic arthritis. Around 36.3% of JPsA patients in the CARRA registry were overweight (calculated body mass index of $\geq$85th percentile for age and sex).[38] This group was older at symptom onset and had worse patient/physician global and Childhood Health Assessment Questionnaire scores when compared with nonoverweight children. The prevalence of overweight in children with JPsA enrolled in the CARRA registry was higher than age-matched RF+ and RF– Poly JIA Registry patients and the general population non-Hispanic White population in the United States. A possible relationship between obesity and medications such as corticosteroids and tumor necrosis factor (TNF) inhibitors (TNFi) was not explored in this study. Several hypotheses for obesity in JPsA exist, such as the contribution of altered gut microbiota, inflammation triggered by obesity, and greater biomechanical stress on weight bearing joints triggering arthritis; however, these hypotheses require further study.

Increased cardiovascular burden in adult AS and psoriatic arthritis is well-established.[39,40] Adults with a history of juvenile arthritis have a significantly increased risk of metabolic syndrome compared with those without arthritis,[41] which could be a contributing factor to long-term cardiovascular risk. In a small cohort study, children with JSpA had possible early signs of right ventricular diastolic dysfunction compared with healthy controls. A possible association between lower left ventricular systolic function and MRI confirmed enthesitis was noted.[42] Future prospective studies on cardiovascular function in JSpA are needed.

GENETIC SUSCEPTIBILITY AND PATHOGENESIS

Highlighting the contribution of genetics to disease development, SpA tends to run within families. The most significant genetic risk factor for axial SpA is HLA-B27.[43,44] Although it is present in about 90% of cases of AS[45] compared with less than 10% of unaffected individuals of northern European ancestry, HLA-B27 contributes only about 20% of overall heritability,[45] underscoring the importance of other genetic and/or environmental modifiers. In fact, risk of disease occurrence is 6- to 16-fold greater in HLA-B27+ family members of an affected individual compared with unrelated healthy HLA-B27+ individuals.[46,47] Further illustrating the importance of genetic factors outside of the MHC region, the disease concordance rate among dizygotic HLA-B27+ twins is significantly lower than for monozygotic HLA-B27+ twins.[45]

Consistent with AS being a complex genetic disease, multiple risk genes beyond HLA-B27 have been identified. Indeed, genome-wide association studies (GWAS) have uncovered multiple pathways contributing to pathogenesis,[48] highlighting similarities between phenotypically overlapping diseases (psoriasis, inflammatory bowel disease, and Behcet's disease),[49,50] as well as the pathogenic role of the IL-23/IL-17 axis.[51] GWAS of AS patients have identified associations with genes responsible for production of IL-23 (CARD9, IL12 B, and PTGER4), development of IL-23 responsive cells (IL27 and IL7R), and responsiveness to IL-23 (TYK2, STAT3, and IL23 R).[52–55] However, well over 100 non-MHC genomic variants identified via GWAS are estimated to contribute only about 7.3% to the heritability of AS.[45,49] This missing heritability may be accounted for by as-yet undiscovered high effect size rare (mean allele frequency <1%) variants, copy number variations, genetic epistasis, or epigenetic changes. Multiple GWAS have been performed on pediatric chronic arthritis patients.[56–60] These studies lumped different forms of JIA together, so were likely underpowered to demonstrate associations specific for ERA, and hence offer limited unique insight into ERA pathogenesis. Indeed, fine mapping of the MHC region highlights the genetic heterogeneity between different subtypes of JIA, with ERA correlating poorly with other subtypes.[61] As with systemic JIA,[62] genetic studies focusing on ERA would likely be more informative. Focusing on pediatric-onset disease, one study examined 2 well-established single nucleotide polymorphisms (SNPs) in IL23R and ERAP1 that confer risk for AS/psoriatic arthritis, across different subtypes of JIA. This study revealed an association between ERAP1 in ERA and IL23R in JPsA, yet failed to demonstrate an expected association between ERA and IL23 R, possibly owing to insufficient power.[63]

Common *IL23R* variants identified through GWAS are also associated with inflammatory bowel disease[64] and psoriasis,[65] highlighting the pathogenic role of the IL-23/IL-17 axis in SpA-related diseases. IL-23 is produced by myeloid cells and promotes differentiation, proliferation, and production of IL-17 from CD4+ Th17 T cells.[66] It also promotes IL-17 production from cells of the innate immune system, including γδ T cells, certain natural killer cells, invariant natural killer T cells, Paneth cells, mast cells, lymphoid tissue inducer cells, and a population of CD4−/CD8−/CD3+ T cells found in the entheses of mice.[67,68] The *IL23R* SNP (rs11209026) that is most strongly associated with protection from AS and inflammatory bowel disease produces a nonsynonymous Arg381Gln substitution in the cytoplasmic region, causing decreased IL-23–induced STAT3 phosphorylation and IL-17 production in Th17 cells.[69–71] In addition to rs11209026, another independent AS-associated SNP, rs11209032, exists within the intergenic region of IL23R–IL12RB2 that may influence T-cell IFN-γ production in the homozygous state,[72] suggesting that a Th1 versus Th17 pathogenic dichotomy may be too simplistic and Th1 immunity may also play a role in SpA pathogenesis.[73] It is important to note that combinatorial effects of risk and susceptibility alleles, rather than isolated effects, likely dictate SpA disease development. Indeed, combinatory SNPs within the IL-23/IL-17 axis influence both Th17 and Th1 immune response development[74] in SpA.

There is significant evidence from human studies that indicates the IL-23/IL-17 axis is activated in SpA.[75] Although serum and synovial fluid levels of IL-17 and/or IL-23 can be elevated across different ages,[76–79] SpA disease activity poorly correlates with serum IL-23 as compared with rheumatoid arthritis.[80] However, serum or synovial fluid cytokine data should be interpreted with caution, because they may not reflect pathologic processes active in the SI joints, vertebral bodies, facet joints, or bone marrow adjacent to sites of axial inflammation. For example, TNF serum levels are not uniformly increased in SpA[81,82] and can even be lower in AS than healthy controls.[83] However, increased expression of TNF has been demonstrated in actively inflamed hip and SI joints,[84,85] and is an established therapeutic target. Several studies have documented the expression of IL-17 and IL-23 at sites of inflammation in SpA. In AS, IL-17+ neutrophils (myeloperoxidase+/CD15+) and mononuclear cells, as well as IL-23+ myeloid cells, are increased in both subchondral bone marrow and facet joints compared with osteoarthritic controls.[86,87] Taken together, and consistent with animal model data, considerable evidence implicates the IL-23/IL-17 axis in the pathogenesis of human axial SpA.

Perhaps the most relevant insights into the pathogenesis of SpA come from clinical trials. The neutralization of IL-17A has demonstrated clear efficacy in AS,[88] psoriasis,[89] and psoriatic arthritis,[90] while causing worsening of Crohn disease[91] possibly owing to protective effects of IL-17A in the gut.[92] Although antibodies targeting IL-23 (risankizumab) or IL-12 and IL-23 (ustekinumab) have demonstrated clear efficacy in plaque psoriasis,[93] psoriatic arthritis,[94] and Crohn disease,[95] they have been surprisingly ineffective in double-blind placebo-controlled trials for AS and axial SpA, respectively,[88,96] despite results from animal models. Interestingly, nonsteroidal anti-inflammatory drugs, which have been used for decades to treat SpA, decrease production of prostaglandin E2, the ligand for prostaglandin E receptor 4, which is encoded by the disease-associated gene *PTGER4*. Interaction between prostaglandin E2 and its receptor on T cells and dendritic cells leads to Th1 expansion, as well as IL-23–mediated Th17 differentiation.[97] In summary, although preclinical data strongly support the role of the IL-23/IL-17 axis in SpA, the surprising failure of IL-23 blockade in axial SpA underscores the complexity of human inflammatory disease, uncouples an absolute need for IL-23 in sustained IL-17 production, and may hint at temporal roles of both IL-23 and IL-17 in different stages of disease pathogenesis.[98]

DIAGNOSTIC IMAGING
Radiography and Ultrasound Examination

Although plain radiographic changes reflecting SI joint damage are essential for diagnosing adult AS, they have limited usefulness in early disease and are not required to diagnose nonradiographic axial SpA. In children, radiographs of the SI joints have limited usefulness as a screening tool[99] because the damage can take considerable time to develop (**Fig. 3**). Ultrasound examination has emerged as an attractive modality to diagnose peripheral arthritis, enthesitis, and tenosynovitis,[100] but it has limited usefulness in diagnosing sacroiliitis perhaps because of its complex anatomy. Uniform definitions for normal appearance of peripheral joints and entheses on ultrasound in the pediatric population and a standardized scoring system are being developed by the CARRA Ultrasound Workgroup and may provide an additional tool for monitoring peripheral disease activity longitudinally.

MRI

MRI is used for diagnosing, classifying, and monitoring both peripheral and axial disease in JSpA. It has greatest usefulness in imaging the SI joint(s), because both clinical examination and plain radiographs lack sufficient sensitivity or specificity for diagnosing sacroiliitis.[21] The ASAS definition for sacroiliitis developed for adults is generally used in clinical practice to define sacroiliitis in both adults and children. According to the ASAS definition, lesions representative of active sacroiliitis are bone marrow edema, capsulitis, synovitis, and enthesitis (**Fig. 4**). Bone marrow edema must be present in 2 consecutive slices or in multiple areas in a single slice.[101] However, the ASAS definition has low sensitivity in JSpA using radiologist's global assessment of sacroiliitis as the gold standard.[102] Active lesions as defined by ASAS are visualized adequately on fluid-sensitive sequences and contrast administration does not add incremental value in evaluating for active sacroiliitis in JSpA.[103] However, in clinical practice contrast MRI of the SI joints is generally used when other causes of back pain mimicking sacroiliitis such as bony tumors, infections, and leukemia are in the differential. It is important to note that developmental changes in the SI joint can be confused with sacroiliitis (**Fig. 5**). Furthermore, nonspecific bone marrow changes occur in young athletes,[104] and radiologists may overcall active sacroiliitis.[105] Chauvin and colleagues[106] recently provided a reference description of normative SI joint MRI

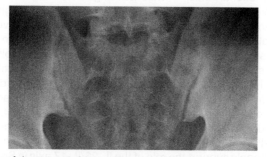

Fig. 3. Radiograph of the SI joints from a 20-year old man who had disease onset at 14 years of age. The radiograph shows bilateral erosion and subchondral sclerosis that is more prominent on the right.

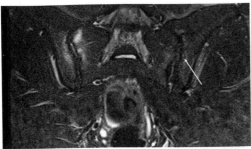

Fig. 4. Coronal oblique short T1 inversion recovery image of the SI joints in an 18-year-old HLA-B27 positive man demonstrating bilateral sacroiliitis. Bone marrow edema on the iliac and sacral side of the right SI joint is indicative of active sacroiliitis. The left SI joint shows chronic appearing changes, including prominent erosive changes and milder bone marrow edema of the iliac and sacral sides of SI joint (*long white arrow*).

findings in children that could help to decrease the variability in interpretation of SI joint imaging. The Spondyloarthritis Research Consortium of Canada Scoring System is a reliable tool for objective quantification of sacroiliitis and measuring responsiveness to change in JSpA.[107] The use of calibration modules increases the reliability of these

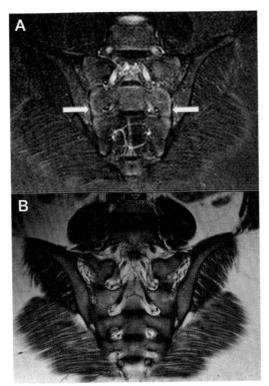

Fig. 5. (*A, B*). Coronal oblique short T1 inversion recovery (*A*) and T1-weighted (*B*) images of the SI joints from an 11-year-old normal girl. Notice the areas of homogeneous bilateral symmetric rims of subchondral short T1 inversion recovery hyperintensity within subarticular bone of the sacrum (*white arrows*).

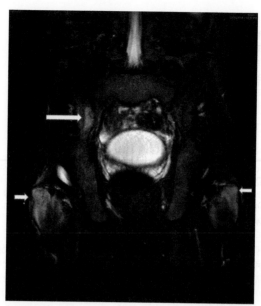

Fig. 6. Short T1 inversion recovery image from whole body MRI of a 15-year-old boy with HLA-B27–positive JSpA depicting the SI and hip joints. There is subchondral bone marrow edema and a focal erosion within the right iliac bone adjacent to inferior aspect of the right SI joint (*long white arrow*). Also note bone marrow edema of the greater trochanters bilaterally (*short white arrows*), reflecting enthesitis.

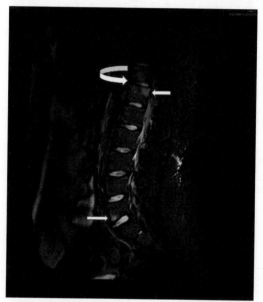

Fig. 7. Short T1 inversion recovery image from whole body MRI of a 15-year-old boy with HLA-B27–negative JSpA. The MRI shows active corner inflammatory lesions of vertebral end plates at multiple levels (*straight white arrows*), and more chronic appearing discovertebral unit changes (*curved white arrow*).

composite measures.[108] There is an increased interest in using whole body MRI to evaluate the overall disease burden in JSpA. Whole body MRI can potentially identify areas of bone marrow edema, synovitis, and enthesitis not apparent on clinical evaluation[109] or validate physical examination findings to aid treatment decisions (**Figs. 6 and 7**).There is an international effort organized through the Outcome Measures in Rheumatology to develop a semiquantitative scoring system for whole body MRI in JIA.[110] Future studies should explore the validity of any proposed scoring systems in initial diagnosis and monitoring longitudinal inflammatory burden in JSpA.

DISEASE ACTIVITY MEASURES

The Juvenile Spondyloarthritis Disease Activity Index is the only validated disease activity measure specific for JSpA. It is a composite measure including history, physical examination, laboratory marker and pain visual analog scale (**Table 2**) where each item is equally weighted and summed. The score can range from 0 to 8, with higher scores indicating greater disease activity.[111] A modified version of this scoring system excluding back mobility was validated in ERA.[112]

Table 2
Elements in the Juvenile Spondyloarthritis Disease Activity Index[a]

Item	Score
Active joint count	0 joints = 0 1–2 joints = 0.5 >2 joints = 1
Active enthesitis count	0 entheses = 0 1–2 entheses = 0.5 >2 enthesis = 1
Pain – VAS (0–10)	0–0 1–2 = 0.5 5–10 = 1
ESR or CRP related to JSpA activity	Normal = 0 1–2 times normal = 0.5 >2 times normal = 1
Morning stiffness (≥15 min)	Absent = 0 Present = 1
Clinical sacroiliitis	Absent = 0 Present = 1
Uveitis	Absent = 0 Present = 1
Back mobility	Normal = 0 Abnormal = 1

Abbreviations: CRP, C-reactive protein; ESR, erythrocyte sedimentation rate; VAS, Visual analog scale.
[a]Each item is equally weighted. The range of possible scores is 0 to 8, with higher scores indicating more disease activity.
Adapted from Weiss PF, Colbert RA, Xiao R, et al. Development and retrospective validation of the juvenile spondyloarthritis disease activity index. *Arthritis care & research.* 2014;66(12):1775-1782.

TREATMENT

The 2019 American College of Rheumatology guidelines for treatment of JIA[113] includes recommendations for sacroiliitis and enthesitis. Initial treatment with nonsteroidal anti-inflammatory drugs is strongly recommended. In the event of a poor response to nonsteroidal anti-inflammatory drugs, the use of TNFi is strongly recommended in those with sacroiliitis and conditionally recommended over conventional disease-modifying antirheumatic drugs in those with enthesitis. Sulfasalazine is conditionally recommended in those who fail TNFi or have contraindications to their use in sacroiliitis. Methotrexate monotherapy is strongly discouraged for the management of sacroiliitis, and glucocorticoids are recommended only as bridging therapy. Intra-articular injection of the SI joints is conditionally recommended as an adjunct therapy. The use of physical therapy is conditionally recommended for both sacroiliitis and enthesitis. Although non-TNFi biologics such as IL-17–blocking agents and small molecules such as JAK inhibitors have shown promise in treatment of adult SpA, they are not currently approved by the US Food and Drug Administration for JSpA.

SUMMARY

JSpA exists on a continuum with adult SpA. Any new nomenclature or classification system should be based on molecular classification. There are genetic factors beyond HLA-B27 that determine heritability and influence the pathogenesis of disease. Enthesitis and sacroiliitis are the most challenging aspects of treatment. Physical examination for evaluation of enthesitis and sacroiliitis lack sensitivity and specificity, and additional imaging is required for longitudinal monitoring. The recent American College of Rheumatology guidelines have helped to address the management of sacroiliitis and enthesitis in JSpA, but additional studies are needed.

CLINICS CARE POINTS

- The effective treatment of JSpA requires prompt recognition and distinction from other forms of juvenile arthritis
- Enthesitis, a key clinical feature of JSpA, must be distinguished from other causes of soft tissue or musculoskeletal tenderness
- Although HLA-B27 is a key predisposing genetic factor, its absence does not rule out JSpA, nor does its presence establish a diagnosis
- Sacroiliitis should be considered even in the absence of prominent symptoms of inflammatory back pain, and may warrant more aggressive treatment
- Considering JSpA on a continuum with adult-onset SpA is strongly supported and facilitates the approach to treatment as well as communication during transition of care.

DISCLOSURE

The authors have nothing to disclose.

ACKNOWLEDGMENTS

The authors to acknowledge Bernadette Redd, MD, for her expertise in helping choose imaging studies and describing the findings.

REFERENCES

1. Colbert RA. Classification of juvenile spondyloarthritis: enthesitis-related arthritis and beyond. Nat Rev Rheumatol 2010;6(8):477–85.
2. Rumsey DG, Laxer RM. The challenges and opportunities of classifying childhood arthritis. Curr Rheumatol Rep 2020;22(1):4.
3. Rosenberg AM. Do we need a new classification of juvenile idiopathic arthritis? Clin Immunol 2020;211:108298.
4. Adrovic A, Sezen M, Barut K, et al. The performance of classification criteria for juvenile spondyloarthropathies. Rheumatol Int 2017;37(12):2013–8.
5. Goirand M, Breton S, Chevallier F, et al. Clinical features of children with enthesitis-related juvenile idiopathic arthritis/juvenile spondyloarthritis followed in a French tertiary care pediatric rheumatology centre. Pediatr Rheumatol Online J 2018;16(1):21.
6. Martini A, Ravelli A, Avcin T, et al. toward new classification criteria for juvenile idiopathic arthritis: first steps, Pediatric Rheumatology International Trials Organization International Consensus. J Rheumatol 2019;46(2):190–7.
7. Nigrovic PA, Colbert RA, Holers VM, et al. Biological classification of childhood arthritis: roadmap to a molecular nomenclature. Nat Rev Rheumatol 2021;17(5):257–69.
8. Rumsey DG, Lougee A, Matsouaka R, et al. Juvenile spondyloarthritis in the CARRA registry: high biologic use, low prevalence of HLA-B27, and equal sex representation in sacroiliitis. Arthritis Care Res 2020;73(7):940–6.
9. Zisman D, Gladman DD, Stoll ML, et al. The Juvenile Psoriatic Arthritis Cohort in the CARRA Registry: clinical characteristics, classification, and outcomes. J Rheumatol 2017;44(3):342–51.
10. Gmuca S, Xiao R, Brandon TG, et al. Multicenter inception cohort of enthesitis-related arthritis: variation in disease characteristics and treatment approaches. Arthritis Res Ther 2017;19(1):84.
11. Kavadichanda CG, Seth G, Kumar G, et al. Clinical correlates of HLA-B*27 and its subtypes in enthesitis-related arthritis variant of juvenile idiopathic arthritis in south Indian Tamil patients. Int J Rheum Dis 2019;22(7):1289–96.
12. Stoll ML, Punaro M. Psoriatic juvenile idiopathic arthritis: a tale of two subgroups. Curr Opin Rheumatol 2011;23(5):437–43.
13. Shenoy S, Aggarwal A. Sonologic enthesitis in children with enthesitis-related arthritis. Clin Exp Rheumatol 2016;34(1):143–7.
14. Hemalatha Srinivasalu SCH, Gina A. Montealegre Sanchez, April D Brundidge, Michael M. Ward and Robert A. Colbert. Whole body magnetic resonance imaging in evaluation of enthesitis in spondyloarthropathy. American College of Rheumatology 2012.
15. Rumsey DG, Guzman J, Rosenberg AM, et al. Characteristics and course of enthesitis in a juvenile idiopathic arthritis inception cohort. Arthritis Care Res 2018;70(2):303–8.
16. Roberton DM, Cabral DA, Malleson PN, et al. Juvenile psoriatic arthritis: followup and evaluation of diagnostic criteria. J Rheumatol 1996;23(1):166–70.
17. Lin C, MacKenzie JD, Courtier JL, et al. Magnetic resonance imaging findings in juvenile spondyloarthropathy and effects of treatment observed on subsequent imaging. Pediatr Rheumatol Online J 2014;12:25.
18. Gensler LS, Ward MM, Reveille JD, et al. Clinical, radiographic and functional differences between juvenile-onset and adult-onset ankylosing spondylitis: results from the PSOAS cohort. Ann Rheum Dis 2008;67(2):233–7.

19. Phatak S, Mohindra N, Zanwar A, et al. Prominent midfoot involvement in children with enthesitis-related arthritis category of juvenile idiopathic arthritis. Clin Rheumatol 2017;36(8):1737–45.

20. Petty RE, Southwood TR, Manners P, et al. International League of Associations for Rheumatology classification of juvenile idiopathic arthritis: second revision, Edmonton, 2001. J Rheumatol 2004;31(2):390–2.

21. Weiss PF, Xiao R, Biko DM, et al. Assessment of sacroiliitis at diagnosis of juvenile spondyloarthritis by radiography, magnetic resonance imaging, and clinical examination. Arthritis Care Res 2016;68(2):187–94.

22. Stoll ML, Bhore R, Dempsey-Robertson M, et al. Spondyloarthritis in a pediatric population: risk factors for sacroiliitis. J Rheumatol 2010;37(11):2402–8.

23. Rusman T, van Vollenhoven RF, van der Horst-Bruinsma IE. Gender differences in axial spondyloarthritis: women are not so lucky. Curr Rheumatol Rep 2018; 20(6):35.

24. McGonagle D. Enthesitis: an autoinflammatory lesion linking nail and joint involvement in psoriatic disease. J Eur Acad Dermatol Venereol 2009; 23(Suppl 1):9–13.

25. Heiligenhaus A, Niewerth M, Mingels A, et al. [Epidemiology of uveitis in juvenile idiopathic arthritis from a national paediatric rheumatologic and ophthalmologic database]. Klin Monbl Augenheilkd 2005;222(12):993–1001.

26. Marino A, Weiss PF, Brandon TG, et al. Juvenile spondyloarthritis: focus on uveitis. Pediatr Rheumatol Online J 2020;18(1):70.

27. Angeles-Han ST, Ringold S, Beukelman T, et al. 2019 American College of Rheumatology/Arthritis Foundation guideline for the screening, monitoring, and treatment of juvenile idiopathic arthritis-associated uveitis. Arthritis Rheumatol 2019; 71(6):864–77.

28. Gracey E, Vereecke L, McGovern D, et al. Revisiting the gut-joint axis: links between gut inflammation and spondyloarthritis. Nat Rev Rheumatol 2020;16(8): 415–33.

29. Mielants H, Veys EM, Goemaere S, et al. Gut inflammation in the spondyloarthropathies: clinical, radiologic, biologic and genetic features in relation to the type of histology. A prospective study. J Rheumatol 1991;18(10):1542–51.

30. Mielants H, Veys EM, Cuvelier C, et al. Gut inflammation in children with late onset pauciarticular juvenile chronic arthritis and evolution to adult spondyloarthropathy–a prospective study. J Rheumatol 1993;20(9):1567–72.

31. Stoll ML, Punaro M, Patel AS. Fecal calprotectin in children with the enthesitis-related arthritis subtype of juvenile idiopathic arthritis. J Rheumatol 2011; 38(10):2274–5.

32. Lamot L, Miler M, Vukojević R, et al. The increased levels of fecal calprotectin in children with active enthesitis related arthritis and MRI signs of sacroiliitis: the results of a single center cross-sectional exploratory study in juvenile idiopathic arthritis patients. Front Med 2021;8:650619.

33. Van Praet L, Jans L, Carron P, et al. Degree of bone marrow oedema in sacroiliac joints of patients with axial spondyloarthritis is linked to gut inflammation and male sex: results from the GIANT cohort. Ann Rheum Dis 2014;73(6): 1186–9.

34. Stoll ML. Gut microbes, immunity, and spondyloarthritis. Clin Immunol 2015; 159(2):134–42.

35. Stoll ML, Weiss PF, Weiss JE, et al. Age and fecal microbial strain-specific differences in patients with spondyloarthritis. Arthritis Res Ther 2018;20(1):14.

36. Stoll ML, Kumar R, Morrow CD, et al. Altered microbiota associated with abnormal humoral immune responses to commensal organisms in enthesitis-related arthritis. Arthritis Res Ther 2014;16(6):486.

37. Aggarwal A, Sarangi AN, Gaur P, et al. Gut microbiome in children with enthesitis-related arthritis in a developing country and the effect of probiotic administration. Clin Exp Immunol 2017;187(3):480–9.

38. Samad A, Stoll ML, Lavi I, et al. Adiposity in juvenile psoriatic arthritis. J Rheumatol 2018;45(3):411–8.

39. Ladehesa-Pineda ML, Arias de la Rosa I, López Medina C, et al. Assessment of the relationship between estimated cardiovascular risk and structural damage in patients with axial spondyloarthritis. Ther Adv Musculoskelet Dis 2020;12. 1759720x20982837.

40. Liew JW, Ramiro S, Gensler LS. Cardiovascular morbidity and mortality in ankylosing spondylitis and psoriatic arthritis. Best Pract Res Clin Rheumatol 2018; 32(3):369–89.

41. Sule S, Fontaine K. Metabolic syndrome in adults with a history of juvenile arthritis. Open access Rheumatol : Res Rev 2018;10:67–72.

42. Yildiz M, Dedeoglu R, Akdeniz B, et al. Systolic and diastolic cardiac functions in juvenile spondyloarthropathies. J Clin Rheumatol 2020. https://doi.org/10.1097/RHU.0000000000001674.

43. Brewerton DA, Hart FD, Nicholls A, et al. Ankylosing spondylitis and HL-A 27. Lancet 1973;1(7809):904–7.

44. Schlosstein L, Terasaki PI, Bluestone R, et al. High association of an HL-A antigen, W27, with ankylosing spondylitis. N Engl J Med 1973;288(14):704–6.

45. Brown MA, Kenna T, Wordsworth BP. Genetics of ankylosing spondylitis–insights into pathogenesis. Nat Rev Rheumatol 2016;12(2):81–91.

46. Calin A, Marder A, Becks E, et al. Genetic differences between B27 positive patients with ankylosing spondylitis and B27 positive healthy controls. Arthritis Rheum 1983;26(12):1460–4.

47. van der Linden S, Valkenburg H, Cats A. The risk of developing ankylosing spondylitis in HLA-B27 positive individuals: a family and population study. Br J Rheumatol 1983;22(4 Suppl 2):18–9.

48. Manolio TA. Genomewide association studies and assessment of the risk of disease. N Engl J Med 2010;363(2):166–76.

49. Ellinghaus D, Jostins L, Spain SL, et al. Analysis of five chronic inflammatory diseases identifies 27 new associations and highlights disease-specific patterns at shared loci. Nat Genet 2016;48(5):510–8.

50. Parkes M, Cortes A, van Heel DA, et al. Genetic insights into common pathways and complex relationships among immune-mediated diseases. Nat Rev Genet 2013;14(9):661–73.

51. Layh-Schmitt G, Colbert RA. The interleukin-23/interleukin-17 axis in spondyloarthritis. Curr Opin Rheumatol 2008;20(4):392–7.

52. Burton PR, Clayton DG, Cardon LR, et al. Association scan of 14,500 nonsynonymous SNPs in four diseases identifies autoimmunity variants. Nat Genet 2007; 39(11):1329–37.

53. Danoy P, Pryce K, Hadler J, et al. Association of variants at 1q32 and STAT3 with ankylosing spondylitis suggests genetic overlap with Crohn's disease. PLoS Genet 2010;6(12):e1001195.

54. Evans DM, Spencer CC, Pointon JJ, et al. Interaction between ERAP1 and HLA-B27 in ankylosing spondylitis implicates peptide handling in the mechanism for HLA-B27 in disease susceptibility. Nat Genet 2011;43(8):761–7.

55. Cortes A, Hadler J, Pointon JP, et al. Identification of multiple risk variants for ankylosing spondylitis through high-density genotyping of immune-related loci. Nat Genet 2013;45(7):730–8.

56. Finkel TH, Li J, Wei Z, et al. Variants in CXCR4 associate with juvenile idiopathic arthritis susceptibility. BMC Med Genet 2016;17:24.

57. López-Isac E, Smith SL, Marion MC, et al. Combined genetic analysis of juvenile idiopathic arthritis clinical subtypes identifies novel risk loci, target genes and key regulatory mechanisms. Ann Rheum Dis 2020;80(3):321–8.

58. McIntosh LA, Marion MC, Sudman M, et al. Genome-wide association meta-analysis reveals novel juvenile idiopathic arthritis susceptibility loci. Arthritis Rheumatol 2017;69(11):2222–32.

59. Hinks A, Barton A, Shephard N, et al. Identification of a novel susceptibility locus for juvenile idiopathic arthritis by genome-wide association analysis. Arthritis Rheum 2009;60(1):258–63.

60. Thompson SD, Marion MC, Sudman M, et al. Genome-wide association analysis of juvenile idiopathic arthritis identifies a new susceptibility locus at chromosomal region 3q13. Arthritis Rheum 2012;64(8):2781–91.

61. Hinks A, Bowes J, Cobb J, et al. Fine-mapping the MHC locus in juvenile idiopathic arthritis (JIA) reveals genetic heterogeneity corresponding to distinct adult inflammatory arthritic diseases. Ann Rheum Dis 2017;76(4):765–72.

62. Ombrello MJ, Arthur VL, Remmers EF, et al. Genetic architecture distinguishes systemic juvenile idiopathic arthritis from other forms of juvenile idiopathic arthritis: clinical and therapeutic implications. Ann Rheum Dis 2017;76(5):906–13.

63. Hinks A, Martin P, Flynn E, et al. Subtype specific genetic associations for juvenile idiopathic arthritis: ERAP1 with the enthesitis related arthritis subtype and IL23R with juvenile psoriatic arthritis. Arthritis Res Ther 2011;13(1):R12.

64. Duerr RH, Taylor KD, Brant SR, et al. A genome-wide association study identifies IL23R as an inflammatory bowel disease gene. Science 2006;314(5804):1461–3.

65. Cargill M, Schrodi SJ, Chang M, et al. A large-scale genetic association study confirms IL12B and leads to the identification of IL23R as psoriasis-risk genes. Am J Hum Genet 2007;80(2):273–90.

66. McGeachy MJ, Chen Y, Tato CM, et al. The interleukin 23 receptor is essential for the terminal differentiation of interleukin 17-producing effector T helper cells in vivo. Nat Immunol 2009;10(3):314–24.

67. Cua DJ, Tato CM. Innate IL-17-producing cells: the sentinels of the immune system. Nat Rev Immunol 2010;10(7):479–89.

68. Sherlock JP, Joyce-Shaikh B, Turner SP, et al. IL-23 induces spondyloarthropathy by acting on ROR-γt+ CD3+CD4-CD8- entheseal resident T cells. Nat Med 2012;18(7):1069–76.

69. Sarin R, Wu X, Abraham C. Inflammatory disease protective R381Q IL23 receptor polymorphism results in decreased primary CD4+ and CD8+ human T-cell functional responses. Proc Natl Acad Sci U S A 2011;108(23):9560–5.

70. Di Meglio P, Di Cesare A, Laggner U, et al. The IL23R R381Q gene variant protects against immune-mediated diseases by impairing IL-23-induced Th17 effector response in humans. PloS One 2011;6(2):e17160.

71. Di Meglio P, Villanova F, Napolitano L, et al. The IL23R A/Gln381 allele promotes IL-23 unresponsiveness in human memory T-helper 17 cells and impairs Th17 responses in psoriasis patients. J Invest Dermatol 2013;133(10):2381–9.

72. Roberts AR, Vecellio M, Chen L, et al. An ankylosing spondylitis-associated genetic variant in the IL23R-IL12RB2 intergenic region modulates enhancer activity and is associated with increased Th1-cell differentiation. Ann Rheum Dis 2016;75(12):2150–6.

73. Vecellio M, Cohen CJ, Roberts AR, et al. RUNX3 and T-Bet in immunopathogenesis of ankylosing spondylitis-novel targets for therapy? Front Immunol 2018;9: 3132.

74. Coffre M, Roumier M, Rybczynska M, et al. Combinatorial control of Th17 and Th1 cell functions by genetic variations in genes associated with the interleukin-23 signaling pathway in spondyloarthritis. Arthritis Rheum 2013; 65(6):1510–21.

75. Smith JA, Colbert RA. Review: the interleukin-23/interleukin-17 axis in spondyloarthritis pathogenesis: Th17 and beyond. Arthritis Rheumatol 2014;66(2): 231–41.

76. Mei Y, Pan F, Gao J, et al. Increased serum IL-17 and IL-23 in the patient with ankylosing spondylitis. Clin Rheumatol 2011;30(2):269–73.

77. Singh R, Aggarwal A, Misra R. Th1/Th17 cytokine profiles in patients with reactive arthritis/undifferentiated spondyloarthropathy. J Rheumatol 2007;34(11): 2285–90.

78. Wendling D, Cedoz JP, Racadot E, et al. Serum IL-17, BMP-7, and bone turnover markers in patients with ankylosing spondylitis. Joint bone Spine 2007; 74(3):304–5.

79. Mahendra A, Misra R, Aggarwal A. Th1 and Th17 predominance in the enthesitis-related arthritis form of juvenile idiopathic arthritis. J Rheumatol 2009;36(8):1730–6.

80. Melis L, Vandooren B, Kruithof E, et al. Systemic levels of IL-23 are strongly associated with disease activity in rheumatoid arthritis but not spondyloarthritis. Ann Rheum Dis 2010;69(3):618–23.

81. Keller C, Webb A, Davis J. Cytokines in the seronegative spondyloarthropathies and their modification by TNF blockade: a brief report and literature review. Ann Rheum Dis 2003;62(12):1128–32.

82. Bal A, Unlu E, Bahar G, et al. Comparison of serum IL-1 beta, sIL-2R, IL-6, and TNF-alpha levels with disease activity parameters in ankylosing spondylitis. Clin Rheumatol 2007;26(2):211–5.

83. Nossent JC, Sagen-Johnsen S, Bakland G. Tumor necrosis factor-α promoter -308/238 polymorphism association with less severe disease in ankylosing spondylitis is unrelated to serum TNF-α and does not predict TNF inhibitor response. J Rheumatol 2014;41(8):1675–82.

84. Braun J, Bollow M, Neure L, et al. Use of immunohistologic and in situ hybridization techniques in the examination of sacroiliac joint biopsy specimens from patients with ankylosing spondylitis. Arthritis Rheum 1995;38(4):499–505.

85. Chen WS, Chen CH, Lin KC, et al. Immunohistological features of hip synovitis in ankylosing spondylitis with advanced hip involvement. Scand J Rheumatol 2009;38(2):154–5.

86. Appel H, Maier R, Bleil J, et al. In situ analysis of interleukin-23- and interleukin-12-positive cells in the spine of patients with ankylosing spondylitis. Arthritis Rheum 2013;65(6):1522–9.

87. Appel H, Maier R, Wu P, et al. Analysis of IL-17(+) cells in facet joints of patients with spondyloarthritis suggests that the innate immune pathway might be of greater relevance than the Th17-mediated adaptive immune response. Arthritis Res Ther 2011;13(3):R95.

88. Baeten D, Sieper J, Braun J, et al. Secukinumab, an Interleukin-17A inhibitor, in ankylosing spondylitis. N Engl J Med 2015;373(26):2534–48.

89. Langley RG, Elewski BE, Lebwohl M, et al. Secukinumab in plaque psoriasis–results of two phase 3 trials. N Engl J Med 2014;371(4):326–38.

90. Mease PJ, McInnes IB, Kirkham B, et al. Secukinumab Inhibition of Interleukin-17A in Patients with Psoriatic Arthritis. N Engl J Med 2015;373(14):1329–39.

91. Hueber W, Sands BE, Lewitzky S, et al. Secukinumab, a human anti-IL-17A monoclonal antibody, for moderate to severe Crohn's disease: unexpected results of a randomised, double-blind placebo-controlled trial. Gut 2012;61(12): 1693–700.

92. Lee JS, Tato CM, Joyce-Shaikh B, et al. Interleukin-23-independent IL-17 production regulates intestinal epithelial permeability. Immunity 2015;43(4):727–38.

93. Gordon KB, Duffin KC, Bissonnette R, et al. A phase 2 trial of guselkumab versus adalimumab for plaque psoriasis. N Engl J Med 2015;373(2):136–44.

94. Deodhar A, Gottlieb AB, Boehncke WH, et al. Efficacy and safety of guselkumab in patients with active psoriatic arthritis: a randomised, double-blind, placebo-controlled, phase 2 study. Lancet 2018;391(10136):2213–24.

95. Feagan BG, Sandborn WJ, Gasink C, et al. Ustekinumab as induction and maintenance therapy for Crohn's disease. N Engl J Med 2016;375(20):1946–60.

96. Deodhar A, Gensler LS, Sieper J, et al. Three multicenter, randomized, double-blind, placebo-controlled studies evaluating the efficacy and safety of ustekinumab in axial spondyloarthritis. Arthritis Rheumatol 2019;71(2):258–70.

97. Yao C, Sakata D, Esaki Y, et al. Prostaglandin E2-EP4 signaling promotes immune inflammation through Th1 cell differentiation and Th17 cell expansion. Nat Med 2009;15(6):633–40.

98. Siebert S, Millar NL, McInnes IB. Why did IL-23p19 inhibition fail in AS: a tale of tissues, trials or translation? Ann Rheum Dis 2019;78(8):1015–8.

99. Weiss PF, Xiao R, Brandon TG, et al. Radiographs in screening for sacroiliitis in children: what is the value? Arthritis Res Ther 2018;20(1):141.

100. Roth J. Emergence of musculoskeletal ultrasound use in pediatric rheumatology. Curr Rheumatol Rep 2020;22(5):14.

101. Sieper J, Rudwaleit M, Baraliakos X, et al. The Assessment of SpondyloArthritis International Society (ASAS) handbook: a guide to assess spondyloarthritis. Ann Rheum Dis 2009;68(Suppl 2):ii1–44.

102. Herregods N, Dehoorne J, Van den Bosch F, et al. ASAS definition for sacroiliitis on MRI in SpA: applicable to children? Pediatr Rheumatol Online J 2017; 15(1):24.

103. Weiss PF, Xiao R, Biko DM, et al. Detection of inflammatory sacroiliitis in children with magnetic resonance imaging: is gadolinium contrast enhancement necessary? Arthritis Rheumatol 2015;67(8):2250–6.

104. Weber U, Jurik AG, Zejden A, et al. MRI of the sacroiliac joints in athletes: recognition of non-specific bone marrow oedema by semi-axial added to standard semi-coronal scans. Rheumatology (Oxford) 2020;59(6):1381–90.

105. Weiss PF, Brandon TG, Bohnsack J, et al. Variability in magnetic resonance imaging interpretation of the pediatric sacroiliac joint. Arthritis Care Res 2020; 73(6):841–8.

106. Chauvin NA, Xiao R, Brandon TG, et al. MRI of the sacroiliac joint in healthy children. AJR Am J Roentgenol 2019;1–7. https://doi.org/10.2214/AJR.18.20708.

107. Panwar J, Tse SML, Lim L, et al. Spondyloarthritis Research Consortium of Canada scoring system for sacroiliitis in juvenile spondyloarthritis/enthesitis-related

arthritis: a reliability, validity, and responsiveness study. J Rheumatol 2019;46(6): 636–44.

108. Weiss PF, Maksymowych WP, Xiao R, et al. Spondyloarthritis Research Consortium of Canada sacroiliac joint inflammation and structural scores: change score reliability and recalibration utility in children. Arthritis Res Ther 2020; 22(1):58.

109. Aquino MR, Tse SM, Gupta S, et al. Whole-body MRI of juvenile spondyloarthritis: protocols and pictorial review of characteristic patterns. Pediatr Radiol 2015; 45(5):754–62.

110. Panwar J, Patel H, Tolend M, et al. Toward developing a semiquantitative whole body-MRI scoring for juvenile idiopathic arthritis: critical appraisal of the state of the art, challenges, and opportunities. Acad Radiol 2021;28(2):271–86.

111. Weiss PF, Colbert RA, Xiao R, et al. Development and retrospective validation of the juvenile spondyloarthritis disease activity index. Arthritis Care Res 2014; 66(12):1775–82.

112. Zanwar A, Phatak S, Aggarwal A. Prospective validation of the Juvenile Spondyloarthritis Disease Activity Index in children with enthesitis-related arthritis. Rheumatology (Oxford) 2018;57(12):2167–71.

113. Ringold S, Angeles-Han ST, Beukelman T, et al. 2019 American College of Rheumatology/Arthritis Foundation guideline for the treatment of juvenile idiopathic arthritis: therapeutic approaches for non-systemic polyarthritis, sacroiliitis, and enthesitis. Arthritis Rheumatol 2019;71(6):846–63.

Pathogenesis and Treatment of Refractory Disease Courses in Systemic Juvenile Idiopathic Arthritis

Refractory Arthritis, Recurrent Macrophage Activation Syndrome and Chronic Lung Disease

Remco Erkens, MD[a,b,1], Ysabella Esteban, MD[c,1], Christopher Towe, MD[d,e], Grant Schulert, MD, PhD[c,e,1], Sebastiaan Vastert, MD, PhD[a,b,*,1]

KEYWORDS

- Systemic JIA • Refractory disease • Translational research • Lung disease
- Macrophage activation syndrome

KEY POINTS

- Patients with sJIA are still at risk for a refractory disease course despite recently approved IL-1 and IL-6 blocking agents for systemic juvenile idiopathic arthritis.
- There is an unmet need for broadly accepted consensus definitions of refractory disease courses in systemic juvenile idiopathic arthritis, to boost international collaborative research.
- Here, we propose preliminary descriptions of 3 refractory disease courses, namely, refractory arthritis (systemic juvenile idiopathic arthritis failing to respond to both IL-1 and IL-6 therapy, defined as continued disease activity requiring maintenance therapy with glucocorticoids); systemic juvenile idiopathic arthritis with recurrent or longstanding signs of macrophage activation syndrome; and systemic juvenile idiopathic arthritis associated with suspected, probable or definite lung disease.

[a] Division of Pediatric Rheumatology & Immunology, Wilhelmina Children's Hospital, University Medical Center Utrecht, the Netherlands; [b] Center for Translational Immunology, University Medical Center Utrecht, University of Utrecht, the Netherlands; [c] Division of Rheumatology, Cincinnati Children's Hospital Medical Center, 3333 Burnet Avenue, Cincinnati, OH 45229, USA; [d] Division of Pulmonary Medicine, Cincinnati Children's Hospital Medical Center, 3333 Burnet Avenue, Cincinnati, OH 45229, USA; [e] Department of Pediatrics, University of Cincinnati College of Medicine, Cincinnati, OH, USA
[1] Shared first and shared last authors.
* Corresponding author. Division of Pediatric Rheumatology & Immunology, Wilhelmina Children's Hospital, University Medical Center Utrecht, PO Box 3500RB, Utrecht, the Netherlands.
E-mail address: b.vastert@umcutrecht.nl

Rheum Dis Clin N Am 47 (2021) 585–606
https://doi.org/10.1016/j.rdc.2021.06.003
0889-857X/21/© 2021 Elsevier Inc. All rights reserved.

rheumatic.theclinics.com

INTRODUCTION

Systemic juvenile idiopathic arthritis (sJIA) is generally seen as the most severe category of JIA. These categories are distinct in their pathobiology, disease course and specific comorbidities. Systemic JIA can manifest varying degrees of arthritis, but is distinct from other JIA categories because of its prominent systemic features reflecting autoinflammation.[1]

The introduction of biologic therapies in the past 20 years has revolutionized treatment and improved outcomes for all children with JIA, but especially for sJIA with the approval of both IL-1 and IL-6 blocking therapies for sJIA in 2012. The widespread use of biologics has not only resulted in improved outcomes and less glucocorticoid (GC) dependency, but also to new insights in the disease mechanisms, with the recognition of a so-called window of opportunity early in the disease course. During this early phase of disease, autoinflammatory mechanisms seem to play a dominant role, and patients seem to be more responsive to targeted therapy by IL-1 blockade.[2]

Registration trials have proven the effectiveness of these therapies and the Childhood Arthritis and Rheumatology Research Alliance (CARRA) and the Pediatric Rheumatology European Society (PReS) have undertaken large longitudinal cohort registry studies that will help to understand how biologic therapies perform in real-life settings. Through these initiatives, as well as other long-term follow-up studies like the Nordic cohort and Canadian ReACCh-Out cohort, it has become clear that, even in 2021, patients with sJIA can be treatment refractory.[3,4] Indeed, a significant number of patients with sJIA show an incomplete response to standard biologic treatments that necessitates sequential trials with multiple biologic and other therapies, and sometimes in combination.[5]

To advance our understanding of these refractory sJIA disease courses, international collaboration is fundamental. The Systemic JIA Foundation (www.systemicjia. org) has been instrumental in boosting such collaborations, not only by organizing focused meetings (NEXTGen) on clinical and research initiatives aiming to gain insight in refractory sJIA, but also by setting up patient driven research initiatives.[6]

This review focuses on refractory disease courses in sJIA. We present the various clinical phenotypes that are recognized as refractory disease, as well as the importance of coming to uniform and widely accepted definitions of these disease states. The epidemiology, mechanisms, and therapeutic options for these refractory disease states are also discussed.

THE NEED FOR DEFINING REFRACTORY DISEASE COURSES IN SYSTEMIC JUVENILE IDIOPATHIC ARTHRITIS

Although significant progress has been made toward identifying specific mechanisms of disease, sJIA is generally seen as a diagnosis per exclusionem, with clinical characteristics prevailing in the current classification criteria.[7,8] Therefore, patients are still at risk for delayed diagnosis and treatment. Moreover, although some progress has been made in understanding the biological differences in refractory disease courses compared with monophasic sJIA,[9] there are currently no biomarker(s) or clinical risk factor(s) that can diagnose or predict the course of sJIA reliably. Finally, patients with refractory sJIA are at high risk for severe side effects from long-term GC treatment, because this modality may be the only therapy that is partially effective. Patients with refractory sJIA are challenging; there is no curative treatment, significant cumulative morbidity exists, and there is an unacceptably high mortality rate. An international consensus on the definition of sJIA refractory disease does not yet exist, but it has been an important topic at conferences and meetings, including the NEXTGen meeting.[6] We urgently need widely accepted definitions of refractory sJIA, to begin international cohort studies of patients meeting these definitions to understand its pathogenesis and treatment. For the current review, we present the preliminary descriptions of 3 refractory disease courses building off the 2019 NEXTGen meeting (**Table 1**).

REFRACTORY SYSTEMIC JUVENILE IDIOPATHIC ARTHRITIS COURSE I: REFRACTORY ARTHRITIS
Background and Prevalence

The disease course for sJIA is notoriously heterogeneous. As of 2014, about 40% of patients had a monophasic disease course (complete remission after a period of months of typical sJIA disease manifestations) and about 7% had a polyphasic course, marked by disease flares and periods of remission. The remaining one-half of patients had a persistent course lasting for at least 2 years.[10] Based on consensus treatment plans developed by CARRA in North America, the initial therapy for sJIA most commonly includes 4 options: starting with GC alone, IL 1 inhibition, IL 6 inhibition, or methotrexate, all with or without GC.[11] We propose to define refractory sJIA arthritis as persistent arthritis without apparent systemic manifestations, despite treatment with both IL-1 and IL-6 inhibitors, and/or patients requiring GC in addition to IL-1 or IL-6 inhibition to control their arthritis.

Mechanisms of Disease in Refractory Arthritis

Refractory arthritis seems to be a complex dance between the innate and adaptive immune systems. The biphasic hypothesis laid out by Nigrovic[12] in 2015 proposes that mechanisms responsible for sJIA at onset differ from those for chronic disease. At onset, autoinflammation is driven by increased levels of cytokines, including IL-1 and IL-6. This state then selects for a T-lymphocyte population—composed of a balance of T-lymphocyte effector and regulatory cells—that perpetuates the pathogenic response for chronic arthritis.[12]

Table 1
Refractory disease courses in sJIA definitions for this review

Description	Proposed Definition
Refractory sJIA arthritis	Patients with sJIA whose arthritis fails to respond to both IL-1 and IL-6 therapy, defined as continued arthritis disease activity requiring maintenance therapy with GC
Refractory sJIA–MAS	sJIA-related MAS, requiring long-term adjunctive therapy with GC, or Recurrent ($\geq$2 episodes of) sJIA related MAS
sJIA LD	Suspected SJIA-LD: Objective findings on clinical examination (including but not limited to tachypnea, cough, or clubbing) or diffuse abnormalities on chest imaging[a] Probable SJIA-LD: both clinical findings and chest imaging findings as in suspected sJIA-LD, or pulmonary hypertension as measured by echocardiogram. Definite SJIA-LD: tissue biopsy consistent with interstitial lung disease, pulmonary alveolar proteinosis/endogenous lipoid pneumonia, or pulmonary artery hypertension.

Abbreviations: LD, lung disease; MAS, macrophage activation syndrome.
[a] Not owing to LD that preexisted sJIA diagnosis, infection, or other identifiable cause.

A potential mechanism for this process was published by Akitsu and colleagues in 2015,[13] who demonstrated the development of arthritis in IL-1 receptor antagonist–deficient mice. This study showed that $CD4^+$ T lymphocytes facilitate localization of $CCR2^+$, $V\gamma6^+$, and $\gamma\delta$ T cells into joints. The subsequent interactions of CCR2 with CCL2 mediated the development of arthritis.[13]

In 2017, Kessel and colleagues[14] found that the cytokine profile in active sJIA could prime $\gamma\delta$T cells and lead to increased IL-17A. A subsequent study published by Henderson and colleagues[15] in 2020 characterized T cells in patients with acute and chronic sJIA. This study showed that patients with acute sJIA exhibited increased activation of T-regulatory cells with a Th17 gene expression signature. In patients with chronic arthritis, this gene expression signature was found in $CD4^+$ T effector cells, as if a shift occurred in Th17 response from T-regulatory cells in acute disease to T effector cells in chronic disease. The use of early IL-1 inhibition offsets the expression of this Th17 signature.

Given these processed, the early use of IL-1 and IL-6 inhibition potentially helps prevent Th17 induction, suggesting the importance of treating within a window of opportunity during early onset disease, as well as further investigations of T cells as potential treatment targets in refractory arthritis.[15] In addition, Henderson and colleagues[15] speculate that therapies aimed at restoring immune tolerance in T-regulatory cells, with medications like abatacept (CTLA4-Ig) or rapamycin, could be of clinical benefit. Further insight in the pathogenesis of chronic sJIA arthritis is needed to frame the underlying rationale for other potential therapies when CG, IL-1 inhibition, and IL-6 inhibition fail to control the disease.

THERAPEUTIC STRATEGIES FOR REFRACTORY ARTHRITIS IN SYSTEMIC JUVENILE IDIOPATHIC ARTHRITIS
Tumor Necrosis Factor Inhibition

Previous studies from the late 1990s and early 2000s showed just fewer than one-half of patients with refractory sJIA responded to etanercept.[16–18] In the initial multicenter, open-label, double-blind, randomized withdrawal study of etanercept in patients with polyarticular JIA (in which patients with sJIA with arthritis and no systemic features were allowed entry), 59% of enrolled patients with sJIA responded in the open-label phase, and flares occurred when etanercept was withdrawn in 44%.[16]

An additional study on small cohorts of patients retrospectively concluded that etanercept therapy could be effective in refractory arthritis and other systemic features of sJIA, if used in combination with other immunosuppressants, including prednisone and/or disease-modifying antirheumatic drugs.[19] More recently, however, it has become clear that etanercept is less effective than IL-6 or IL-1 inhibition using American College of Rheumatology response criteria and the Juvenile Arthritis Disease Activity Score based on 10 joints (JADAS-10).[20–22]

Abatacept

As suggested by Henderson and colleagues,[15] abatacept could have a role in restoring immune tolerance specifically by changing the environment to which T-regulatory cells are exposed in early sJIA. Indeed, the successful use of abatacept in patients with sJIA has been reported in patients with refractory arthritis without systemic features. Twenty percent of total enrolled patients in a phase III, double-blind, randomized controlled withdrawal trial of abatacept in JIA conducted across Europe, Latin America, and the United States had sJIA without persistent systemic symptoms. Arthritis flared in 20% of patients remaining on abatacept during the withdrawal period, compared with one-half of the patients who received the placebo.[23] Based on these data, the authors concluded that abatacept was a safe and effective alternative treatment for children with JIA, including sJIA without systemic features.[24] Combination anakinra and abatacept therapy was reported in a retrospective case series of 4 patients with refractory sJIA, all of whom were GC dependent.[25] The combination therapy resulted in improvement of arthritis and systemic features, and facilitated decreasing doses of anakinra and GC.

JAK Inhibitors

The advent of JAK inhibitor therapy brings new therapeutic options for sJIA. The US Food and Drug Administration (FDA) approved tofacitinib for use in polyarticular course JIA, including patients with sJIA without active systemic features.[26] Although only the results of the initial phase I trial have been published, this initial study did not include patients with sJIA.[27] There is an ongoing clinical trial of tofacitinib in patients with sJIA with active systemic features (NCT03000439). However, 1 case report showed improvement of arthritis and systemic features in a patient with sJIA.[28] There are also published case series exploring the use of tofacitinib and baricitinib in patients with adult-onset Still's disease (AOSD) with refractory arthritis.[29–31]

IL-17 and IL-17A Inhibition

The proposed pathogenesis of refractory arthritis in sJIA begs a question about the efficacy of IL-17/IL-17A inhibition in this disease. However, at the time of this writing, there is nothing in the literature evaluating the use of these medications in sJIA.

Other Agents

An open-label, multicenter, dose-escalating phase II clinical trial was published in 2018 regarding the use of IL-18 inhibition, tadekinig alfa, in patients with AOSD who failed GCs, conventional disease-modifying antirheumatic drugs, and biologic disease-modifying antirheumatic drugs. Tadekinig alfa was shown to have a favorable safety profile and to demonstrate early efficacy in these patients.[32] However, more clinical trials need to be conducted to confirm efficacy.

In summary, when patients fail initial standard biologic therapy for sJIA, and require maintenance therapy with GC, other biologics can be tried to treat refractory arthritis. Based on the authors' clinical experience and current existing data, abatacept or etanercept may be considered in cases where recalcitrant arthritis without systemic features predominates. The recent FDA approval of tofacitinib in patients with polyarticular course JIA is promising and, although results of the clinical trial of this drug in sJIA with systemic features have not been completed, JAK inhibitors could prove to be viable candidates for treatment of refractory arthritis in sJIA (**Table 2**).

REFRACTORY SYSTEMIC JUVENILE IDIOPATHIC ARTHRITIS COURSE II: RECURRENT MACROPHAGE ACTIVATION SYNDROME
Background and Prevalence

Macrophage activation syndrome (MAS) is a puzzling and potentially life-threatening complication of sJIA and its adult counterpart AOSD.[49–51] MAS is characterized by systemic inflammation presenting with a high unremitting fever, as opposed to the typical quotidian fever in sJIA.[52] Patients may have generalized lymphadenopathy and develop hepatomegaly and splenomegaly that can also be found in active sJIA.[52–55] MAS typically evolves in a sepsis-like clinical picture and can lead to rapid clinical deterioration with organ failure and central nervous system involvement.[53–55] Owing to liver involvement and disseminated coagulopathy, patients are prone to

Table 2
General dosing of medications used in sJIA

Medication	Dosing	Comments
Anakinra	Typical: 2–4 mg/kg/d[11,33,34]	In cases of refractory disease/MAS, higher dosing can be recommended. Anakinra may not be as effective in treating arthritis as it is for systemic features.[35]
Canakinumab	Typical: 4 mg/kg every 4 wk[36]	
Tocilizumab	Typical: IV: <30 kg: 12 mg/kg every 14 d; ≥30 kg: 8 mg/kg every 14 d[11] Subcutaneous: <30 kg: 162 mg every 14 d; ≥30 kg: 162 mg every 7 d[37]	–
Etanercept	Typical: 0.4 mg/kg twice weekly; maximum 50 mg/wk[16]	Patients with sJIA excluded from the clinical trial, which examined 0.8 mg/kg weekly dosing[38]
Abatacept	<75 kg: 10 mg/kg IV on weeks 0, 2, 4 then every 4 wk 75–100 kg: 750 mg IV on weeks 0, 2, and 4, then every 4 wk >100 kg: 1000 mg IV on weeks 0, 2, and 4, then every 4 wk[23]	
Tofacitinib	5 to <7 kg: 2 mg PO BID 7 to <10 kg: 2.5 mg PO BID 10 to <15 kg: 3 mg PO BID 15 to <25 kg: 3.5 mg PO BID 25 to <40 kg: 4 mg PO BID 40 kg: 5 mg PO BID	Based on the clinical trial for patients with polyarticular course JIA[27]
The following medications have been used-off label (limited literature available)		
IVIG	2 m/kg (≤100 g) IV monthly	Based on case reports for refractory sJIA and MAS[39,40]
Ruxolitinib	Up to 1 mg/kg/d	Single case report of improvement in sJIA-LD[41]
Baricitinib	Initial: 2mg BID	Higher doses may be needed based on data from patients with autoinflammatory interferonopathy[42–44]
Cyclosporine A	4–7 mg/kg/d PO divided BID	Little guidance regarding target levels for MAS or sJIA-LD[45]
Mycophenolic acid	600 mg/m² BID up to 1 g BID	Case reports in MAS flares, primarily in lupus[46]
Infliximab	Typical: 6–10 mg/kg/infusion on weeks 0, 2, and 6, then every 4–8 wk[47]	Dosing for patients >75 kg is based on clinical trials in adult patients with rheumatoid arthritis Generally used in combination therapy with methotrexate
Emapalumab	6 mg/kg initial dose 3 mg/kg every 72 h	Currently in trial for refractory sJIA-MAS[48]

Abbreviations: BID, twice per day; IVIG, intravenous immunoglobulin; MAS, macrophage activation syndrome; PO, by mouth; sJIA-LD, sJIA with lung disease.

develop hemorrhages, petechiae, and disseminated intravascular coagulation.[52–55] MAS can be triggered by a flare of the underlying disease or (usually viral) infections including Epstein–Barr virus, cytomegalovirus, or the influenza virus.[51–53,56] Typical laboratory features of MAS include relative cytopenia (specifically, decreasing leukocyte and platelet counts in patients with sJIA who typically have high counts) and marked hyperferritinemia.[52–55] Contemporary studies indicate a mortality rate of 8% to 12%.[39,53–55] The prevalence of MAS among patients with sJIA has been estimated to be 10% to 15%. However, multiple reports suggest that subclinical MAS may occur in as many as 30% to 40% of patients with sJIA.[52,57,58]

A substantial number of MAS (22%–53%) presents at sJIA onset[53–55] and not all episodes of MAS constitute refractory disease. However, some patients have a treatment-resistant, sometimes smoldering, MAS or have recurrent MAS episodes. These disease courses represent a subset of patients with sJIA with refractory disease. MAS is also proposed as a risk factor for the development of sJIA with lung disease (sJIA-LD),[59,60] as discussed elsewhere in this article. Large cohort studies on the frequency of MAS recurrence and persistence unfortunately are lacking.

Diagnosis of Macrophage Activation Syndrome in Systemic Juvenile Idiopathic Arthritis

It is of crucial importance to quickly recognize MAS and promptly initiate therapy. There is no single pathognomonic clinical or laboratory parameter to diagnose MAS. Although not intended to be diagnostic criteria, the PReS/European League Against Rheumatism/American College of Rheumatology developed classification criteria in 2016 that have improved clinical monitoring for MAS in (active) sJIA[52] and facilitate early recognition and initiation of appropriate therapy. Because the use of biologics such as tocilizumab can obscure some of the features of MAS,[50,61,62] clinical vigilance remains imperative. Biomarkers such as ferritin, IL-18, IFN-γ, CXCL9, soluble tumor necrosis factor receptor, soluble CD163, and ADA2 may aid in its diagnosis.[63–68]

Mechanisms of Disease in Systemic Juvenile Idiopathic Arthritis–Associated Macrophage Activation Syndrome

MAS is caused by the hyperactivation and expansion of cytolytic T cells and hemophagocytic macrophages resulting in hypersecretion of proinflammatory cytokines leading to a so-called cytokine storm.[51,69,70] There are multiple disease mechanisms underlying this cytokine storm in sJIA-MAS. First, depressed natural killer (NK) cell cytolytic function has been reported in sJIA-associated MAS[51,71–73] and is also a cardinal feature of primary or familial hemophagocytic lymphohistiocytosis, which is caused by mutations in genes involved in the perforin-mediated degranulation pathway.[50,51,74–77] The pathophysiology of sJIA-MAS most likely involves related pathogenic pathways to hemophagocytic lymphohistiocytosis,[69,70] because there is in a subset of patients overlap in genes involved.[78,79] Some patients with sJIA with functional defects in the exosome degranulation pathway of NK and CD8 T cells display heterozygous mutations in hemophagocytic lymphohistiocytosis–associated genes.[71–73,80–82] Second, findings in mouse models of MAS suggest that aberrant stimulation of Toll-like receptors (TLR) such as TLR9 might lead to a MAS like disease.[83] This finding is interesting, because Epstein–Barr virus, one of the most common viral triggers identified in MAS,[53] is a potent stimulator of TLR9.[84] In support of this line of reasoning, sJIA-MAS has been associated with abnormal TLR-induced gene expression patterns.[85] Third, the specific cytokine milieu in active sJIA renders patients susceptible to developing MAS. It is clear that sJIA-MAS is often associated with a surge in both IL-18 and IFN-γ.[86,87] Animal models and human data have shown that IFN-γ is a key cytokine driver of hemophagocytic lymphohistiocytosis/MAS pathology.[51,69,88,89] IL-18 is a driver of IFN-γ production and might be the link between sJIA and MAS.[90] IL-18 correlates with sJIA disease activity and its levels are often increased even more during MAS.[61,91–93] IL-18 is normally a strong activator for NK cells. However, in sJIA, even in the presence of very high IL-18, NK cell cytolytic function remains impaired, possibly owing to reversible defects in phosphorylation of the IL-18 receptor.[90,92,94–96] The important role of IL-18 in MAS is further illustrated by patients with a gain-of-function mutation in NLRC4, a NOD-like receptor that activates the inflammasome and caspase 1. These patients have persistently high IL-18 and IL-1β levels and suffer from recurrent episodes of MAS.[97] Altogether, genetic and induced cytolytic impairment of the response to environmental and autologous triggers may be contributing to the development of MAS in sJIA.

Treatment of (Refractory) Systemic Juvenile Idiopathic Arthritis–Associated Macrophage Activation Syndrome

So far, no controlled studies on the treatment of sJIA associated MAS are available. The main goal for the initial treatment is to quickly control the hyperinflammation and address any identified triggers. The Histiocyte Society contributed to the standardization of hemophagocytic lymphohistiocytosis treatment over the years, with treatment protocols including the hemophagocytic lymphohistiocytosis–2004 protocol.[98] Currently, high-dose GC (sometimes with cyclosporine A added) are still the mainstay of the treatment.[53–55] Increased insight in the mechanisms underlying both active sJIA and sJIA-associated MAS have resulted in the use of targeted therapy in combination with GC.[99,100] The introduction of biologic drugs blocking the action of key cytokines in sJIA, including anakinra, canakinumab, and tociluzimab, has dramatically improved SJIA treatment and decreased the need for GC.[49] Surprisingly however, canakinumab and tocilizumab seem not to decrease the risk of developing MAS in sJIA.[50,61,101–103] High-dose anakinra on the other hand does show promising results in treating sJIA-MAS as an alternative to cyclosporine A in combination with GC and, therefore, is increasingly used.[50,53,74,76,104,105] A recent report that included 44 patients with secondary hemophagocytic lymphohistiocytosis, of which 13 had sJIA/MAS, showed that anakinra was most effective when given early and to patients with sJIA-MAS.[106] An ongoing clinical trial NCT02780583 is investigating the safety and efficacy of anakinra treatment in MAS.

As mentioned elsewhere in this article, IFN-γ and IL-18 are key cytokines in MAS. Emapalumab, a monoclonal antibody directed against IFN-γ, administered together with dexamethasone has an overall high response rate in patients with primary or familial hemophagocytic lymphohistiocytosis[107,108] and induced complete remission in a patient with therapy-resistant AOSD-associated MAS.[109,110] An ongoing study (NCT03311854) is being conducted in patients with sJIA-MAS who failed standard of care with promising preliminary results; all 9 patients enrolled so far showed a complete response and resolution of MAS symptoms.[48] Finally, an IL-18 pathway–blocking therapy might be an interesting therapeutic option. Indeed recombinant IL-18 binding protein has been used successfully in treating primary or familial hemophagocytic lymphohistiocytosis,[111] AOSD,[32] and refractory MAS in a patient with sJIA.[112]

An alternative to direct cytokine blockade is inhibiting the downstream signaling pathways, shared by various ligands, through JAK inhibition, which are administered orally and well-tolerated[113,114] and has FDA approval for other inflammatory conditions.[115] Mouse models have shown that JAK inhibition can be effective in secondary hemophagocytic lymphohistiocytosis and synthesizes CD8 T cells for dexamethasone induced apoptosis.[116–118] Verweyen and colleagues[119] showed that JAK-1/3 inhibition can significantly decrease IL-18 serum levels in MAS murine models and in a patient with treatment refractory MAS. The 2 most studied JAK-inhibitors in hemophagocytic lymphohistiocytosis/MAS are ruxolitinib, which inhibits JAK-1/2,[113,120] and tofacitinib, which targets JAK-1/3 and has been shown to be effective in inducing remission in cases of refractory AOSD complicated by MAS[121] and refractory sJIA.[28]

In summary, targeted biologic therapy and JAK-inhibition are promising new treatments for (refractory) MAS. Collaborative translational research initiatives,[6] aiming for a deeper understanding of the pathophysiology and therapy mechanisms in refractory disease is urgently needed to advance care for these patients.

REFRACTORY SYSTEMIC JUVENILE IDIOPATHIC ARTHRITIS COURSE III: SYSTEMIC JUVENILE IDIOPATHIC ARTHRITIS–ASSOCIATED LUNG DISEASE
Background and Prevalence

Over the past decade, children with SJIA have been increasingly recognized to have clinically significant lung disease (sJIA-LD), coincident with changing patterns in sJIA treatment, including the widespread use of anti–IL-1 and anti–IL-6 biologics as first-line therapy.[122] Kimura and colleagues[123] reported 25 children with interstitial LD, pulmonary artery hypertension, and/or pulmonary alveolar proteinosis (PAP). Compared with children with sJIA without LD, those with sJIA-LD had increased exposure to anti-cytokine biologics, a high incidence of MAS, and more than two-thirds had died. A large international cohort study confirmed and expanded these observations, including highlighting patterns of LD associated with biologic exposure including acute clubbing and digital erythema, radiographic findings of septal thickening, and histologic evidence of PAP and endogenous lipoid pneumonia.[59] This report also noted that many patients with sJIA-LD experienced reactions to biologics (most notably tocilizumab), and some met criteria for drug reaction with eosinophilia and systemic symptoms. Indeed, a recent preprint reports a specific HLA association (HLA DRB1*15) in children with SJIA and features of drug reaction with eosinophilia and systemic symptoms with and without LD.[124] A large single-center study from Cincinnati Children's Hospital[60] noted that sJIA-LD may be present in 5% or more of children with sJIA and, compared with patients with sJIA without LD, were generally younger at diagnosis, had higher IL-18 levels, and were more likely to have had MAS and adverse drug events. Indeed, most patients with sJIA-LD had failed biologic therapy and/or had signs of persistent systemic inflammation including elevated ferritin, lactate dehydrogenase, or S100 alarmin proteins. This study also provided the first pathophysiological description of sJIA-LD (Fig. 1), finding no evidence of primary or congenital PAP but high levels of IL-18 in bronchoalveolar lavage (BAL) fluid and increased expression of IFN-γ–associated pathways and T-cell activation in lung tissue. Together these findings suggest possible overlapping disease mechanisms in MAS and sJIA-LD.

Diagnosis and Patient Evaluation Overview

Often, sJIA-LD presents in the first 6 to 12 months after sJIA diagnosis, with initially subtle respiratory symptoms such as cough or tachypnea with normal oxygen saturation.[60] A frequent and early sign of sJIA-LD is acute development of digital clubbing and/or erythema.[59,60] Patients with risk factors for development of LD, such as early age of onset and recurrent MAS, should be monitored closely for sJIA-LD development with pulse oximetry including overnight oximetry studies, pulmonary function tests, and potentially, screening chest radiography and echocardiograms. Patients with any signs or symptoms concerning for sJIA-LD development should undergo

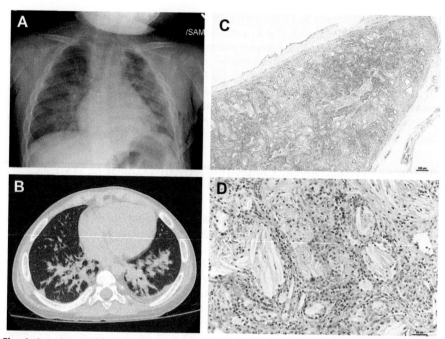

Fig. 1. Imaging and histopathologic findings in sJIA-LD. (*A*) Chest radiograph showing ill-defined opacities in each lung with a basilar predominance. (*B*) Chest computed tomography scan showing characteristic findings of sJIA-LD, including pleural thickening, septal thickening, and tree-in-bud opacities. (*C, D*) Histopathology from open lung biopsy showing PAP with chronic inflammation, numerous macrophages and cholesterol clefts with focal cholesterol granulomas (hematoxylin-eosin, original magnification, 100x (*C*) and 400x (*D*).

high resolution chest computed tomography scans to confirm the LD diagnosis (see **Fig. 1**).[60] In agreement with the American Thoracic Society guidelines for childhood interstitial lung disease,[125] patients with newly diagnosed sJIA-LD should undergo a complete evaluation including pulmonary function tests, echocardiogram, and bronchoscopy with BAL to evaluate for infection. In addition, children with atypical or progressive LD should undergo surgical lung biopsy to confirm the diagnosis.

Mechanisms of Disease and Treatment Options

Medical treatment for sJIA-LD can be divided broadly into options that are specific for the LD and those directed at the underlying sJIA and/or MAS. As noted, at the time of sJIA-LD diagnosis, most patients have evidence of active systemic inflammation as evidenced by clinical or laboratory features of sJIA or MAS requiring adjunctive therapy. In general, our practice has been to discontinue biologic therapy that has been ineffective or if there is any concern for a drug reaction, while considering adding other agents when biologics are well-tolerated but full disease control has not been attained. Notably, we have several patients with sJIA-LD whose LD improved while remaining on biologics and other therapies.

One medication class to consider is JAK inhibitors. As discussed elsewhere in this article, tofacitinib has been recently approved in the United States for the treatment of a polyarticular course JIA,[26] with ongoing clinical trials in sJIA with systemic features. There are published case reports of successful use of tofacitinib in children with refractory sJIA,[28] as well as refractory AOSD[29]; however, none of these patients had known LD. There is also a report of successful treatment of a child with sJIA-LD with ruxolitinib 1 mg/kg/d, including interval improvement in chest CT findings.[41] Finally, baricitinib has been used successfully in monogenic systemic interferonopathies with similarity to sJIA-LD, with available dosing guidance in those conditions.[42–44] The clinical and immunologic overlap between MAS and sJIA-LD suggests a key role for IFN-γ, and whether blockade with emapalumab could be effective. As noted elsewhere in this article, this medication has been shown to be effective in hemophagocytic lymphohistiocytosis,[107] and there are ongoing clinical trials in MAS with promising early results.[48] We have used emapalumab for the treatment of MAS in several patients with sJIA-LD and observed stabilization of the LD (Schulert, Towe, and colleagues, unpublished results, 2020). Several case reports also support the usefulness of intravenous immunoglobulin as an adjunctive treatment in children with refractory sJIA and/or MAS.[39,40] There is also 1 report of progressive sJIA-LD where the disease was stabilized using several cycles of plasma exchange.[126] Other treatment options for sJIA-LD include agents used in other autoimmune conditions and childhood interstitial LD, including mycophenolic acid or calcineurin inhibitors (cyclosporine A and tacrolimus).[46] Finally, cytotoxic chemotherapy can be considered as salvage therapy in children with progression to life-threatening disease. Cyclophosphamide bolus therapy (monthly 500 mg/m^2) has been reported to improve patients with refractory sJIA.[45] Moderately dosed etoposide (50–100 mg/m^2 once weekly) has also been shown to be effective in a series of children with MAS, including 3 patients with sJIA-LD.[127]

Lung-directed medical therapies include those that decrease inflammation and those that prevent infectious complications. The frequent pathologic findings of lymphoplasmacytic infiltrates[60] suggest that widely used anti-inflammatory therapies such as inhaled GC[128] and/or chronic azithromycin may be beneficial. Specifically, chronic azithromycin deserves further study in sJIA-LD, because it has been shown to improve lymphocytic airway inflammation in lung transplant recipients.[129] Finally, inhaled granulocyte macrophage colony stimulating factor (molgramostim) has recently been shown to be highly effective in patients with primary autoimmune PAP.[130] However, children with sJIA-LD do not have evidence of impairment in granulocyte macrophage colony stimulating factor responsiveness,[60] and the high levels of granulocyte macrophage colony stimulating factor seen in MAS raise the at least theoretic concern that such therapy could trigger disease flares. We would recommend caution, because there are no reports of the use of this medication in sJIA-LD.

Antimicrobial prophylaxis against *Pneumocystis jirovecii* pneumonia is often used in patients on immunosuppressive medications and should be considered in sJIA-LD.[131] The incidence of *Pneumocystis jirovecii* pneumonia in patients with sJIA-LD is unknown, but initial reports of sJIA-LD co-infection with *Pneumocystis jirovecii* pneumonia was suggested as a risk factor for mortality.[132]

Nonpharmacologic or Surgical and Interventional Treatment Options

Nonpharmacologic supportive care should be given in sJIA-LD, similar to other patients with interstitial lung disease. Chronic home oxygen therapy and potentially positive pressure ventilation should be prescribed as needed and titrated as per published guidelines.[133] Chest physiotherapy is a common treatment in patients with cystic fibrosis[134] and non–cystic fibrosis bronchiectasis,[135] but because bronchiectasis is not a common feature in patients with sJIA-LD, its role is less clear.

Whole lung lavage is a risky but common treatment for patients with autoimmune and congenital PAP.[136] Here, the architecture of the distal airways and alveoli are preserved, with lymphocytic infiltration and fibrosis being less common. BAL samples from these patients contain large foamy macrophages and large acellular, eosinophilic bodies in the background. In contrast, sJIA-LD is often characterized by a significant lymphocytic infiltration of the airways and alveoli, and the BAL samples most often contain significantly fewer lipid-laden macrophages compared with the patients with autoimmune and patients with congenital PAP with disrupted granulocyte macrophage colony stimulating factor signaling. Therefore, although many patients with PAP benefit, albeit transiently, from whole lung lavage, the majority of patients with sJIA-LD would not be expected to receive the same degree of benefit. Furthermore, the minor potential benefits are likely outweighed by the significant procedural risks given the young age and small size of the typical patient with sJIA-LD.[137]

SUMMARY AND FUTURE DIRECTIONS

This article has reviewed our current understanding of refractory disease courses in sJIA, as well as discussed potential treatment approaches. Given the lack of clinical trial data in these disease subsets, treatment guidance largely consists of expert opinion supported by case reports and small case series. The optimal treatment approach must be individualized for each patient, given the overlapping nature of these disease states and accounting for previously failed agents, drug interactions, and patient/family preference.

In addition to these modalities, cellular therapies including bone marrow transplantation and mesenchymal stroma cell transplantation are emerging therapies for refractory (s)JIA.[138–140] The small phase Ib study of bone marrow derived mesenchymal stem cell transplantation in refractory JIA included 1 patient with sJIA who developed MAS again at 7 weeks after mesenchymal stem cell infusion, but this was curtailed after 3 days of pulse GC therapy and subsequently restarted tocilizumab. Overall, the mesenchymal stem cell transplantations in this cohort were considered safe.[139] Autologous stem cell transplantation has been documented in patients with refractory sJIA.[138,141] However, 4 of 22 patients died during transplant or follow-up, and many patients ultimately had disease relapse.[138] More recently, allogeneic stem cell transplantation has been increasingly used for refractory sJIA, with a recent case series including 11 patients, 6 with recurrent MAS and 5 with chronic dependence on GC and other medications.[140] This study reported that 2 of 16 patients (12.5%) died, but more than 75% were in complete remission off medication at last the follow-up. Although this treatment has the potential for durable complete remission, it must be balanced against the substantial risk of morbidity and mortality of allogeneic stem cell transplantation.

With modern treatment, disease outcomes for many patients with sJIA are improving drastically. However, there is an unmet need for a better understanding and definition of refractory disease courses in sJIA. Accepted definitions will then enable collaborative research aimed at understanding the disease mechanisms in patients with sJIA fitting these definitions. This knowledge can then be translated into targeted therapeutic strategies, which are urgently needed to improve the outcomes and daily life of these patients.

CLINICS CARE POINTS

Refractory arthritis
  Provisional diagnosis
  • Patients with sJIA whose arthritis fails to respond to both IL-1 and IL-6 therapy, defined as continued arthritis disease activity requiring maintenance therapy with GC

Treatment
- Abatacept or etanercept may be considered in cases where recalcitrant arthritis without systemic features predominates
- JAK inhibitors could prove to be viable candidates for treatment of refractory arthritis in sJIA.

Refractory MAS
Provisional diagnosis
- sJIA-related MAS, requiring long term adjunctive therapy with GC or recurrent (≥ 2 episodes of) sJIA-related MAS
- Biologic therapy can obscure MAS symptoms
  Treatment
- Treatments for refractory MAS can include corticosteroids, cyclosporine A, intravenous immunoglobulin, cytokine blockade (anakinra, emapalumab, tadekinig alpha), or JAK inhibitors

sJIA-LD
Provisional diagnosis
- Patients should be suspected of having SJIA-LD if they develop objective findings on clinical examination (including but not limited to tachypnea, cough, or clubbing) and/or diffuse abnormalities on chest imaging not owing to other identifiable cause.
Treatment
- Although the optimal treatment for SJIA-LD is unknown, we recommend discontinuing (biologic) therapy that has been ineffective or any concern for drug hypersensitivity and consider adding other agents including calcineurin inhibitors, mycophenolate mofetil, JAK inhibitors, or emapalumab
- Supportive care, including chronic home oxygen therapy, positive pressure ventilation, chest physiotherapy, and whole lung lavage, may be considered in consultation with experts in childhood interstitial lung diseases

ACKNOWLEDGMENTS

The authors thank Dr Kathryn Wikenheiser-Brokamp, Division of Pathology and Laboratory Medicine, Cincinnati Children's Hospital Medical Center and University of Cincinnati College of Medicine, for providing histopathological images. Dr. Schulert was supported by the National Institutes of Arthritis and Musculoskeletal and Skin Diseases, National Institutes of Health (K08-AR072075).

DISCLOSURE

Dr. Schulert has received consulting fees from Novartis.

REFERENCES

1. Mellins ED, MacAubas C, Grom AA. Pathogenesis of systemic juvenile idiopathic arthritis: some answers, more questions. Nat Rev Rheumatol 2011;7(7): 416–26. Available at: http://www.embase.com/search/results?subaction= viewrecord&from=export&id=L51464339.
2. Nigrovic PA. Review: is there a window of opportunity for treatment of systemic juvenile idiopathic arthritis? Arthritis Rheumatol 2014;66(6):1405–13.
3. Chhabra A, Robinson C, Houghton K, et al. Long-term outcomes and disease course of children with juvenile idiopathic arthritis in the ReACCh-Out cohort: a two-centre experience. Reumatology (Oxford) 2020. https://doi.org/10.1093/rheumatology/keaa118.
4. Glerup M, Rypdal V, Arnstad ED, et al. Long-term outcomes in juvenile idiopathic arthritis: eighteen years of follow-up in the population-based Nordic

Juvenile Idiopathic Arthritis cohort. Arthritis Care Res 2020. https://doi.org/10. 1002/acr.23853.

5. Brunner HI, Schanberg LE, Kimura Y, et al. New medications are needed for children with juvenile idiopathic arthritis. Arthritis Rheumatol 2020. https://doi. org/10.1002/art.41390.

6. Canna SW, Schulert GS, De Jesus A, et al. Proceedings from the 2ndNext Gen Therapies for Systemic Juvenile Idiopathic Arthritis and Macrophage Activation Syndrome symposium held on October 3-4, 2019. Pediatr Rheumatol 2020. https://doi.org/10.1186/s12969-020-00444-7.

7. Petty RE, Southwood TR, Manners P, et al. International League of Associations for Rheumatology classification of juvenile idiopathic arthritis: second revision, Edmonton, 2001. J Rheumatol 2004;31(2):390–2.

8. Martini A, Ravelli A, Avcin T, et al. Toward new classification criteria for juvenile idiopathic arthritis: first steps, pediatric rheumatology international trials organization international consensus. J Rheumatol 2019;46(2):190–7.

9. Gohar F, McArdle A, Jones M, et al. Molecular signature characterisation of different inflammatory phenotypes of systemic juvenile idiopathic arthritis. Ann Rheum Dis 2019;78(8):1107–13.

10. Correll CK, Binstadt BA. Advances in the pathogenesis and treatment of systemic juvenile idiopathic arthritis. Pediatr Res 2014. https://doi.org/10.1038/pr. 2013.187.

11. Dewitt EM, Kimura Y, Beukelman T, et al. Consensus treatment plans for new-onset systemic juvenile idiopathic arthritis. Arthritis Care Res 2012. https://doi. org/10.1002/acr.21625.

12. Nigrovic PA. Autoinflammation and autoimmunity in systemic juvenile idiopathic arthritis. Proc Natl Acad Sci U S A 2015. https://doi.org/10.1073/pnas. 1521837113.

13. Akitsu A, Ishigame H, Kakuta S, et al. IL-1 receptor antagonist-deficient mice develop autoimmune arthritis due to intrinsic activation of IL-17-producing CCR2 + Vγ6 + γδT cells. Nat Commun 2015. https://doi.org/10.1038/ ncomms8464.

14. Kessel C, Lippitz K, Weinhage T, et al. Proinflammatory Cytokine Environments Can Drive Interleukin-17 Overexpression by gamma/delta T Cells in Systemic Juvenile Idiopathic Arthritis. Arthritis Rheumatol 2017;69(7):1480–94.

15. Henderson LA, Hoyt KJ, Lee PY, et al. Th17 reprogramming of T cells in systemic juvenile idiopathic arthritis. JCI Insight 2020. https://doi.org/10.1172/jci.insight. 132508.

16. Lovell DJ, Giannini EH, Reiff A, et al. Etanercept in Children with Polyarticular Juvenile Rheumatoid Arthritis. N Engl J Med 2000. https://doi.org/10.1056/ nejm200003163421103.

17. Kimura Y, Pinho P, Walco G, et al. Etanercept treatment in patients with refractory systemic onset juvenile rheumatoid arthritis. J Rheumatol 2005;32(5): 935–42.

18. Lovell DJ, Reiff A, Jones OY, et al. Long-term safety and efficacy of etanercept in children with polyarticular-course juvenile rheumatoid arthritis. Arthritis Rheum 2006. https://doi.org/10.1002/art.21885.

19. Hu X, Yuan F, Zhang J, et al. Effect of etanercept on refractory systemic-onset juvenile idiopathic arthritis. World J Pediatr 2016. https://doi.org/10.1007/ s12519-015-0009-3.

20. Horneff G, Schulz AC, Klotsche J, et al. Experience with etanercept, tocilizumab and interleukin-1 inhibitors in systemic onset juvenile idiopathic arthritis patients

from the BIKER registry. Arthritis Res Ther 2017. https://doi.org/10.1186/s13075-017-1462-2.

21. Katsicas MM, Russo RAG. Use of infliximab in patients with systemic juvenile idiopathic arthritis refractory to etanercept. Clin Exp Rheumatol 2005;23(4): 545–8.

22. Russo RAG, Katsicas MM. Clinical remission in patients with systemic juvenile idiopathic arthritis treated with anti-tumor necrosis factor agents. J Rheumatol 2009. https://doi.org/10.3899/jrheum.090952.

23. Ruperto N, Lovell DJ, Quartier P, et al. Abatacept in children with juvenile idiopathic arthritis: a randomised, double-blind, placebo-controlled withdrawal trial. Lancet 2008. https://doi.org/10.1016/S0140-6736(08)60998-8.

24. Ruperto N, Lovell DJ, Quartier P, et al. Long-term safety and efficacy of abatacept in children with juvenile idiopathic arthritis. Arthritis Rheum 2010;62(6): 1792–802.

25. Record JL, Beukelman T, Cron RQ. Combination therapy of abatacept and anakinra in children with refractory systemic juvenile idiopathic arthritis: a retrospective case series. J Rheumatol 2011;38(1):180–1.

26. Pfizer. U.S. FDA Approves Pfizer's XELJANZ® (tofacitinib) for the treatment of ACTIVE POLYARTICULAR COURSE Juvenile IDIOPATHIC ARTHRITIS. 2020. Available at: https://www.pfizer.com/news/press-release/press-release-detail/us-fda-approves-pfizers-xeljanzr-tofacitinib-treatment. Accessed April 15, 2021.

27. Ruperto N, Brunner HI, Zuber Z, et al. Pharmacokinetic and safety profile of tofacitinib in children with polyarticular course juvenile idiopathic arthritis: results of a phase 1, open-label, multicenter study. Pediatr Rheumatol Online J 2017; 15(1):86.

28. Huang Z, Lee PY, Yao X, et al. Tofacitinib treatment of refractory systemic juvenile idiopathic arthritis. Pediatrics 2019. https://doi.org/10.1542/peds.2018-2845.

29. Hu Q, Wang M, Jia J, et al. Tofacitinib in refractory adult-onset Still's disease: 14 cases from a single centre in China. Ann Rheum Dis 2020. https://doi.org/10.1136/annrheumdis-2019-216699.

30. Kacar M, Fitton J, Gough AK, et al. Mixed results with baricitinib in biological-resistant adult-onset Still's disease and undifferentiated systemic autoinflammatory disease. RMD Open 2020. https://doi.org/10.1136/rmdopen-2020-001246.

31. Ladhari C, Jorgensen C, Pers YM. Treatment of refractory adult onset Still's disease with combination anakinra and baricitinib therapy. Rheumatology (Oxford) 2019. https://doi.org/10.1093/rheumatology/key414.

32. Gabay C, Fautrel B, Rech J, et al. Open-label, multicentre, dose-escalating phase II clinical trial on the safety and efficacy of tadekinig alfa (IL-18BP) in adult-onset Still's disease. Ann Rheum Dis 2018;77(6):840–7.

33. Nigrovic PA, Mannion M, Prince FHM, et al. Anakinra as first-line disease-modifying therapy in systemic juvenile idiopathic arthritis: report of forty-six patients from an international multicenter series. Arthritis Rheum 2011. https://doi.org/10.1002/art.30128.

34. Vastert SJ, De Jager W, Noordman BJ, et al. Effectiveness of first-line treatment with recombinant interleukin-1 receptor antagonist in steroid-naive patients with new-onset systemic juvenile idiopathic arthritis: results of a prospective cohort study. Arthritis Rheumatol 2014. https://doi.org/10.1002/art.38296.

35. Gattorno M, Piccini A, Lasigliè D, et al. The pattern of response to anti-interleukin-1 treatment distinguishes two subsets of patients with systemic-

onset juvenile idiopathic arthritis. Arthritis Rheum 2008. https://doi.org/10.1002/art.23437.

36. Ruperto N, Brunner HI, Quartier P, et al. Two Randomized Trials of Canakinumab in Systemic Juvenile Idiopathic Arthritis. N Engl J Med 2012. https://doi.org/10.1056/nejmoa1205099.

37. Ruperto N, Brunner HI, Ramanan AV, et al. Subcutaneous dosing regimens of tocilizumab in children with systemic or polyarticular juvenile idiopathic arthritis. Rheumatology 2021. https://doi.org/10.1093/rheumatology/keab047.

38. Horneff G, Ebert A, Fitter S, et al. Safety and efficacy of once weekly etanercept 0.8 mg/kg in a multicentre 12 week trial in active polyarticular course juvenile idiopathic arthritis. Rheumatology 2009. https://doi.org/10.1093/rheumatology/kep122.

39. Minoia F, Davì S, Horne A, et al. Dissecting the heterogeneity of macrophage activation syndrome complicating systemic juvenile idiopathic arthritis. J Rheumatol 2015. https://doi.org/10.3899/jrheum.141261.

40. Aizawa-Yashiro T, Oki E, Tsuruga K, et al. Intravenous immunoglobulin therapy leading to dramatic improvement in a patient with systemic juvenile idiopathic arthritis and severe pericarditis resistant to steroid pulse therapy. Rheumatol Int 2012. https://doi.org/10.1007/s00296-010-1413-6.

41. Bader-Meunier B, Hadchouel A, Berteloot L, et al. Effectiveness and safety of ruxolitinib for the treatment of refractory systemic idiopathic juvenile arthritis like associated with interstitial lung disease: a case report. Ann Rheum Dis 2020. https://doi.org/10.1136/annrheumdis-2020-216983.

42. Kim H, Brooks KM, Tang CC, et al. Pharmacokinetics, pharmacodynamics, and proposed dosing of the oral JAK1 and JAK2 inhibitor baricitinib in pediatric and young adult CANDLE and SAVI patients. Clin Pharmacol Ther 2018. https://doi.org/10.1002/cpt.936.

43. de Jesus AA, Hou Y, Brooks S, et al. Distinct interferon signatures and cytokine patterns define additional systemic autoinflammatory diseases. J Clin Invest 2020. https://doi.org/10.1172/JCI129301.

44. Montealegre Sanchez GA, Reinhardt A, Ramsey S, et al. JAK1/2 inhibition with baricitinib in the treatment of autoinflammatory interferonopathies. J Clin Invest 2018. https://doi.org/10.1172/JCI98814.

45. Chen CY, Chen LC, Yeh KW, et al. Sequential changes to clinical parameters and adhesion molecules following intravenous pulse cyclophosphamide and methylprednisolone treatment of refractory juvenile idiopathic arthritis. Clin Exp Rheumatol 2004;22(2):259–64.

46. Breuer O, Schultz A. Side effects of medications used to treat childhood interstitial lung disease. Paediatr Respir Rev 2018. https://doi.org/10.1016/j.prrv.2018.03.002.

47. Tambralli A, Beukelman T, Weiser P, et al. High doses of infliximab in the management of juvenile idiopathic arthritis. J Rheumatol 2013. https://doi.org/10.3899/jrheum.130133.

48. De Benedetti F, Brogan P, Bracaglia C, et al. OP0290 Emapalumab (anti-interferon-gamma monoclonal antibody) in patients with macrophage activation syndrome (MAS) complicating systemic juvenile idiopathic arthritis (SJIA). Ann Rheum Dis 2020. https://doi.org/10.1136/annrheumdis-2020-eular.3169.

49. Vastert SJ, Jamilloux Y, Quartier P, et al. Anakinra in children and adults with Still's disease. Rheumatology (Oxford) 2019;58. https://doi.org/10.1093/rheumatology/kez350.

50. Grom AA, Horne A, De Benedetti F. Macrophage activation syndrome in the era of biologic therapy. Nat Rev Rheumatol 2016;12(5):259–68.

51. Schulert GS, Grom AA. Pathogenesis of macrophage activation syndrome and potential for cytokine-directed therapies. Annu Rev Med 2015. https://doi.org/10.1146/annurev-med-061813-012806.

52. Ravelli A, Minoia F, Davi S, et al. 2016 classification criteria for macrophage activation syndrome complicating systemic juvenile idiopathic arthritis: a European League Against Rheumatism/American College of Rheumatology/Paediatric Rheumatology International Trials Organisation Collaborat. Arthritis Rheumatol 2016;68(3):566–76.

53. Minoia F, Davì S, Horne A, et al. Clinical features, treatment, and outcome of macrophage activation syndrome complicating systemic juvenile idiopathic arthritis: a multinational, multicenter study of 362 patients. Arthritis Rheumatol 2014. https://doi.org/10.1002/art.38802.

54. Zou LX, Zhu Y, Sun L, et al. Clinical and laboratory features, treatment, and outcomes of macrophage activation syndrome in 80 children: a multi-center study in China. World J Pediatr 2020. https://doi.org/10.1007/s12519-019-00256-0.

55. Aytaç S, Batu ED, Ünal Ş, et al. Macrophage activation syndrome in children with systemic juvenile idiopathic arthritis and systemic lupus erythematosus. Rheumatol Int 2016. https://doi.org/10.1007/s00296-016-3545-9.

56. Schulert GS, Zhang M, Fall N, et al. Whole-exome sequencing reveals mutations in genes linked to hemophagocytic lymphohistiocytosis and macrophage activation syndrome in fatal cases of H1N1 influenza. J Infect Dis 2016. https://doi.org/10.1093/infdis/jiv550.

57. Bleesing J, Prada A, Siegel DM, et al. The diagnostic significance of soluble CD163 and soluble interleukin-2 receptor alpha-chain in macrophage activation syndrome and untreated new-onset systemic juvenile idiopathic arthritis. Arthritis Rheum 2007;56(3):965–71. https://doi.org/10.1002/art.22416.

58. Behrens EM, Beukelman T, Paessler M, et al. Occult macrophage activation syndrome in patients with systemic juvenile idiopathic arthritis. J Rheumatol 2007;34(5):1133–8.

59. Saper VE, Chen G, Deutsch GH, et al. Emergent high fatality lung disease in systemic juvenile arthritis. Ann Rheum Dis 2019. https://doi.org/10.1136/annrheumdis-2019-216040.

60. Schulert GS, Yasin S, Carey B, et al. systemic juvenile idiopathic arthritis–associated lung disease: characterization and risk factors. Arthritis Rheumatol 2019. https://doi.org/10.1002/art.41073.

61. Schulert GS, Minoia F, Bohnsack J, et al. Effect of biologic therapy on clinical and laboratory features of macrophage activation syndrome associated with systemic juvenile idiopathic arthritis. Arthritis Care Res 2018. https://doi.org/10.1002/acr.23277.

62. Shimizu M, Mizuta M, Okamoto N, et al. Tocilizumab modifies clinical and laboratory features of macrophage activation syndrome complicating systemic juvenile idiopathic arthritis. Pediatr Rheumatol 2020. https://doi.org/10.1186/s12969-020-0399-1.

63. Lee PY, Schulert GS, Canna SW, et al. Adenosine deaminase 2 as a biomarker of macrophage activation syndrome in systemic juvenile idiopathic arthritis. Ann Rheum Dis 2019. https://doi.org/10.1136/annrheumdis-2019-216030.

64. Eloseily EMA, Minoia F, Crayne CB, et al. Ferritin to erythrocyte sedimentation rate ratio: simple measure to identify macrophage activation syndrome in

systemic juvenile idiopathic Arthritis. ACR Open Rheumatol 2019. https://doi.org/10.1002/acr2.11048.

65. Sakumura N, Shimizu M, Mizuta M, et al. Soluble CD163, a unique biomarker to evaluate the disease activity, exhibits macrophage activation in systemic juvenile idiopathic arthritis. Cytokine 2018. https://doi.org/10.1016/j.cyto.2018.05.017.

66. Takakura M, Shimizu M, Irabu H, et al. Comparison of serum biomarkers for the diagnosis of macrophage activation syndrome complicating systemic juvenile idiopathic arthritis. Clin Immunol 2019. https://doi.org/10.1016/j.clim.2019.108252.

67. Irabu H, Shimizu M, Kaneko S, et al. Comparison of serum biomarkers for the diagnosis of macrophage activation syndrome complicating systemic juvenile idiopathic arthritis during tocilizumab therapy. Pediatr Res 2020. https://doi.org/10.1038/s41390-020-0843-4.

68. Guo L, Xu Y, Qian X, et al. Sudden Hypotension and Increased Serum IFN-γ and IL-10 Predict Early Macrophage Activation Syndrome in Systemic Juvenile Idiopathic Arthritis Patients. J Pediatr 2021. https://doi.org/10.1016/j.jpeds.2021.02.008.

69. Crayne CB, Albeituni S, Nichols KE, et al. The immunology of macrophage activation syndrome. Front Immunol 2019. https://doi.org/10.3389/fimmu.2019.00119.

70. Ravelli A, Grom AA, Behrens EM, et al. Macrophage activation syndrome as part of systemic juvenile idiopathic arthritis: diagnosis, genetics, pathophysiology and treatment. Genes Immun 2012. https://doi.org/10.1038/gene.2012.3.

71. Grom AA, Villanueva J, Lee S, et al. Natural killer cell dysfunction in patients with systemic-onset juvenile rheumatoid arthritis and macrophage activation syndrome. J Pediatr 2003;142(3):292–6.

72. Vastert SJ, van Wijk R, D'Urbano LE, et al. Mutations in the perforin gene can be linked to macrophage activation syndrome in patients with systemic onset juvenile idiopathic arthritis. Rheumatology (Oxford) 2010;49(3):441–9.

73. Villanueva J, Lee S, Giannini EH, et al. Natural killer cell dysfunction is a distinguishing feature of systemic onset juvenile rheumatoid arthritis and macrophage activation syndrome. Arthritis Res Ther 2005;7(1):R30–7.

74. Henderson LA, Cron RQ. Macrophage activation syndrome and secondary hemophagocytic lymphohistiocytosis in childhood inflammatory disorders: diagnosis and management. Pediatr Drugs 2020. https://doi.org/10.1007/s40272-019-00367-1.

75. Schulert GS, Cron RQ. The genetics of macrophage activation syndrome. Genes Immun 2020. https://doi.org/10.1038/s41435-020-0098-4.

76. Griffin G, Shenoi S, Hughes GC. Hemophagocytic lymphohistiocytosis: an update on pathogenesis, diagnosis, and therapy. Best Pract Res Clin Rheumatol 2020. https://doi.org/10.1016/j.berh.2020.101515.

77. Filipovich AH. Hemophagocytic lymphohistiocytosis (HLH) and related disorders. Hematol Am Soc Hematol Educ Program 2009. https://doi.org/10.1182/asheducation-2009.1.127.

78. Kaufman KM, Linghu B, Szustakowski JD, et al. Whole-Exome Sequencing Reveals Overlap Between Macrophage Activation Syndrome in Systemic Juvenile Idiopathic Arthritis and Familial Hemophagocytic Lymphohistiocytosis. Arthritis Rheumatol 2014. https://doi.org/10.1002/art.38793.

79. Zhang M, Behrens EM, Atkinson TP, et al. Genetic Defects in Cytolysis in Macrophage Activation Syndrome. Curr Rheumatol Rep 2014. https://doi.org/10.1007/s11926-014-0439-2.

80. Zhang K, Biroschak J, Glass DN, et al. Macrophage activation syndrome in patients with systemic juvenile idiopathic arthritis is associated with MUNC13-4 polymorphisms. Arthritis Rheum 2008;58(9):2892–6.

81. Hazen MM, Woodward AL, Hofmann I, et al. Mutations of the hemophagocytic lymphohistiocytosis-associated gene UNC13D in a patient with systemic juvenile idiopathic arthritis. Arthritis Rheum 2008. https://doi.org/10.1002/art.23199.

82. Vandenhaute J, Wouters CH, Matthys P. Natural killer cells in systemic autoinflammatory diseases: a focus on systemic juvenile idiopathic arthritis and macrophage activation syndrome. Front Immunol 2020. https://doi.org/10.3389/fimmu.2019.03089.

83. Behrens EM, Canna SW, Slade K, et al. Repeated TLR9 stimulation results in macrophage activation syndrome: like disease in mice. J Clin Invest 2011. https://doi.org/10.1172/JCI43157.

84. Zauner L, Nadal D. Understanding TLR9 action in Epstein Barr virus infection. Front Biosci 2012. https://doi.org/10.2741/3982.

85. Fall N, Barnes M, Thornton S, et al. Gene expression profiling of peripheral blood from patients with untreated new-onset systemic juvenile idiopathic arthritis reveals molecular heterogeneity that may predict macrophage activation syndrome. Arthritis Rheum 2007. https://doi.org/10.1002/art.22981.

86. Bracaglia C, de Graaf K, Pires Marafon D, et al. Elevated circulating levels of interferon-gamma and interferon-gamma-induced chemokines characterise patients with macrophage activation syndrome complicating systemic juvenile idiopathic arthritis. Ann Rheum Dis 2017;76(1):166–72.

87. Put K, Avau A, Brisse E, et al. Cytokines in systemic juvenile idiopathic arthritis and haemophagocytic lymphohistiocytosis: tipping the balance between interleukin-18 and interferon-γ. Rheumatology (Oxford) 2015. https://doi.org/10.1093/rheumatology/keu524.

88. Jordan MB, Hildeman D, Kappler J, et al. An animal model of hemophagocytic lymphohistiocytosis (HLH): CD8 + T cells and interferon gamma are essential for the disorder. Blood 2004. https://doi.org/10.1182/blood-2003-10-3413.

89. Xu XJ, Tang YM, Song H, et al. Diagnostic accuracy of a specific cytokine pattern in hemophagocytic lymphohistiocytosis in children. J Pediatr 2012. https://doi.org/10.1016/j.jpeds.2011.11.046.

90. Yasin S, Fall N, Brown RA, et al. IL-18 as a biomarker linking systemic juvenile idiopathic arthritis and macrophage activation syndrome. Rheumatology (Oxford) 2020. https://doi.org/10.1093/rheumatology/kez282.

91. de Jager W, Hoppenreijs EPAH, Wulffraat NM, et al. Blood and synovial fluid cytokine signatures in patients with juvenile idiopathic arthritis: a cross-sectional study. Ann Rheum Dis 2007;66(5):589–98.

92. Shimizu M, Nakagishi Y, Inoue N, et al. Interleukin-18 for predicting the development of macrophage activation syndrome in systemic juvenile idiopathic arthritis. Clin Immunol 2015. https://doi.org/10.1016/j.clim.2015.06.005.

93. Vastert S, Prakken B. Update on research and clinical translation on specific clinical areas: from bench to bedside: how insight in immune pathogenesis can lead to precision medicine of severe juvenile idiopathic arthritis. Best Pract Res Clin Rheumatol 2014;28(2). https://doi.org/10.1016/j.berh.2014.05.0024.

94. Weiss ES, Girard-Guyonvarc'h C, Holzinger D, et al. Interleukin-18 diagnostically distinguishes and pathogenically promotes human and murine macrophage activation syndrome. Blood 2018;131(13):1442–55.

95. Takakura M, Shimizu M, Yokoyama T, et al. Transient natural killer cell dysfunction associated with interleukin-18 overproduction in systemic juvenile idiopathic arthritis. Pediatr Int 2018. https://doi.org/10.1111/ped.13679.

96. De Jager W, Vastert SJ, Beekman JM, et al. Defective phosphorylation of interleukin-18 receptor β causes impaired natural killer cell function in systemic-onset juvenile idiopathic arthritis. Arthritis Rheum 2009;60(9). https://doi.org/10.1002/art.24750.

97. Canna SW, de Jesus AA, Gouni S, et al. An activating NLRC4 inflammasome mutation causes autoinflammation with recurrent macrophage activation syndrome. Nat Genet 2014;46(10):1140–6.

98. Henter JI, Horne AC, Aricó M, et al. HLH-2004: diagnostic and therapeutic guidelines for hemophagocytic lymphohistiocytosis. Pediatr Blood Cancer 2007. https://doi.org/10.1002/pbc.21039.

99. Ravelli A, Davì S, Minoia F, et al. Macrophage Activation Syndrome. Hematol Oncol Clin North Am 2015. https://doi.org/10.1016/j.hoc.2015.06.010.

100. Tang S, Li S, Zheng S, et al. Understanding of cytokines and targeted therapy in macrophage activation syndrome. Semin Arthritis Rheum 2021. https://doi.org/10.1016/j.semarthrit.2020.12.007.

101. Grom AA, Ilowite NT, Pascual V, et al. Rate and Clinical Presentation of Macrophage Activation Syndrome in Patients with Systemic Juvenile Idiopathic Arthritis Treated with Canakinumab. Arthritis Rheumatol 2016. https://doi.org/10.1002/art.39407.

102. Yokota S, Itoh Y, Morio T, et al. Macrophage activation syndrome in patients with systemic juvenile idiopathic arthritis under treatment with tocilizumab. J Rheumatol 2015. https://doi.org/10.3899/jrheum.140288.

103. De Benedetti F, Brunner HI, Ruperto N, et al. Randomized trial of tocilizumab in systemic juvenile idiopathic arthritis. N Engl J Med 2012;367(25):2385–95.

104. Sönmez HE, Demir S, Bilginer Y, et al. Anakinra treatment in macrophage activation syndrome: a single center experience and systemic review of literature. Clin Rheumatol 2018. https://doi.org/10.1007/s10067-018-4095-1.

105. Miettunen PM, Narendran A, Jayanthan A, et al. Successful treatment of severe paediatric rheumatic disease-associated macrophage activation syndrome with interleukin-1 inhibition following conventional immunosuppressive therapy: case series with 12 patients. Rheumatology 2011. https://doi.org/10.1093/rheumatology/keq218.

106. Eloseily EM, Weiser P, Crayne CB, et al. Benefit of anakinra in treating pediatric secondary hemophagocytic lymphohistiocytosis. Arthritis Rheumatol 2020. https://doi.org/10.1002/art.41103.

107. Locatelli F, Jordan MB, Allen C, et al. Emapalumab in children with primary hemophagocytic lymphohistiocytosis. N Engl J Med 2020. https://doi.org/10.1056/nejmoa1911326.

108. Vallurupalli M, Berliner N. Emapalumab for the treatment of relapsed/refractory hemophagocytic lymphohistiocytosis. Blood 2019. https://doi.org/10.1182/blood.2019002289.

109. Gabr J Ben, Liu E, Mian S, et al. Successful treatment of secondary macrophage activation syndrome with emapalumab in a patient with newly diagnosed adult-onset Still's disease: case report and review of the literature. Ann Transl Med 2020. https://doi.org/10.21037/atm-20-3127.

110. Al-Salama ZT. Emapalumab: first global approval. Drugs 2019. https://doi.org/10.1007/s40265-018-1046-8.

111. Canna SW, Girard C, Malle L, et al. Life-threatening NLRC4-associated hyperinflammation successfully treated with IL-18 inhibition. J Allergy Clin Immunol 2017. https://doi.org/10.1016/j.jaci.2016.10.022.

112. Yasin S, Solomon K, Canna SW, et al. IL-18 as therapeutic target in a patient with resistant systemic juvenile idiopathic arthritis and recurrent macrophage activation syndrome. Rheumatology (Oxford) 2020;59(2):442–5.

113. Keenan C, Nichols KE, Albeituni S. Use of the JAK inhibitor ruxolitinib in the treatment of hemophagocytic lymphohistiocytosis. Front Immunol 2021. https://doi.org/10.3389/fimmu.2021.614704.

114. Ruperto N, Brunner HI, Zuber Z, et al. Pharmacokinetic and safety profile of tofacitinib in children with polyarticular course juvenile idiopathic arthritis: results of a phase 1, open-label, multicenter study. Pediatr Rheumatol 2017. https://doi.org/10.1186/s12969-017-0212-y.

115. Kerrigan SA, McInnes IB. JAK inhibitors in rheumatology: implications for paediatric syndromes? Curr Rheumatol Rep 2018. https://doi.org/10.1007/s11926-018-0792-7.

116. Das R, Guan P, Sprague L, et al. Janus kinase inhibition lessens inflammation and ameliorates disease in murine models of hemophagocytic lymphohistiocytosis. Blood 2016. https://doi.org/10.1182/blood-2015-12-684399.

117. Maschalidi S, Sepulveda FE, Garrigue A, et al. Therapeutic effect of JAK1/2 blockade on the manifestations of hemophagocytic lymphohistiocytosis in mice. Blood 2016. https://doi.org/10.1182/blood-2016-02-700013.

118. Meyer LK, Verbist KC, Albeituni S, et al. JAK/STAT pathway inhibition sensitizes CD8 T cells to dexamethasone-induced apoptosis in hyperinflammation. Blood 2020. https://doi.org/10.1182/BLOOD.2020006075.

119. Verweyen E, Holzinger D, Weinhage T, et al. Synergistic signaling of TLR and IFNα/β facilitates escape of IL-18 expression from endotoxin tolerance. Am J Respir Crit Care Med 2020. https://doi.org/10.1164/rccm.201903-0659OC.

120. Wang J, Zhang R, Wu X, et al. Ruxolitinib-combined doxorubicin-etoposide-methylprednisolone regimen as a salvage therapy for refractory/relapsed haemophagocytic lymphohistiocytosis: a single-arm, multicentre, phase 2 trial. Br J Haematol 2021. https://doi.org/10.1111/bjh.17331.

121. Honda M, Moriyama M, Kondo M, et al. Tofacitinib-induced remission in refractory adult-onset Still's disease complicated by macrophage activation syndrome. Scand J Rheumatol 2020. https://doi.org/10.1080/03009742.2020.1729405.

122. Lee JJY, Schneider R. Systemic juvenile idiopathic arthritis. Pediatr Clin North Am 2018. https://doi.org/10.1016/j.pcl.2018.04.005.

123. Kimura Y, Weiss JE, Haroldson KL, et al. Pulmonary hypertension and other potentially fatal pulmonary complications in systemic juvenile idiopathic arthritis. Arthritis Care Res 2013. https://doi.org/10.1002/acr.21889.

124. Hollenbach JA, Ombrello MJ, Tremoulet AH, et al. IL-1 and IL-6 inhibitor hypersensitivity link to common HLA-DRB1*15 alleles. medRxiv 2021. https://doi.org/10.1101/2020.08.10.20172338.

125. Kurland G, Deterding RR, Hagood JS, et al. An official American Thoracic Society clinical practice guideline: classification, evaluation, and management of childhood interstitial lung disease in infancy. Am J Respir Crit Care Med 2013. https://doi.org/10.1164/rccm.201305-0923ST.

126. Sato S, Hosokawa T, Kawashima H. Successful treatment of plasma exchange for refractory systemic juvenile idiopathic arthritis complicated with macrophage activation syndrome and severe lung disease. Ann Rheum Dis 2020. https://doi.org/10.1136/annrheumdis-2020-217390.

127. Horne A, von Bahr Greenwood T, Chiang SCC, et al. Efficacy of moderately dosed etoposide in macrophage activation syndrome - hemophagocytic lymphohistiocytosis (MAS-HLH). J Rheumatol 2021. https://doi.org/10.3899/jrheum.200941.

128. de Benedictis FM, Carloni I, Guidi R. Safety of anti-inflammatory drugs in children with asthma. Curr Opin Allergy Clin Immunol 2021. https://doi.org/10.1097/ACI.0000000000000730.

129. Vos R, Verleden SE, Ruttens D, et al. Azithromycin and the treatment of lymphocytic airway inflammation after lung transplantation. Am J Transplant 2014. https://doi.org/10.1111/ajt.12942.

130. Trapnell BC, Inoue Y, Bonella F, et al. Inhaled molgramostim therapy in autoimmune pulmonary alveolar proteinosis. N Engl J Med 2020. https://doi.org/10.1056/nejmoa1913590.

131. Schmajuk G, Jafri K, Evans M, et al. Pneumocystis jirovecii pneumonia (PJP) prophylaxis patterns among patients with rheumatic diseases receiving high-risk immunosuppressant drugs. Semin Arthritis Rheum 2019. https://doi.org/10.1016/j.semarthrit.2018.10.018.

132. Cushion MT, Limper AH, Porollo A, et al. The 14th International Workshops on Opportunistic Protists (IWOP 14). J Eukaryot Microbiol 2018. https://doi.org/10.1111/jeu.12631.

133. Hayes D, Wilson KC, Krivchenia K, et al. Home oxygen therapy for children an official American Thoracic Society clinical practice guideline. Am J Respir Crit Care Med 2019. https://doi.org/10.1164/rccm.201812-2276ST.

134. Turcios NL. Cystic fibrosis lung disease: an overview. Respir Care 2020. https://doi.org/10.4187/respcare.06697.

135. Chang AB, Fortescue R, Grimwood K, et al. Task force report: European Respiratory Society guidelines for the management of children and adolescents with bronchiectasis. Eur Respir J 2021. https://doi.org/10.1183/13993003.02990-2020.

136. Trapnell BC, Whitsett JA, Nakata K. Pulmonary alveolar proteinosis. N Engl J Med 2003;349(26):2527–39.

137. Towe C, Trapnell B. Whole-Lung Lavage. In: Goldfarb S, Piccione J, editors. Diagnostic and interventional bronchoscopy in children. Switzerland: Springer Nature; 2021. p. 443–51.

138. Brinkman DM, de Kleer IM, ten Cate R, et al. Autologous stem cell transplantation in children with severe progressive systemic or polyarticular juvenile idiopathic arthritis: long-term follow-up of a prospective clinical trial. Arthritis Rheum 2007;56(7):2410–21.

139. Swart JF, De Roock S, Nievelstein RAJ, et al. Bone-marrow derived mesenchymal stromal cells infusion in therapy refractory juvenile idiopathic arthritis patients. Rheumatology (Oxford) 2019. https://doi.org/10.1093/rheumatology/kez157.

140. M F Silva J, Ladomenou F, Carpenter B, et al. Allogeneic hematopoietic stem cell transplantation for severe, refractory juvenile idiopathic arthritis. Blood Adv 2018;2(7):777–86.

141. De Kleer IM, Brinkman DMC, Ferster A, et al. Autologous stem cell transplantation for refractory juvenile idiopathic arthritis: analysis of clinical effects, mortality, and transplant related morbidity. Ann Rheum Dis 2004;63(10):1318–26.

The Temporomandibular Joint in Juvenile Idiopathic Arthritis

Peter Stoustrup, DDS, PhD[a], Melissa A. Lerman, MD, PhD, MSCE[b],
Marinka Twilt, MD, PhD, MSCE[c],*

KEYWORDS

- Juvenile idiopathic arthritis • Temporomandibular joint
- Temporomandibular joint arthritis • Temporomandibular joint involvement
- Treatment

KEY POINTS

- The temporomandibular joint (TMJ) is an under-recognized complication of juvenile idiopathic arthritis (JIA) that needs more attention in clinical decision making and clinical trials.
- Late diagnosis of TMJ arthritis leads to delayed treatment and subsequent long-term orofacial consequences.
- Routine standardized clinical functional evaluation of the TMJ should be integrated into clinical practice.
- Treatment of TMJ arthritis and the orofacial consequences warrants a multidisciplinary approach.

INTRODUCTION

Juvenile idiopathic arthritis (JIA) is the most common joint disease in childhood and is currently classified according to the International League of Associations for Rheumatology (ILAR).[1] Involvement of the temporomandibular joint (TMJ) was first described by Sir Frederick Still in his first report on childhood arthritis in 1897;[2] yet for over a century, the TMJ was a largely forgotten joint in rheumatology despite the fact that it can cause severe functional limitations and physical deformities. In the last 2 decades, however, TMJ involvement in JIA (JIA-TMJ) has become more widely recognized and increasingly studied. International efforts are underway to further increase the awareness of JIA-TMJ.

[a] Section of Orthodontics, Department of Dentistry and Oral Health, Aarhus University, Vennelyst Blvd 9, 8000 Aarhus, Denmark; [b] Department of Pediatrics, Division of Rheumatology, Perelman School of Medicine at the University of Pennsylvania, Children's Hospital of Philadelphia, 3401 Civic Center Blvd, Philadelphia, PA 19104, USA; [c] Department of Pediatrics, Alberta Children's Hospital, Cumming School of Medicine, University of Calgary, 28 Oki Drive NW, Calgary, T3B6A8 Alberta, Canada
* Corresponding author.
E-mail address: marinka.twilt@ahs.ca

Rheum Dis Clin N Am 47 (2021) 607–617
https://doi.org/10.1016/j.rdc.2021.06.004
0889-857X/21/© 2021 Elsevier Inc. All rights reserved.

The frequency of JIA-TMJ varies significantly in the literature and has been estimated to affect up to 87% depending on the JIA category investigated and the clinical measure and/or radiological method used to assess TMJ involvement.[3–5] JIA-TMJ can be present at diagnosis or may develop during the course of the disease. JIA-TMJ can lead to decreased growth of the mandible and micrognathia.[6,7] The TMJ can be the initial and only joint involved during the disease course.[8–10] Isolated TMJ arthritis remains controversial and presents a diagnostic problem, as MRI and cone-beam computed tomography (CT) appearance overlaps with other mechanical diseases of the TMJ.[11]

International multidisciplinary groups such as TMJaw (previously known as euro-TMjoint) and the Childhood Arthritis and Rheumatology Research Alliance (CARRA) TMJ Work Group have advanced the field by involving researchers across disciplines and developing consensus-based standards.[12–14] New and effective biologic treatments for JIA have become available in recent decades, but the effectiveness of these treatments on JIA-TMJ has not been studied. Although the TMJ is included in the joint evaluation during clinical trials, no specific consensus parameters to define either TMJ involvement or response to systemic treatment have been included in trials. Through the efforts by the TMJaw group, interdisciplinary consensus-based standardized terminology has been established for JIA-TMJ and the related consequences.[12] This article reviews the unique challenges of the TMJ in JIA.

JUVENILE IDIOPATHIC ARTHRITIS-ASSOCIATED TEMPOROMANDIBULAR JOINT TERMINOLOGY

The terminology used within the review adheres to the TMJaw consensus-based standardized terminology.[12] TMJ arthritis indicates the presence of active TMJ inflammation. In contrast, TMJ involvement includes all TMJ abnormalities presumed to be the result of current or previous TMJ arthritis. The terms TMJ deformity and dentofacial deformity refer to the osseous changes caused by TMJ involvement (**Table 1**).

Table 1
Recommended standardized temporomandibular joint terminology for juvenile idiopathic arthritis-associated temporomandibular joint arthritis

Terminology	Definition
TMJ arthritis	Active inflammation in the TMJ
TMJ involvement	Abnormalities presumed to be result of TMJ arthritis
TMJ management	Diagnosis, treatment, and monitoring of TMJ arthritis and involvement
Dentofacial deformity	Abnormality in growth, development, structure, and/or alignment of the facial bones and dentition
TMJ deformity	Abnormality in growth, development, or structure of the osseous and/or soft-tissue components of the TMJ
TMJ symptoms	Patient- or parent-reported conditions related to TMJ arthritis or involvement
TMJ dysfunction	Physician-reported functional examination abnormalities related to TMJ arthritis or involvement

Adapted from Stoustrup P, Resnick CM, Pedersen TK, Abramowicz S, Michelotti A, Küseler A, et al. Standardizing Terminology and Assessment for Orofacial Conditions in Juvenile Idiopathic Arthritis: International, Multidisciplinary Consensus-based Recommendations. J Rheumatol. 2019 May;46(5):518–22.

REPERCUSSIONS OF TEMPOROMANDIBULAR JOINT INVOLVEMENT IN JUVENILE IDIOPATHIC ARTHRITIS

Orofacial Symptoms and Quality of Life

Studies have shown a relationship between orofacial pain, orofacial health, and quality of life with TMJ involvement, and a relationship of these factors with JIA in general, independent of the presence of TMJ involvement. Carlsson and colleagues[15] showed associations between stress, psychosocial distress, jaw dysfunction, and loss of activities of daily living with orofacial pain, although TMJ imaging was not included in the study. Isola and colleagues[16] demonstrated that those with TMJ arthritis had a longer duration of JIA, had higher peripheral disease activity, and showed lower oral health-related quality of life scores.[16] A systematic review and meta-analysis on oral health in children and adolescents with JIA described more periodontal disease and temporomandibular disorders in patients with JIA compared with healthy peers.[17] A Danish 3-year regional cohort study observed an increase over time in orofacial symptoms and dysfunction.[18] In the Nordic JIA cohort, in which an extensive orofacial protocol was performed at 17-year follow-up, 1 of 3 JIA patients reported at least 1 orofacial symptom; JIA patients more often reported TMJ pain, TMJ morning stiffness, and limitation on chewing.[7] Recent studies have shown long-term symptomatic consequences of JIA-TMJ into young adulthood[6,7,19]

Dentofacial Deformities

Dentofacial deformities secondary to JIA are often under-recognized, even though many patients develop dentofacial abnormalities, including mandibular asymmetry, mandibular posterior rotation, or micrognathia and retrognathia (**Figs. 1** and **2**).[3,18] Which morphometric measures best correlate with TMJ arthritis is being actively

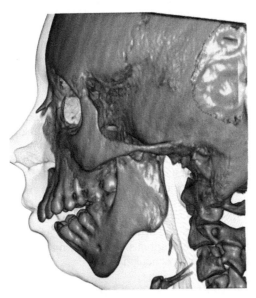

Fig. 1. Cone beam CT 3-dimensional reconstruction of a 12-year-old girl with dentofacial deformity related to long-term bilateral temporomandibular joint involvement, reduced vertical mandibular development causing mandibular micrognathia with an anterior open bite, and an unstable occlusion and reduced upper airway volume.

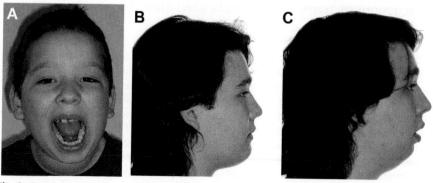

Fig. 2. Patient with extended oligoarticular JIA since age 2 years and 10 months. (*A*) TMJ issues detected at age 8 years with asymmetry on maximal opening. (*B*) At 20 years of age with micrognathia and open bite. (*C*) One month later, after orthognathic surgery Lefort I osteotomy with bilateral sagittal osteotomy mandible and anterior mandibular osteotomy.

studied. An interdisciplinary consensus study identified 7 highly recommended radiological morphometric measures for assessment of JIA-related dentofacial deformity.[20] In a Danish cohort study one-third of the cohort had apparent dentofacial deformities at the 36 months follow-up.[18]

CLINICAL SIGNS AND SYMPTOMS OF TEMPOROMANDIBULAR JOINT ARTHRITIS

TMJ arthritis can be asymptomatic at presentation, but other patients can also present with symptoms of TMJ discomfort early in the disease course.[18] Identifying clinical signs and symptoms of JIA-TMJ can be challenging. Many studies have unsuccessfully tried to identify reliable clinical predictors of JIA-TMJ.[3,21,22] Several studies have shown that decreased mouth opening is associated with JIA-TMJ.[3,7,22] To complicate matters, patients with TMJ involvement (damage) may present with TMJ symptoms and discomfort, but may not have any active signs of arthritis on MRI.[23] In these cases, the TMJ symptoms and dysfunction may arise from poor mechanical loading in joints with sequelae from previous TMJ inflammation.[20] Therefore, a careful orofacial examination is an important aspect of the general clinical JIA joint examination.

A systematic review of clinical predictors of JIA-TMJ showed a low level of evidence and high degree of study heterogeneity.[23] This led to the development of consensus-based standardized orofacial examination recommendations.[14] Five domains were proposed for the orofacial examination in JIA: medical history, orofacial symptoms, muscle and TMJ function, orofacial function, and dentofacial growth.[14] Stoustrup and colleagues developed a 3-minute screening protocol of the orofacial examination for use in routine clinical examination and future research (**Table 2**).[13,14] Over the years, many studies did not include concurrent MRI, which is unfortunate, because the lack of reliable clinical signs and symptoms showed that distinguishing between the differential diagnoses of TMJ arthritis cannot be made by clinical examination alone and requires confirmation by imaging[13,14,24,25]

IMAGING OF TEMPOROMANDIBULAR JOINT ARTHRITIS

Various methods have been used to detect JIA-TMJ, complicating the ability to compare frequency and severity of TMJ involvement in different populations. Imaging of the TMJ can be performed to confirm the presence of active arthritis, assess the

Table 2
Recommendations for the clinical orofacial examination in subjects with juvenile idiopathic arthritis according to the consensus-based standards

Domains	Items
Overarching principle	The clinical orofacial examination is an important component in the general health assessment of individuals diagnosed with JIA.
Assessment of orofacial symptoms	• Location • Intensity • Frequency • Character • Situations in which symptoms occur
Clinical examination – signs of TMJ arthritis	• TMJ pain on palpation • Masticatory muscle pain on palpation (Masseter and temporalis muscle) • TMJ pain on mandibular movement
Clinical examination – TMJ function	• Maximal mouth opening capacity • Mouth opening deviation • Condylar movements (during mandibular protrusion, laterotrusion) • Condylar head translation during opening • TMJ sounds during opening
Facial morphology and symmetry	• Mandibular sagittal position (convexity of profile) • Lower face asymmetry in frontal plane

Data from Stoustrup P, Herlin T, Spiegel L, Rahimi H, Koos B, Pedersen TK, et al. Standardizing the Clinical Orofacial Examination in Juvenile Idiopathic Arthritis: An Interdisciplinary, Consensus-based, Short Screening Protocol. J Rheumatol. 2020 Sep 1;47(9):1397–404 and Stoustrup P, Twilt M, Spiegel L, Kristensen KD, Koos B, Pedersen TK, et al. Clinical Orofacial Examination in Juvenile Idiopathic Arthritis: International Consensus-based Recommendations for Monitoring Patients in Clinical Practice and Research Studies. J Rheumatol. 2017 Mar;44(3):326–33.

degree of osseous deformities, or planning surgical intervention. The ideal imaging modality depends on the goal.

Currently the gold standard for detecting active TMJ arthritis is gadolinium-enhanced MRI (Gd-MRI).[12] The Gd-MRI can detect both inflammatory and osseous changes, where other techniques are superior in detailing osseous changes. Performing Gd-MRI poses particular challenges in younger patients, because of the length of the examination, often requiring sedation in younger patients, and interference created by metal braces. Despite these challenges, it is the most effective imaging modality in detecting the inflammation of early TMJ arthritis in new-onset JIA patients.[25–27]

Although TMJ-MRI is the gold standard, the sensitivity of an abnormal TMJ-MRI has been questioned. Stoll and colleagues[28] showed that changes consistent with minimal active TMJ arthritis were equally likely in children with JIA compared with controls. The authors caution interpreting small amounts of effusion or contrast enhancement as TMJ arthritis, in the absence of chronic changes.[28] Leschied and colleagues[29] compared TMJ-MRI findings with arthroscopy findings. Significant correlation was found between joint space width and hyperplastic synovitis and between synovitis and enhancement ratio of synovium on MRI and hyperplastic synovitis on arthroscopy, but not between synovitis on MRI and active synovitis on arthroscopy.[29]

Work is ongoing to develop consensus on the interpretation and scoring of TMJ-MRIs. Three TMJ-MRI scoring systems have been published (Swiss, German, and US).[30–32] The Outcome Measures in Rheumatoid Arthritis and Clinical Trials (OMERACT) JIA special interest group is developing a consensus-based TMJ-MRI scoring system.[33] Tolend and colleagues[33] published the first results of the OMERACT consensus-based TMJ-MRI scoring system, which includes 8 items: bone marrow edema and enhancement, condylar flattening, effusions, erosions, synovial enhancement and thickening, and disk abnormalities. Recently this group performed a discrete choice experiment to determine item weightings and grades of the previously proposed consensus-based scoring system.[34] In the inflammatory domain, higher weights were given to synovial thickening and joint enhancement compared with bone marrow items and effusion, while in the damage domain, erosions and condylar flattening were given higher weights compared with disk abnormalities.[34] Kellenberger and colleagues[35] developed an MRI pictorial atlas for detecting and grading the TMJ-MRI in JIA, including the appearance at different ages.[35]

Cone-beam CT (CBCT) is a 3-dimensional morphometric imaging modality. It is inferior to MRI in identifying active TMJ arthritis, but is superior in evaluating dentofacial morphology.[36,37]

Panoramic radiographs are widely used in the dental field. Dental professionals should be aware that radiographic abnormalities detected should warrant further evaluation by more advanced imaging.[38,39]

LOCAL AND SYSTEMIC TREATMENT

Ideally, treatment decisions for TMJ arthritis should be based on clinical JIA disease activity. A standardized clinical orofacial examination should be performed and can drive treatment choices if new orofacial functional limitations or abnormalities are observed.[13,14] However, in many cases, clinicians depend on the MRI. Hauser and colleagues[26] showed treatment was adjusted for most new-onset patients after TMJ-MRI results showed TMJ arthritis. In 62% of cases, detection of TMJ arthritis led to changes in treatment.[26]

The objectives of TMJ arthritis management are to reduce TMJ inflammation, reduce orofacial signs and symptoms related to current TMJ arthritis or the sequelae of previous TMJ arthritis, normalize dentofacial growth and development in growing patients with TMJ involvement, and address JIA-related dentofacial deformities. Timely diagnosis of TMJ arthritis and related orofacial manifestations is a prerequisite for optimal management.[20] TMJ treatment options include local treatments, systemic treatments, orthopedic devices, and surgical interventions. An interdisciplinary consensus-based project on guidelines/recommendations for treatment of active arthritis is currently being performed.

For many years, intra-articular corticosteroid injections (IACS) were performed to treat JIA-TMJ, particularly when no other joints were involved.[40–43] One systematic review reported that IACS helped reduce reported pain and improve mouth opening capacity, although huge variation was found in different studies.[44] Lochbuhler and colleagues[45] demonstrated that repeated TMJ IACS did not prevent progression of osseous deformities and did not normalize mandibular ramus growth in children with JIA. Another review showed that the level of evidence of efficacy only allowed minimal conclusions and alluded to potential detrimental effects of IACS on mandibular growth.[40] In 2011, Ringold and colleagues[46] and Stoll and colleagues[47] described heterotopic ossification in patients with JIA-TMJ. This was associated with severe TMJ arthritis, joint destruction, and pannus formation, and appeared to be more likely in those with repeated TMJ IACS and younger age at diagnosis.[47] As a result, there has been a shift to avoid IACS, specifically in skeletally immature patients.[48]

Arthrocentesis alone, without steroid injection, has been shown to result in significant improvement in pain and maximal mouth opening.[49,50] Olsen-Bergem and colleagues[49] showed that there was no difference in improvement between arthrocentesis with or without corticosteroid injection.

Prospective studies on systemic treatments for JIA unfortunately do not describe TMJ outcomes. Although it may be included in the joint count, involvement is based on clinical examination of the TMJ (eg, pain, limited range of motion), as for other joints and does not include MRI findings. In a retrospective study, Bollhalder and colleagues[51] showed a decrease in degree of inflammation on MRI, preservation of osseous TMJ morphology, and maintenance of normal mandibular growth in JIA-TMJ treated with systemic therapy. None of the patients received any IACS before or during the study period. However, comparative effectiveness studies of systemic treatments for active TMJ arthritis have not been done and are greatly needed.

ORTHOPEDIC DEVICES AND SURGERY

Oral splints can be used to alleviate orofacial symptoms from JIA-TMJ and normalize mandibular and dentofacial development in skeletally immature patients. Stabilization splints had a positive effect on orofacial pain frequency and intensity in an 8-week splint treatment study.[52] Another study showed comparable favorable effects on mouth opening and orofacial symptoms after introduction of an orthopedic splint.[53]

The TMJaw surgical task force developed and presented an algorithm for the management of dentofacial deformity resulting from JIA to be used as a conceptual framework.[54] Stoustrup and colleagues[20] emphasized the need for interdisciplinary management of dentofacial deformity in JIA and discussed the use of different orthopedic devices.

Severe dentofacial deformities or functional limitation can be treated by oral maxillofacial surgery (see **Fig. 2**). Frid and colleagues[55] performed a systematic literature review on surgical correction of dentofacial deformities. Extrapolated evidence supports orthognathic surgery in skeletally mature patients with controlled or quiescent JIA and a stable dentofacial deformity. Distraction osteogenesis was recommended for severe deformities. Alloplastic TMJ reconstruction is effective but should be used with caution in skeletally immature patients.[55]

SUMMARY

JIA-TMJ is frequent and can lead to dentofacial deformities and longstanding reduced orofacial health and quality of life that may persist into adulthood. Diagnosis remains difficult and should include a focused history, standardized clinical examination, and imaging with Gd-MRI. JIA treatment decision making should include considerations regarding the TMJ. Studies have suggested that systemic therapies decrease TMJ inflammation and may limit long-term dentofacial deformity. Local intra-articular joint injections with corticosteroids should be used with caution and be avoided in skeletally immature patients if possible. The integration of functional appliances (oral splints) into the care of growing patients with JIA is advised. Surgical interventions are a possibility for patients with severe dentofacial deformities. The optimal management of JIA-associated TMJ arthritis should be a coordinated effort by a multi-interdisciplinary team and should include a rheumatologist, a radiologist, an orthodontist, an oral maxillofacial surgeon, a physiotherapist, and dental professionals.

CLINICS CARE POINTS

- Active TMJ arthritis is diagnosed by Gd-MRI.
- Intra-articular corticosteroids injections should be used with caution.
- JIA-associated TMJ arthritis warrants a multidisciplinary approach.

DISCLOSURE

The authors have nothing to disclose.

REFERENCES

1. Petty RE, Southwood TR, Manners P, et al. International league of associations for rheumatology classification of juvenile idiopathic arthritis: second revision, Edmonton, 2001. J Rheumatol 2004;31(2):390–2.
2. Still GF, Garrod AE. On a form of chronic joint disease in children. J R Soc Med 1897;MCT-80:47–59.
3. Twilt M, Mobers SMLM, Arends LR, et al. Temporomandibular involvement in juvenile idiopathic arthritis. J Rheumatol 2004;31(7):1418–22.
4. Küseler A, Pedersen TK, Gelineck J, et al. A 2 year followup study of enhanced magnetic resonance imaging and clinical examination of the temporomandibular joint in children with juvenile idiopathic arthritis. J Rheumatol 2005;32(1): 162–9.
5. Pedersen TK, Küseler A, Gelineck J, et al. A prospective study of magnetic resonance and radiographic imaging in relation to symptoms and clinical findings of the temporomandibular joint in children with juvenile idiopathic arthritis. J Rheumatol 2008;35(8):1668–75.
6. Kalaykova S, Klitsie A, Visscher C, et al. A retrospective study on possible predictive factors for long-term temporomandibular joint degeneration and impaired mobility in juvenile arthritis patients. J Oral Facial Pain Headache 2017;31:: 165–71.
7. Glerup M, Stoustrup P, Matzen LH, et al. Longterm outcomes of temporomandibular joints in juvenile idiopathic arthritis: 17 years of followup of a Nordic juvenile idiopathic arthritis cohort. J Rheumatol 2020;47:730–8.
8. Scolozzi P, Bosson G, Jaques B. Severe isolated temporomandibular joint involvement in juvenile idiopathic arthritis. J Oral Maxillofac Surg 2005;63(9): 1368–71.
9. Martini G, Bacciliero U, Tregnaghi A, et al. Isolated temporomandibular synovitis as unique presentation of juvenile idiopathic arthritis. J Rheumatol 2001;28(7): 1689–92.
10. Hügle B, Spiegel L, Hotte J, et al. Isolated arthritis of the temporomandibular joint as the initial manifestation of juvenile idiopathic arthritis. J Rheumatol 2017; 44(11):1632–5.
11. Alimanovic D, Pedersen TK, Matzen LH, et al. Comparing clinical and radiological manifestations of adolescent idiopathic condylar resorption and juvenile idiopathic arthritis in the temporomandibular joint. J Oral Maxillofac Surg 2021;79(4): 774–85.
12. Stoustrup P, Resnick CM, Pedersen TK, et al. Standardizing terminology and assessment for orofacial conditions in juvenile idiopathic arthritis: international,

multidisciplinary consensus-based recommendations. J Rheumatol 2019;46(5):518–22.

13. Stoustrup P, Herlin T, Spiegel L, et al. Standardizing the clinical orofacial examination in juvenile idiopathic arthritis: an interdisciplinary, consensus-based, short screening protocol. J Rheumatol 2020;47(9):1397–404.

14. Stoustrup P, Twilt M, Spiegel L, et al. Clinical orofacial examination in juvenile idiopathic arthritis: international consensus-based recommendations for monitoring patients in clinical practice and research studies. J Rheumatol 2017;44(3):326–33.

15. Dimitrijevic Carlsson A, Wahlund K, Kindgren E, et al. Orofacial pain in juvenile idiopathic arthritis is associated with stress as well as psychosocial and functional limitations. Pediatr Rheumatol Online J 2019;17(1):83.

16. Isola G, Perillo L, Migliorati M, et al. The impact of temporomandibular joint arthritis on functional disability and global health in patients with juvenile idiopathic arthritis. Eur J Orthod 2019;41(2):117–24.

17. Skeie MS, Gil EG, Cetrelli L, et al. Oral health in children and adolescents with juvenile idiopathic arthritis - a systematic review and meta-analysis. BMC Oral Health 2019;19(1):285.

18. Stoustrup P, Glerup M, Bilgrau AE, et al. Cumulative incidence of orofacial manifestations in early juvenile idiopathic arthritis: a regional, three-year cohort study. Arthritis Care Res 2020;72(7):907–16.

19. Arvidsson LZ, Fjeld MG, Smith H-J, et al. Craniofacial growth disturbance is related to temporomandibular joint abnormality in patients with juvenile idiopathic arthritis, but normal facial profile was also found at the 27-year follow-up. Scand J Rheumatol 2010;39(5):373–9.

20. Stoustrup P, Pedersen TK, Nørholt SE, et al. Interdisciplinary management of dentofacial deformity in juvenile idiopathic arthritis. Oral Maxillofacial Surg Clin N Am 2020;32(1):117–34.

21. Fischer J, Skeie MS, Rosendahl K, et al. Prevalence of temporomandibular disorder in children and adolescents with juvenile idiopathic arthritis - a Norwegian cross-sectional multicentre study. BMC Oral Health 2020;20(1):282.

22. von Schuckmann L, Klotsche J, Suling A, et al. Temporomandibular joint involvement in patients with juvenile idiopathic arthritis: a retrospective chart review. Scand J Rheumatol 2020;49(4):271–80.

23. Kristensen KD, Stoustrup P, Küseler A, et al. Clinical predictors of temporomandibular joint arthritis in juvenile idiopathic arthritis: a systematic literature review. Semin Arthritis Rheum 2016;45(6):717–32.

24. Koos B, Twilt M, Kyank U, et al. Reliability of clinical symptoms in diagnosing temporomandibular joint arthritis in juvenile idiopathic arthritis [Internet]. J Rheumatol 2014;41:1871–7.

25. Keller H, Müller LM, Markic G, et al. Is early TMJ involvement in children with juvenile idiopathic arthritis clinically detectable? Clinical examination of the TMJ in comparison with contrast enhanced MRI in patients with juvenile idiopathic arthritis. Pediatr Rheumatol 2015;13::56.

26. Hauser RA, Schroeder S, Cannizzaro E, et al. How important is early magnetic resonance imaging of the temporomandibular joint for the treatment of children with juvenile idiopathic arthritis: a retrospective analysis. Pediatr Rheumatol 2014;12::36.

27. Sonesson M, Al-Qabandi F, Månsson S, et al. Orthodontic appliances and MR image artefacts: an exploratory in vitro and in vivo study using 1.5-T and 3-T scanners. Imaging Sci Dentistry 2021;51::63.

28. Stoll ML, Guleria S, Mannion ML, et al. Defining the normal appearance of the temporomandibular joints by magnetic resonance imaging with contrast: a comparative study of children with and without juvenile idiopathic arthritis. Pediatr Rheumatol Online J 2018;16(1):8.
29. Leschied JR, Smith EA, Baker S, et al. Contrast-enhanced MRI compared to direct joint visualization at arthroscopy in pediatric patients with suspected temporomandibular joint synovitis. Pediatr Radiol 2019;49(2):196–202.
30. Vaid YN, Dunnavant FD, Royal SA, et al. Imaging of the temporomandibular joint in juvenile idiopathic arthritis. Arthritis Care Res 2014;66(1):47–54.
31. Kellenberger CJ, Arvidsson LZ, Larheim TA. Magnetic resonance imaging of temporomandibular joints in juvenile idiopathic arthritis [Internet]. Semin Orthod 2015;21::111–20.
32. Koos B, Tzaribachev N, Bott S, et al. Classification of temporomandibular joint erosion, arthritis, and inflammation in patients with juvenile idiopathic arthritis. J Orofac Orthop 2013;74(6):506–19.
33. Tolend MA, Twilt M, Cron RQ, et al. Toward establishing a standardized magnetic resonance imaging scoring system for temporomandibular joints in juvenile idiopathic arthritis. Arthritis Care Res 2018;70::758–67.
34. Tolend M, Junhasavasdikul T, Cron RQ, et al. Discrete choice experiment on a magnetic resonance imaging scoring system for temporomandibular joints in juvenile idiopathic arthritis. Arthritis Care Res 2021. https://doi.org/10.1002/acr.24577.
35. Kellenberger CJ, Junhasavasdikul T, Tolend M, et al. Temporomandibular joint atlas for detection and grading of juvenile idiopathic arthritis involvement by magnetic resonance imaging. Pediatr Radiol 2018;48(3):411–26.
36. Stoustrup P, Iversen CK, Kristensen KD, et al. Assessment of dentofacial growth deviation in juvenile idiopathic arthritis: reliability and validity of three-dimensional morphometric measures. PLoS One 2018;13:e0194177.
37. Stoustrup PB, Ahlefeldt-Laurvig-Lehn N, Kristensen KD, et al. No association between types of unilateral mandibular condylar abnormalities and facial asymmetry in orthopedic-treated patients with juvenile idiopathic arthritis. Am J Orthod Dentofacial Orthop 2018;153(2):214–23.
38. Piancino MG, Cannavale R, Dalmasso P, et al. Condylar asymmetry in patients with juvenile idiopathic arthritis: could it be a sign of a possible temporomandibular joints involvement? Semin Arthritis Rheum 2015;45:208–13.
39. Abramowicz S, Simon LE, Susarla HK, et al. Are panoramic radiographs predictive of temporomandibular joint synovitis in children with juvenile idiopathic arthritis? J Oral Maxillofac Surg 2014;72(6):1063–9.
40. Stoustrup P, Kristensen KD, Verna C, et al. Intra-articular steroid injection for temporomandibular joint arthritis in juvenile idiopathic arthritis: a systematic review on efficacy and safety [Internet]. Semin Arthritis Rheum 2013;43:63–70.
41. Stoustrup P, Kristensen KD, Küseler A, et al. Temporomandibular joint steroid injections in patients with juvenile idiopathic arthritis: an observational pilot study on the long-term effect on signs and symptoms. Pediatr Rheumatol 2015;13:62..
42. Frid P, Augdal TA, Larheim TA, et al. Efficacy and safety of intraarticular corticosteroid injections in adolescents with juvenile idiopathic arthritis in the temporomandibular joint: a Norwegian 2-year prospective multicenter pilot study. Pediatr Rheumatol Online J 2020;18(1):75.
43. Ringold S, Torgerson TR, Egbert MA, et al. Intraarticular corticosteroid injections of the temporomandibular joint in juvenile idiopathic arthritis. J Rheumatol 2008;35(6):1157–64.

44. Antonarakis GS, Blanc A, Courvoisier DS, et al. Effect of intra-articular corticosteroid injections on pain and mouth opening in juvenile idiopathic arthritis with temporomandibular involvement: a systematic review and meta-analysis. J Craniomaxillofac Surg 2020;48(8):772–8.

45. Lochbühler N, Saurenmann RK, Müller L, et al. Magnetic resonance imaging assessment of temporomandibular joint involvement and mandibular growth following corticosteroid injection in juvenile idiopathic arthritis. J Rheumatol 2015;42:1514–22.

46. Ringold S, Thapa M, Shaw EA, et al. Heterotopic ossification of the temporomandibular joint in juvenile idiopathic arthritis. J Rheumatol 2011;38(7):1423–8.

47. Stoll ML, Amin D, Powell KK, et al. Risk factors for intraarticular heterotopic bone formation in the temporomandibular joint in juvenile idiopathic arthritis. J Rheumatol 2018;45(9):1301–7.

48. Stoustrup P, Twilt M, Resnick CM. Management of temporomandibular joint arthritis in JIA: tradition-based or evidence-based? J Rheumatol 2018;45(9):1205–7.

49. Olsen-Bergem H, Bjørnland T. A cohort study of patients with juvenile idiopathic arthritis and arthritis of the temporomandibular joint: outcome of arthrocentesis with and without the use of steroids. Int J Oral Maxillofac Surg 2014;43::990–5.

50. Antonarakis GS, Courvoisier DS, Hanquinet S, et al. Benefit of temporomandibular joint lavage with intra-articular steroids versus lavage alone in the management of temporomandibular joint involvement in juvenile idiopathic arthritis. J Oral Maxillofac Surg 2018;76:1200–6.

51. Bollhalder A, Patcas R, Eichenberger M, et al. Magnetic resonance imaging followup of temporomandibular joint inflammation, deformation, and mandibular growth in juvenile idiopathic arthritis patients receiving systemic treatment. J Rheumatol 2020;47(6):909–16.

52. Stoustrup P, Kristensen KD, Küseler A, et al. Management of temporomandibular joint arthritis-related orofacial symptoms in juvenile idiopathic arthritis by the use of a stabilization splint. Scand J Rheumatol 2014;43:137–45.

53. Isola G, Ramaglia L, Cordasco G, et al. The effect of a functional appliance in the management of temporomandibular joint disorders in patients with juvenile idiopathic arthritis. Minerva Stomatol 2017;66(1):1–8.

54. Resnick CM, Frid P, Norholt SE, et al. An algorithm for management of dentofacial deformity resulting from juvenile idiopathic arthritis: results of a multinational consensus conference. J Oral Maxillofac Surg 2019;77(6):1152.e1–33.

55. Frid P, Resnick C, Abramowicz S, et al, Temporomandibular Joint Juvenile Arthritis Work Group TMJaw. Surgical correction of dentofacial deformities in juvenile idiopathic arthritis: a systematic literature review. Int J Oral Maxillofac Surg 2019;48(8):1032–42.

Uveitis in Children and Adolescents

Margaret H. Chang, MD, PhD[a,1], Jessica G. Shantha, MD[b,1], Jacob J. Fondriest, MD[c,d], Mindy S. Lo, MD, PhD[a], Sheila T. Angeles-Han, MD, MSc[e,f,g,h,*]

KEYWORDS

- Pediatrics • Uveitis • Rheumatology • Ophthalmology • Autoimmune

KEY POINTS

- Childhood uveitis can lead to sight-threatening complications.
- Ophthalmic screening of children with JIA at risk for uveitis needs to be performed per recommended schedules.
- Ophthalmic evaluation of children with uveitis is important to monitor disease activity, treatment response, and development of complications.
- Prolonged courses of glucocorticoids (GC) should not be used as sole therapy.
- Early and timely treatment with systemic immunosuppression improves vision outcomes.

OVERVIEW
Epidemiology

Uveitis is an inflammatory ocular disease that can lead to sight-threatening complications. Early detection and timely treatment optimize visual outcomes. Childhood uveitis has an incidence of 4.3 per 100,000, and a prevalence of 27.9 per 100,000.[1] It occurs in isolation, as in idiopathic uveitis, but is also associated with infectious and

[a] Division of Immunology, Boston Children's Hospital, Harvard Medical School, Fegan 6, 300 Longwood Avenue, Boston, MA 02115, USA; [b] Department of Ophthalmology, Emory University, Emory Eye Center, 1365 Clifton Road, Clinic Building B, Atlanta, GA 30326, USA; [c] Department of Internal Medicine, Summa Health System, Internal Medicine Center, 55 Arch Street, Suite 1B, Akron, OH 44304, USA; [d] Rush Eye Center, 1725 West Harrison Street, Suite 945, Chicago, IL 60612, USA; [e] Division of Rheumatology, Cincinnati Children's Hospital Medical Center, 3333 Burnett Avenue, Cincinnati, OH 45229, USA; [f] Department of Pediatrics, University of Cincinnati, Cincinnati, OH, USA; [g] Division of Ophthalmology, Cincinnati Children's Hospital Medical Center, Cincinnati, OH, USA; [h] Department of Ophthalmology, University of Cincinnati, Cincinnati, OH, USA
[1] Co-first authors.
* Corresponding author. Division of Rheumatology, Cincinnati Children's Hospital Medical Center, 3333 Burnett Avenue, Cincinnati, OH 45229.
E-mail address: sheila.angeles-han@cchmc.org
Twitter: STHanMD (S.T.A.-H.)

Rheum Dis Clin N Am 47 (2021) 619–641
https://doi.org/10.1016/j.rdc.2021.07.005
0889-857X/21/© 2021 Elsevier Inc. All rights reserved.

noninfectious etiologies. Broadly, males and females are equally affected, and uveitis is most common in non-Hispanic White and Black children. Idiopathic anterior uveitis comprises approximately 29% of all pediatric diagnoses, followed by juvenile idiopathic arthritis-associated uveitis (JIA-U) (21%), pars planitis (17%), and infectious uveitis (6%).[2] Classification is by site of inflammation, with anterior location being most common. This review focuses on noninfectious causes of uveitis.

Pathophysiology

In noninfectious uveitis, inflammation arises from an immune response triggered against antigens within the eye. This process is induced by T cells and mediated by B cells and other immune cells that propagate inflammation (**Fig. 1**).[3,4]

The eye is an immune-privileged site. There are several mechanisms in place that protect against intraocular inflammation, including blood-retinal barriers and immunosuppressive properties of the eye microenvironment, such as anterior chamber (AC)-associated immune deviation.[3–6] AC-associated immune deviation is an active regulatory process in which introduction of foreign antigen into the eye leads to specific, systemic immune tolerance. However, these systems are overcome when autoimmunity develops.

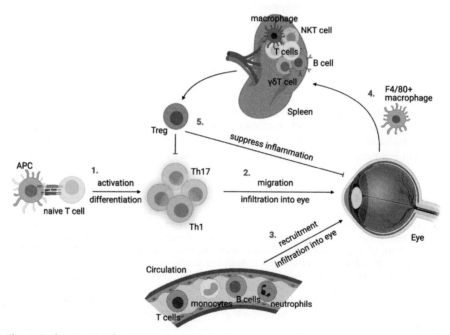

Fig. 1. Pathogenesis of autoimmune uveitis. (1) Autoreactive T cells in the periphery are activated and polarized to Th1 and Th17 cells. (2) Activated T cells migrate to the eye, triggering local release of inflammatory cytokines and permeabilization of the retina-blood barrier. (3) Chemokines released from local inflammation recruits circulating leukocytes to the eye. (4) Macrophages carry ocular antigens to the spleen where they interact with T cells, B cells, natural killer T cells, and γδT cells to generate Tregs. (5) Antigen-specific Tregs suppress effector T-cell proliferation and local inflammation in the eye, promoting remission. Created with BioRender.com.

Autoimmune uveitis arises when an immune response is triggered against native intraocular antigens, either in the setting of trauma or through molecular mimicry of infectious pathogens.[7,8] It is largely regarded as a T cell–driven disease because T cells specific to ocular antigens are found in the peripheral blood of patients with uveitis,[9] and many therapies are T cell–directed. Furthermore, the most widely studied rodent model of uveitis is experimental autoimmune uveitis, a T cell–dependent model of chorioretinitis.[10] B cells and plasma cells are also found in the eye, and autoantibodies from the serum of patients with JIA-U bind to structures within the eye.[11–13] However, no animal model of uveitis to date has shown uveitis conferred from autoantibodies or induced by B-cell activity alone.[14–16]

Genetic and epigenetic factors also influence immune regulation and have been associated with uveitis in children. Polymorphisms in HLA molecules have been linked with uveitis risk and are thought to reflect recognition of particular antigens or epitopes (**Table 1**).[10] Several single-nucleotide polymorphisms and epigenetic factors, such as DNA methylation and microRNA expression, which influence gene expression patterns, have also been associated with uveitis risk.[17–20]

Uveitis biomarkers, such as s100 proteins, cytokines, and chemokines, are differentially expressed in the aqueous humor and serum of adults and children with uveitis.[21–26] They are also detected in tears from patients with uveitis and correlate with disease activity.[27–30] Further work is needed to discover sensitive biomarkers that diagnose and monitor uveitis, using noninvasive methods that are reproducible in the clinical setting.

COMMON UVEITIS SYNDROMES
Noninfectious Uveitis

Anterior uveitis
Anterior uveitis constitutes 45% of pediatric cases, where idiopathic chronic anterior uveitis is most common.[1] JIA-U occurs in up to 25% of children with oligoarthritis.[1,2,31–34] JIA-U is typically asymptomatic with a chronic and relapsing course. Acute anterior uveitis (AAU), which is typically symptomatic and unilateral, is most common in enthesitis-related arthritis and HLA-B27-positive patients with juvenile spondyloarthropathy. The American Academy of Pediatrics and other groups recommend regular ophthalmic screening of children with JIA for prompt detection of uveitis.[35–39] Children at highest uveitis risk are those with the oligoarthritis, polyarthritis rheumatoid factor–negative, psoriatic, and undifferentiated JIA categories who are also less than 7 years old at JIA onset, antinuclear antibody positive, and have less than or equal to 4 years duration of JIA.[36,40] They need screening every 3 months. Other risk factors studied, but not included in the recommendations, are female sex and White race. At their initial ophthalmology visit, up to 45% of those with JIA-U already have ocular complications, such as cataracts and glaucoma.[34,36,41–43]

Nonanterior uveitis
Nonanterior uveitis occurs less frequently. Pars planitis, an idiopathic form of intermediate uveitis, is most common.[2,44] Mean age of onset is 7.8 years.[45,46] Patients with haplotypes HLA-DR2 or HLA-DR15, and pars planitis/periphlebitis on examination have an increased risk of developing multiple sclerosis.[47,48] Children diagnosed before age 7 have a worse visual prognosis.[49] Female sex and Hispanic ethnicity may predict greater rates of remission.[50] Prognosis varies, and treatment includes glucocorticoids (GC), systemic immunomodulatory therapy, and, in select patients, pars plana vitrectomy and panretinal photocoagulation.[45,51,52]

Table 1
HLA associations in uveitis

Disease	Genetic Associations	Location of Inflammation
Juvenile idiopathic arthritis–associated uveitis	DRB1*1104, DRB1*08, DRB1*09, DRB1*13, DPB1*0201, DR5	Anterior
Tubulointerstitial nephritis and uveitis	DQA1, DQB1, DRB1	Anterior
Spondyloarthritis-associated uveitis	B27, DR8	Anterior
Pars planitis	DR2, DR3, DR15, DR51, DR17, B8, B51	Intermediate
Behçet disease	B51	Panuveitis
Birdshot chorioretinopathy	A29	Panuveitis
Sarcoidosis	B8, DRB1*1101, DRB3*0101	Panuveitis
Vogt-Koyanagi-Harada disease	DRB1*04, DQB1*04, DQA1*03, DPB1*05	Panuveitis

Behçet disease is a systemic vasculitis most common in individuals age 10 to 30, causing severe recurrent nongranulomatous uveitis and hypopyon, with recurrent aphthous and genital ulcers.[53–55] Onset age less than 25 years and male sex are risk factors for uveitis, and males have worse visual prognosis.[56–58] Posterior uveitis is associated with more sight-threatening complications, and can manifest as an occlusive retinal vasculitis of arteries and veins causing macular edema and retinal neovascularization.[59]

Blau syndrome and sarcoidosis are similar entities characterized by noncaseating granulomas affecting multiple organ systems. Inflammation occurs in any part of the uvea. Blau syndrome, caused by mutations in *NOD2*, classically presents with a triad of rash, arthritis, and uveitis before age 5.[46,60–63] Pediatric sarcoidosis has two distinct patterns. Early onset sarcoidosis is clinically indistinguishable from Blau syndrome except for the absence of a family history.[46,64] Later-onset sarcoidosis in children resembles adult sarcoidosis, with pulmonary involvement.[65] Elevated angiotensin-converting enzyme and lysozyme levels may support a diagnosis of sarcoidosis, although angiotensin-converting enzyme levels can normally be elevated in children.[66,67]

Vogt-Koyanagi-Harada disease is a bilateral granulomatous panuveitis most common in patients of Hispanic, Asian, Native American, Middle-Eastern, and Asian-Indian ancestry.[68–70] The pathogenesis is likely an autoimmune reaction to a melanin-associated antigen.[71,72] Approximately 8% to 16% of cases affect children younger than 16.[73,74] The initial prodromal phase presents with flulike symptoms, orbital pain, meningismus, sensorineural hearing loss, and tinnitus.[75] The acute uveitic stage follows with bilateral blurry vision, anterior uveitis, optic disk hyperemia, and subretinal fluid.[75] The convalescent stage includes vitiligo, poliosis, and choroid depigmentation. The chronic, recurrent phase, manifests as bouts of AAU.[76]

Tubulointerstitial nephritis and uveitis syndrome typically presents as a bilateral nongranulomatous anterior uveitis, although one-third of patients have vitreous cell and optic nerve hyperemia.[77] Nephritis precedes uveitis in 65% of cases, and antecedent flulike symptoms occur in 50%. Median age of onset is 15 years, and 75% are female. Uveitis is typically mild and nephritis self-limited, only rarely progressing to require dialysis.[78] The diagnosis is strongly supported by elevated urine β_2-microglobulin.[46,77–79]

Infectious Uveitis

Infections are important but less common causes of childhood uveitis. In the United States, infections account for 3% to 8% of pediatric cases.[80,81] In other regions, infections account for approximately 30% of cases.[41,82–85] Toxoplasmosis and toxocariasis are most common, causing posterior uveitis or panuveitis, either unilateral or bilateral. Herpes simplex virus, cytomegalovirus, varicella zoster virus, tuberculosis, and Lyme disease are less common. *Bartonella henselae*, implicated in cat-scratch disease, may cause neuroretinitis. A thorough history and assessment for risk factors are important because laboratory investigations are useful. In select cases, polymerase chain reaction testing of intraocular fluid confirms the diagnosis.[86]

Masquerade Syndromes

Masquerade syndromes can mimic uveitis but do not represent true autoimmune or infectious processes. These include retinal detachments and intraocular tumors. Retinoblastoma is uncommon but is the most common intraocular childhood malignancy and should be considered based on presentation of leukocoria and family history of retinoblastoma.[87]

OCULAR COMPLICATIONS

Ocular complications are common, especially with uncontrolled inflammation or prolonged treatment with topical GC.[34,88,89] They can develop in any eye compartment, may be mild and transient, or lead to severe permanent vision loss. Temporary vision loss can affect the developing visual pathway especially in younger children and cause permanent amblyopia.[90] Up to 80% of patients with JIA-U develop cataracts (23%–83% of cases), glaucoma (17%–28%), synechiae (18%–44%), band keratopathy (14%–46%), cystoid macular edema (2%–30%), and hypotony (3%–10%).[2,91–93] Approximately 5% to 15% of patients experience blindness.[2,92] **Table 2** and **Fig. 2** describe various ocular complications.

Surgery is performed in 15% to 19% of children, including cataract extraction, glaucoma surgery, or vitrectomy.[2,92] Inflammation should be controlled for a minimum of 3 months before surgery to reduce postoperative complications. GC is used in the preoperative, intraoperative, and postoperative period, administered locally or systemically.[94–96] Dose and duration vary, and taper depends on the postoperative clinical course. Usual systemic treatment should be maintained.

OPHTHALMIC WORK-UP
Assessment of Disease Activity

In 2005, the Standardization of Uveitis Nomenclature (SUN) working group described a systematic way to classify uveitis based on anatomic involvement, disease course, and disease activity.[44] Anterior uveitis is inflammation of the AC, intermediate uveitis involves the vitreous, and posterior uveitis involves the retina and/or choroid. Presence of complications, such as vascular sheathing and macular edema, does not affect anatomic classification. In severe anterior uveitis, there may be spillover of cells into the vitreous. Acute uveitis is described as sudden in onset, lasting less than or equal to 3 months. Chronic uveitis is persistent inflammation with recurrence within 3 months of discontinuing treatment. Recurrent uveitis is multiple episodes of uveitis separated by more than 3 months in the absence of treatment. Uveitis may be limited or persistent, with a cutoff of 3 months, and subjectively described as sudden or insidious. Disease activity in anterior uveitis is graded by AC cell and flare from 0 to 4. AC cell reflects the number of cells counted in a 1 mm × 1 mm slit lamp beam. AC flare reflects the degree to which the lens and iris are obscured by protein flare. In nonanterior uveitis, vitreous haze is graded from 0 to 5, reflecting the degree to which the posterior pole is obscured. There is no standardized nomenclature for grading vitreous cell.

Ophthalmic Examination Components

1. *Bedside examination* is an assessment of the ocular vitals and a dilated examination with an indirect ophthalmoscope to assess the posterior segment of the eye (**Table 3**).
2. *Slit lamp examination* assesses and grades inflammation. Precise intraocular pressure measurement with Goldmann applanation tonometry, assessment of corneal pathology, and the use of a gonioscope to evaluate the AC angle may be performed. Dilated examinations are performed at the slit lamp.
3. *Special tests* require specialized machinery to assess visual function and complications, as in visual field testing. Optical coherence tomography (OCT) assesses for macular edema and glaucomatous progression. Fluorescein angiography evaluates for retinal vasculitis or other signs of inflammation that are not detected by the ophthalmic examination.

Innovations in the Ophthalmic Work-up

Ophthalmic imaging and technology are rapidly changing, with advances in anterior and posterior segment imaging. Detection of anterior segment inflammation by anterior segment OCT and laser flare photometry enables standardized quantitative metrics for AC cell and flare, respectively.[97,98] Furthermore, OCT of the retina noninvasively measures blood flow through different levels of the retina. Quantitative metrics including measure of the foveal avascular zone area and vessel density can be acquired. A small retrospective cohort study reported a decrease in vessel density in childhood uveitic patients compared with control subjects.[99] As technologies improve and become available, there may be better end points for clinical disease measurement and clinical trials.

THERAPEUTIC OPTIONS

Timely local and/or systemic immunosuppression is critical. Recommendations for treatment have been country-specific until recently.[100,101] Guidelines developed by pediatric rheumatologists and ophthalmologists in North America and Europe include the American College of Rheumatology/Arthritis Foundation (ACR/AF) and the Single Hub and Access point for pediatric Rheumatology in Europe (SHARE) recommendations.[38,102]

Glucocorticoids

Topical ophthalmic drops, periocular GC, and intraocular GC are used as sole treatment or in conjunction with systemic therapies.[103,104] Mode of administration is based on disease activity, ocular complications, and patient preference/cooperation. Prednisolone acetate 1% is the first-line topical GC for anterior uveitis. Difluprednate is more potent and reserved for severe inflammation, such as intermediate uveitis or treatment of cystoid macular edema. Limitations in difluprednate use are cost and side effects, such as ocular hypertension. Thorne and colleagues[105] report that

Table 2
Complications of childhood uveitis

Complication	Description	Location/Findings	Treatment
Band keratopathy	Calcium deposits in the cornea, if within the visual axis, can cause vision loss Often a sign of chronic inflammation	Cornea/anterior segment	Local chelation Photorefractive keratotomy
Hypotony	Ciliary body shutdown in certain types of uveitis may cause intraocular pressure to become low Can be transient or chronic	Corneal folds Optic nerve edema Choroidal folds Macular edema	*Depends on etiology* Corticosteroids may be beneficial in certain types of uveitis
Peripheral anterior synechiae	Iris adhesions onto the trabecular meshwork, which can block aqueous outflow and lead to angle closure and ocular hypertension	Anterior segment	Treat underlying cause Cycloplegic drops If ocular hypertension, treat accordingly (topical drops and/or glaucoma surgery)
Posterior synechiae	Iris adhesions to anterior surface of lens, these adhesions can limit view of posterior segment structures If severe may cause angle closure and iris bombe	Anterior segment	Cycloplegic drops Surgical release of adhesions
Cataract	Clouding of the lens	Anterior segment	Surgical removal ± intraocular lens placement
Vitreous cell/opacities	Infiltration of inflammatory cells into the vitreous cavity	Vitreous cavity	Treatment of inflammation by oral corticosteroids or systemic immunosuppression Local steroid injection Topical drops are less efficacious in penetrating the vitreous cavity
Epiretinal membrane	Thickening of the inner retina, which is associated with vitreous traction, macular hole formation, or macular edema	Retina/posterior segment	Pars plana vitrectomy with membrane peel if symptomatic

(continued on next page)

Table 2
(continued)

Complication	Description	Location/Findings	Treatment
Cystoid macular edema	Retinal thickening, edema, and/or subretinal fluid	Retina/posterior segment	Treatment of inflammation with topical drops, oral corticosteroids, and/or systemic immunosuppression Local corticosteroid injections
Glaucoma	Permanent damage to the optic nerve associated with high intraocular pressures and visual field loss	Optic nerve/retinal nerve fiber layer	Eyedrops Surgery Treat underlying cause

Uncontrolled uveitis may lead to reversible and irreversible complications. Not all complications listed are seen in all types of uveitis.

prednisolone acetate 1% administered at less than or equal to two drops per day may not increase risk for cataract formation, although guidelines recommend discontinuing topical GC as a goal.[37,38]

Local GC injections are used when more aggressive therapy is necessary and/or systemic therapy is failing or not an option. Careful consideration is required because of the risk of ocular hypertension, glaucoma, and cataract. Young children can have difficulty cooperating. Periocular GC injections are given in the sub-Tenon space (virtual space between the capsule and sclera) with triamcinolone acetonide. Intravitreal GC injections (injection into the vitreous cavity), such as intravitreal triamcinolone acetonide and dexamethasone, are administered as GC implants or direct injection. The PeriOcular versus INTravitreal GC for uveitic macular edema (POINT) trial was a multicenter randomized controlled trial in adults, which showed that intravitreal therapies were superior to periocular triamcinolone acetonide injections in treating uveitic macular edema.[106]

Oral and intravenous GC are prescribed in nonanterior uveitis or severe ocular inflammation. Prolonged courses of GC as sole therapy are not recommended and systemic immunosuppression should be initiated in chronic uveitis. In general, GC are used as short-term bridging therapy while awaiting efficacy of GC-tapering therapy, for control of severe disease, or in children with macular edema.[38,102,107] The CARRA uveitis consensus treatment plan suggests that steroid taper begin no later than 2 weeks after initiation of a steroid-sparing agent.

Conventional Synthetic Disease-Modifying Antirheumatic Drugs and Tumor Necrosis Factor Monoclonal Antibodies as First-Line Agents

Methotrexate

Methotrexate (MTX) has been considered first-line GC-sparing medication, regardless of uveitis category or cause. In children with severe disease and sight-threatening complications at presentation, simultaneous use of tumor necrosis factor monoclonal antibodies (TNF mAb) is recommended.[102,107] Despite decades of experience with MTX, there is scant literature on its effectiveness in childhood uveitis. The earliest case series in 1998 reported six of seven children with JIA-U significantly reduced

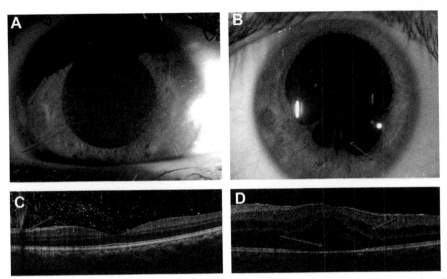

Fig. 2. Anterior segment complications of uveitis include band keratopathy (*A, arrows*) and posterior synechiae (*B, arrow*). Optical coherence tomography displays posterior segment complications of images of the retina with vitreous opacities (*C, arrow*) and cystoid macular edema with subretinal fluid (*D, arrows*).

or discontinued topical GC.[108] A retrospective study of 38 patients with JIA-U describes 25 treated with MTX for uveitis.[109] The other 13 patients only required 3 months of GC therapy. Most patients treated with MTX showed full or partial response; 6 of the 25 (24%) achieved remission over 12 months, whereas 4 of the 25 (16%) did not respond to MTX.

Meta-analysis of MTX studies in childhood uveitis, not limited to JIA-U, estimated that approximately 73% of children respond to MTX, defined as improvement in uveitis activity per SUN criteria. However, the durability of response varied across studies.[52] Most studies included only patients with JIA-U, thus likely representing anterior uveitis. A large multicenter cohort of adult and pediatric patients with uveitis found significantly higher rates of response with anterior and intermediate uveitis as compared with posterior or panuveitis.[110] Furthermore, children were less likely to respond to MTX compared with adults (adjusted hazard ratio for control of inflammation, 0.33; 95% confidence interval, 0.2–0.55).

The ACR/AF guideline recommends a threshold of 3 months for adding or changing systemic therapy. Earlier changes may be needed based on ophthalmic examination, duration of topical and systemic therapy, and ocular complications. The significant number of children who do not respond to MTX, and the proportion experiencing intolerable side effects, necessitate additional therapies.

Tumor necrosis factor inhibitors

Biologic disease-modifying antirheumatic drugs (DMARDs), such as TNF mAb, are commonly used for uveitis. Food and Drug Administration approval was granted for adalimumab for the treatment of noninfectious intermediate, posterior, and panuveitis in adult patients in 2016 and pediatric patients in 2018. A randomized controlled trial in 2017 describes patients with active uveitis on a stable dose of MTX randomized to either adalimumab or placebo.[111] Primary end point was time to treatment failure.

Table 3
Components of the ophthalmic examination

Category	Examination	Notes
Bedside examination	History	Assess history of photophobia
		Ask parents if the child ever has their eyes misaligned
		For children 1–2 y of age, does the child grip objects well?
		For children older than 5 y of age, does the child watch television from an appropriate distance?
	Visual acuity testing	Patients should be positioned 20 feet (6 m) from the chart
		Testing should be performed using glasses of the correct prescription
		Consider picture card for ages 2–3; tumbling "E" or HOTV for preliterate children older than 3 y of age
		The unused eye should be occluded or patched to prevent peeking
	Pupillary examination	Advanced cases of posterior synechiae may be grossly visible
		A relative afferent pupillary defect may suggest optic nerve pathology (eg, severe glaucoma, optic neuritis)
		Patients with active anterior uveitis may demonstrate consensual photophobia
	Extraocular motility and alignment	The presence of strabismus may raise concern for amblyopia
	Confrontational visual fields	May detect large visual field defects suggestive of glaucoma
		Formal machine-based visual field testing remains the gold standard
	Corneal and external examination	Redness and ciliary flush may support a diagnosis of anterior uveitis
		In some cases, band keratopathy may be visible
		Fluorescein staining may be used to evaluate for corneal pathology
	Intraocular pressure	The eye pressure can be taken by various types of commercial hand-held tools
	Direct ophthalmoscopy	May be used to assess the optic nerve
		Assessment of the red reflex can evaluate for cataract or retinoblastoma
	Indirect ophthalmoscopy	May be used to evaluate for vitreous haze, optic nerve edema, retinal vascular pathology

(continued on next page)

Category	Examination	Notes
		Assessment of the red reflex can evaluate for cataract or retinoblastoma
Slit lamp examination	Anterior chamber cell and flare	Quantify the degree of inflammation in the anterior chamber
	Goldmann applanation tonometry	Increased intraocular pressure is associated with increased risk for permanent glaucomatous vision loss
		Goldmann applanation tonometry performed at the slit lamp is the gold standard, but is difficult to perform in children
	Corneal and external examination	Redness and ciliary flush may support a diagnosis of anterior uveitis
		Allows for detailed diagnosis of corneal pathology
	Gonioscopy	Used to visualize the anterior chamber angle to assess for angle closure and glaucoma risk
		May visualize peripheral anterior synechiae that may otherwise be difficult to see
	Dilated fundoscopic examination	Allows for the most detailed direct visualization of the posterior segment
		Evaluate for vitreous cell and haze, retinal or choroidal inflammation, vasculitis, optic nerve pathology, macular edema
Special tests	Visual field testing	Formal machine-based visual field testing is necessary to diagnose visual field loss
		Visual field deficits are often related to glaucoma
		Testing requires maintained concentration and is difficult in young patients
	Optical coherence tomography	High-resolution image, which delineates the layers of the retina
		Retinal nerve fiber layer thickness and optic nerve morphology correlate with glaucomatous progression
		May reliably detect and monitor macular edema

(continued on next page)

Table 3
(continued)

Table 3 (continued)		
Category	**Examination**	**Notes**
	Fluorescein angiography	Use of intravenous fluorescein to visualize and diagnose retinal vasculature pathology
		Assess posterior segment inflammation, including optic disk hyperfluorescence, macular edema, and retinal vascular leakage
	Retinoscopy	Most commonly used to assess refractive error in preverbal children younger than 2 y of age
		Requires cycloplegic eyedrops to suppress accommodation for accurate results

The study, which enrolled 60 patients in the adalimumab arm, was stopped early because of the significantly different rates of treatment failure (27% in the adalimumab group vs 60% in the placebo group). The ADJUVITE trial was another randomized, placebo-controlled trial of adalimumab in patients with idiopathic or JIA-U and inadequate response to MTX.[112] Patients on adalimumab were more than twice as likely to have improvement in inflammation compared with the placebo group after 2 months.

Etanercept (which is a soluble TNF receptor and not an mAb) is not recommended for JIA-U, based on studies showing less benefit in treating or reducing risk of new uveitis as compared with TNF inhibitor (TNFi) mAb.[113–115] Infliximab is frequently used, but neither infliximab nor other commercially available TNFi mAb have Food and Drug Administration approval at present for the indication of uveitis. Although the intravenous administration of infliximab has benefits in certain situations (ie, when adherence is an issue), adalimumab may be superior. In one prospective study of adalimumab versus infliximab in 33 children with uveitis, nearly all achieved remission within a year, but there were fewer flares in the group who received adalimumab.[116] Another study used standard treatment protocols for JIA-U, beginning with GC, then MTX or cyclosporine, then adalimumab or infliximab. At 2 years of follow-up, 60% of patients on adalimumab were in remission, compared with 20% on infliximab.[117] Finally, in an open-label comparison in adults with Behçet-related uveitis, although remission rates after 1 year were similar between adalimumab and infliximab, Best corrected visual acuity and other parameters were better in the adalimumab group.[118] Although these collective results seem compelling, the infliximab dose used in these European studies ranged from 5 mg/kg every 6 to 12 weeks in the two pediatric studies, and 3 to 5 mg/kg every 4 to 8 weeks in the Behçet disease study. These doses are lower than those used by North American practitioners, who may advance doses as high as 20 mg/kg every 4 weeks.[119] Thus, patients who fail either adalimumab or infliximab may still benefit from switching to another TNFi mAb or increasing dose.

Beyond Methotrexate and Traditional Tumor Necrosis Factor Inhibitors

Fewer studies have examined treatment after standard therapy. Guidelines recommend several options. Approximately 30% or more patients have severe uveitis refractory to TNFi mAb and conventional synthetic DMARDs.[120]

Tocilizumab

Tocilizumab, an anti-interleukin-6 receptor mAb, is promising for JIA-U and other types of uveitis in multiple case series.[121–123] The APTITUDE trial was a multicenter phase 2 trial evaluating subcutaneous tocilizumab in patients with JIA-U who failed standard therapy with TNF mAb and MTX.[124] The primary outcome was treatment response at Week 12; of 21 patients enrolled, seven (33%) met this outcome. Only six patients on tocilizumab continued past 12 weeks of treatment. Treatment nonresponse was the most common reason for discontinuing tocilizumab. Thus, the trial did not meet its primary end point.[124] As the authors noted, however, tocilizumab was effective for a subset of patients with refractory uveitis. Three of four patients with baseline macular edema improved. With few evidence-based options, tocilizumab may be a reasonable therapeutic option.

Abatacept

Abatacept, a CTLA-4-Ig fusion protein that blocks T-cell costimulation, showed promising results in small case series of TNFi-refractory patients.[125,126] However, another case series found that although 11 (52%) out of 21 patients with refractory JIA-U responded to abatacept, the response was not sustained for 8 out of the 11.[127] When used as first-line therapy, abatacept was effective for 57% of patients with JIA-U.[128]

Rituximab

Rituximab, an mAb against CD20, has been trialed with varying success for posterior uveitis, panuveitis, and uveitis associated with systemic conditions.[129–131] Miserocchi and colleagues[132] reported eight adults with long-standing, refractory JIA-U who achieved durable remission with a mean follow-up time of more than 44 months. All patients had oligoarticular persistent or extended JIA with ocular complications from uveitis damage or GC treatment. Although promising, little data support the use of rituximab in uveitis.

Janus kinase inhibitors

Janus kinase (JAK) inhibitors are targeted synthetic DMARDs that are small molecular inhibitors, which target multiple cytokine pathways and are being used in the treatment of multiple autoimmune and autoinflammatory conditions. Miserocchi and colleagues[133] reported four patients with JIA-U who were treated successfully with JAK inhibitors, either baricitinib or tofacitinib. Bauermann and colleagues[134] reported excellent response to tofacitinib in an adult with severe JIA-U. Currently, tofacitinib is the only JAK inhibitor approved for use in children, and is indicated for polyarticular JIA. A phase 3 trial of baricitinib in childhood uveitis is in progress (NCT04088409).

TREATMENT WITHDRAWAL

Long-term systemic immunosuppressive therapy is critical, because uveitis recurrence is high. In Behçet-associated uveitis, 43% to 57% of patients flare, regardless of treatment duration.[135–137] In Vogt-Koyanagi-Harada disease, 39% to 72% of patients relapse, although this varies by ethnicity.[138–140] In JIA-U, 43% to 82% relapse off of medications, with a median time of 12 to 24 months.[49,141–146] Idiopathic uveitis may have a better prognosis than JIA-U, because one study reported 62% of 94 children with idiopathic uveitis remained in remission 4 years after discontinuing therapy compared with 17% of JIA-U.[144] Furthermore, those with JIA-U relapsed more quickly.[145] Some studies suggest that patients who initiated systemic immunomodulatory therapy within the first year of uveitis diagnosis and achieved remission within

6 months had a higher success of remaining in remission off of medications.[143,144] Longer duration of therapy may be important, because patients in remission on MTX for at least 2 years had improved success in weaning off medication than those in remission for a shorter duration.[147,148] Thus, guidelines recommend at least 2 years of remission on immunomodulatory therapy before attempting to wean medications.[38,102]

SUMMARY

Recommendations from SHARE and ACR/AF can guide treatment of children with JIA-U. SHARE recommends: (1) establishment of no cells in the AC as a goal for uveitis-directed therapy, (2) initiation of systemic therapy if uveitis cannot be controlled on topical GC within 3 months, (3) 2 years of uveitis inactivity off topical GC before tapering systemic therapy, and (4) recognition that patients on arthritis-directed systemic therapy may be at risk for uncovering uveitis when therapy is discontinued. MTX is recommended as the first-choice DMARD, followed by TNF mAb.[38] The ACR/AF issued similar recommendations regarding step-up therapy in JIA-U with MTX followed by TNF mAb, and further recommended (1) subcutaneous MTX over oral MTX, (2) starting MTX and TNF mAb simultaneously for severe uveitis, and (3) increasing TNF mAb dose to above-standard dosing for uncontrolled uveitis before switching to another agent.[102] The Childhood Arthritis and Rheumatology Research Alliance (CARRA) developed consensus treatment plans to suggest standardized treatment options for chronic anterior uveitis, either JIA-U or idiopathic. These include either subcutaneous or oral MTX, and adalimumab or infliximab. Standardizing patient care and data collection using the CARRA Registry may allow for better comparison of treatment approaches and uveitis outcomes.[107]

No standardized treatment approach of other types of childhood uveitis exists, such as in HLA-B27-associated AAU or pars planitis. Management of these conditions is often led by ophthalmologists. The presence of an underlying rheumatic condition may influence selection of systemic therapy, but MTX and TNFi mAb remain the agents of choice.

Close collaboration among rheumatologists, ophthalmologists, and other eye care specialists is critical.[39] Ophthalmology specialists perform ophthalmic examinations to assess uveitis activity and ocular complications, which inform systemic treatment prescribed by pediatric rheumatologists. Continued and regular communication among all subspecialists optimizes vision outcomes of these children.

CLINICS CARE POINTS

- Vision loss profoundly impacts a child's quality of life and visual functioning, making an urgent need for improved strategies to diagnose uveitis early, before the development of irreversible ocular damage.

- In children at risk for uveitis (ie, JIA), regular ophthalmic screening is important for prompt detection and initiation of therapy.

- In children diagnosed with uveitis, ophthalmic monitoring should include standardized evaluations of uveitis activity, disease course, and development of new or recurring complications to direct therapy.

- Treatment initially consists of local or systemic GC for a short period. Prolonged GC should not be used, and systemic treatment should be initiated in children with refractory chronic disease.

- Methotrexate, infliximab, and adalimumab are the mainstays of therapy in noninfectious uveitis. Combination therapy or higher doses are often needed to control inflammation.
- Treatment of children with refractory uveitis includes golimumab, tocilizumab, abatacept, rituximab, and JAK inhibitors. Because there are few randomized controlled trials, we rely on CARRA consensus treatment plans and guidelines from expert opinion and retrospective studies.
- Duration of treatment is at least 2 years after uveitis is well controlled (no GC, no flares) because of high risk for remission and relapse.
- Goal of treatment is to control inflammation with minimal GC use, to prevent vision-threatening complications.
- Close collaboration and communication among rheumatologists, ophthalmologists, and other eye care specialists optimizes vision outcomes.

DISCLOSURE

Dr M.H. Chang is supported by a Rheumatology Research Foundation Scientist Development Award, NIH/NICHD K12HD052896, and a Joint Biology Consortium microgrant off parent grant NIH/NIAMS P30AR070253. Dr J.G. Shantha is supported by the National Eye Institute of the National Institutes of Health under award number K23 EY030158. Dr S.T. Angeles-Han is supported by the NIH National Eye Institute under Award Number R01EY030521.

REFERENCES

1. Ravelli A, Martini A. Juvenile idiopathic arthritis. Lancet 2007;369(9563):767–78.
2. Smith JA, Mackensen F, Sen HN, et al. Epidemiology and course of disease in childhood uveitis. Ophthalmology 2009;116(8):1544–51, 1551.e1.
3. Caspi RR. Understanding autoimmune uveitis through animal models. The Friedenwald Lecture. Invest Ophthalmol Vis Sci 2011;52(3):1872–9.
4. Wildner G, Diedrichs-Mohring M. Resolution of uveitis. Semin Immunopathol 2019;41(6):727–36.
5. Shechter R, London A, Schwartz M. Orchestrated leukocyte recruitment to immune-privileged sites: absolute barriers versus educational gates. Nat Rev Immunol 2013;13(3):206–18.
6. Streilein JW. Ocular immune privilege: the eye takes a dim but practical view of immunity and inflammation. J Leukoc Biol 2003;74(2):179–85.
7. Arevalo JF, Garcia RA, Al-Dhibi HA, et al. Update on sympathetic ophthalmia. Middle East Afr J Ophthalmol 2012;19(1):13–21.
8. Wildner G, Diedrichs-Mohring M. Molecular mimicry and uveitis. Front Immunol 2020;11:580636.
9. de Smet MD, Dayan M, Nussenblatt RB. A novel method for the determination of T-cell proliferative responses in patients with uveitis. Ocul Immunol Inflamm 1998;6(3):173–8.
10. Caspi RR. A look at autoimmunity and inflammation in the eye. J Clin Invest 2010;120(9):3073–83.
11. Walscheid K, Hennig M, Heinz C, et al. Correlation between disease severity and presence of ocular autoantibodies in juvenile idiopathic arthritis-associated uveitis. Invest Ophthalmol Vis Sci 2014;55(6):3447–53.
12. Uchiyama RC, Osborn TG, Moore TL. Antibodies to iris and retina detected in sera from patients with juvenile rheumatoid arthritis with iridocyclitis by indirect

immunofluorescence studies on human eye tissue. J Rheumatol 1989;16(8): 1074–8.

13. Busch M, Wefelmeyer KL, Walscheid K, et al. Identification of ocular autoantigens associated with juvenile idiopathic arthritis-associated uveitis. Front Immunol 2019;10:1793.

14. Merriam JC, Chylack LT Jr, Albert DM. Early-onset pauciarticular juvenile rheumatoid arthritis. A histopathologic study. Arch Ophthalmol 1983;101(7): 1085–92.

15. Kalinina Ayuso V, van Dijk MR, de Boer JH. Infiltration of plasma cells in the iris of children with ANA-positive anterior uveitis. Invest Ophthalmol Vis Sci 2015; 56(11):6770–8.

16. Parikh JG, Tawansy KA, Rao NA. Immunohistochemical study of chronic non-granulomatous anterior uveitis in juvenile idiopathic arthritis. Ophthalmology 2008;115(10):1833–6.

17. Hou S, Li N, Liao X, et al. Uveitis genetics. Exp Eye Res 2020;190:107853.

18. Xiang Q, Chen L, Fang J, et al. TNF receptor-associated factor 5 gene confers genetic predisposition to acute anterior uveitis and pediatric uveitis. Arthritis Res Ther 2013;15(5):R113.

19. Hughes T, Ture-Ozdemir F, Alibaz-Oner F, et al. Epigenome-wide scan identifies a treatment-responsive pattern of altered DNA methylation among cytoskeletal remodeling genes in monocytes and CD4+ T cells from patients with Behcet's disease. Arthritis Rheumatol 2014;66(6):1648–58.

20. Hou S, Ye Z, Liao D, et al. miR-23a, miR-146a and miR-301a confer predisposition to Vogt-Koyanagi-Harada syndrome but not to Behcet's disease. Sci Rep 2016;6:20057.

21. Haasnoot AM, Kuiper JJ, Hiddingh S, et al. Ocular fluid analysis in children reveals interleukin-29/interferon-lambda1 as a biomarker for juvenile idiopathic arthritis-associated uveitis. Arthritis Rheumatol 2016;68(7):1769–79.

22. Walscheid K, Heiligenhaus A, Holzinger D, et al. Elevated S100A8/A9 and S100A12 serum levels reflect intraocular inflammation in juvenile idiopathic arthritis-associated uveitis: results from a pilot study. Invest Ophthalmol Vis Sci 2015;56(13):7653–60.

23. Kalinina Ayuso V, de Boer JH, Byers HL, et al. Intraocular biomarker identification in uveitis associated with juvenile idiopathic arthritis. Invest Ophthalmol Vis Sci 2013;54(5):3709–20.

24. Sijssens KM, Rijkers GT, Rothova A, et al. Distinct cytokine patterns in the aqueous humor of children, adolescents and adults with uveitis. Ocul Immunol Inflamm 2008;16(5):211–6.

25. Sijssens KM, Rijkers GT, Rothova A, et al. Cytokines, chemokines and soluble adhesion molecules in aqueous humor of children with uveitis. Exp Eye Res 2007;85(4):443–9.

26. Tappeiner C, Klotsche J, Sengler C, et al. Risk factors and biomarkers for the occurrence of uveitis in juvenile idiopathic arthritis: data from the inception cohort of newly diagnosed patients with juvenile idiopathic arthritis study. Arthritis Rheumatol 2018;70(10):1685–94.

27. Angeles-Han ST, Yeh S, Patel P, et al. Discovery of tear biomarkers in children with chronic non-infectious anterior uveitis: a pilot study. J Ophthalmic Inflamm Infect 2018;8(1):17.

28. Angeles-Han ST, Miraldi Utz V, Thornton S, et al. S100 proteins, cytokines, and chemokines as tear biomarkers in children with juvenile idiopathic arthritis-

associated uveitis. Ocul Immunol Inflamm 2020;1–5. https://doi.org/10.1080/09273948.2020.1758731.

29. Carreno E, Portero A, Herreras JM, et al. Cytokine and chemokine tear levels in patients with uveitis. Acta Ophthalmol 2017;95(5):e405–14.

30. Shirinsky IV, Biryukova AA, Kalinovskaya NY, et al. Tear cytokines as potential biomarkers in non-infectious uveitis: post hoc analysis of a randomised clinical trial. Graefes Arch Clin Exp Ophthalmol 2020;258(8):1813–9.

31. Foster CS. Diagnosis and treatment of juvenile idiopathic arthritis-associated uveitis. Curr Opin Ophthalmol 2003;14(6):395–8.

32. Holland GN, Denove CS, Yu F. Chronic anterior uveitis in children: clinical characteristics and complications. Am J Ophthalmol 2009;147(4):667–78.e5.

33. Angeles-Han ST, McCracken C, Yeh S, et al. Characteristics of a cohort of children with juvenile idiopathic arthritis and JIA-associated uveitis. Pediatr Rheumatol Online J 2015;13:19.

34. Thorne JE, Woreta F, Kedhar SR, et al. Juvenile idiopathic arthritis-associated uveitis: incidence of ocular complications and visual acuity loss. Am J Ophthalmol 2007;143(5):840–6.

35. American Academy of Pediatrics Section on Rheumatology and Section on Ophthalmology: guidelines for ophthalmologic examinations in children with juvenile rheumatoid arthritis. Pediatrics 1993;92(2):295–6.

36. Heiligenhaus A, Niewerth M, Ganser G, et al, German Uveitis in Childhood Study G. Prevalence and complications of uveitis in juvenile idiopathic arthritis in a population-based nation-wide study in Germany: suggested modification of the current screening guidelines. Rheumatology (Oxford) 2007;46(6):1015–9.

37. Angeles-Han ST, Ringold S, Beukelman T, et al. 2019 American College of Rheumatology/Arthritis Foundation guideline for the screening, monitoring, and treatment of juvenile idiopathic arthritis-associated uveitis. Arthritis Rheumatol 2019; 71(6):864–77.

38. Constantin T, Foeldvari I, Anton J, et al. Consensus-based recommendations for the management of uveitis associated with juvenile idiopathic arthritis: the SHARE initiative. Ann Rheum Dis 2018;77(8):1107–17.

39. Angeles-Han ST, Imundo L, Lo MS, et al. Screening for early detection of ocular disorders in two populations: children with juvenile idiopathic arthritis and children being treated with hydroxychloroquine. Pediatrics, in press.

40. Angeles-Han ST, Pelajo CF, Vogler LB, et al. Risk markers of juvenile idiopathic arthritis-associated uveitis in the Childhood Arthritis and Rheumatology Research Alliance (CARRA) Registry. J Rheumatol 2013;40(12):2088–96.

41. Kump LI, Cervantes-Castaneda RA, Androudi SN, et al. Analysis of pediatric uveitis cases at a tertiary referral center. Ophthalmology 2005;112(7):1287–92.

42. Paroli MP, Speranza S, Marino M, et al. Prognosis of juvenile rheumatoid arthritis-associated uveitis. Eur J Ophthalmol 2003;13(7):616–21.

43. Ozdal PC, Vianna RN, Deschenes J. Visual outcome of juvenile rheumatoid arthritis-associated uveitis in adults. Ocul Immunol Inflamm 2005;13(1):33–8.

44. Jabs DA, Nussenblatt RB, Rosenbaum JT, Standardization of Uveitis Nomenclature Working G. Standardization of uveitis nomenclature for reporting clinical data. Results of the First International Workshop. Am J Ophthalmol 2005; 140(3):509–16.

45. Ozdal PC, Berker N, Tugal-Tutkun I. Pars planitis: epidemiology, clinical characteristics, management and visual prognosis. J Ophthalmic Vis Res 2015;10(4): 469–80.

46. Tugal-Tutkun I. Pediatric uveitis. J Ophthalmic Vis Res 2011;6(4):259–69.

47. Tang WM, Pulido JS, Eckels DD, et al. The association of HLA-DR15 and intermediate uveitis. Am J Ophthalmol 1997;123(1):70–5.
48. Malinowski SM, Pulido JS, Folk JC. Long-term visual outcome and complications associated with pars planitis. Ophthalmology 1993;100(6):818–24 [discussion: 825].
49. Kalinina Ayuso V, ten Cate HA, van den Does P, et al. Young age as a risk factor for complicated course and visual outcome in intermediate uveitis in children. Br J Ophthalmol 2011;95(5):646–51.
50. Kempen JH, Gewaily DY, Newcomb CW, et al. Remission of intermediate uveitis: incidence and predictive factors. Am J Ophthalmol 2016;164:110–7.e2.
51. Foster CS, Vitale AT. Diagnosis & treatment of uveitis. New Delhi, India: JP Med Ltd; 2013.
52. Simonini G, Taddio A, Cattalini M, et al. Superior efficacy of adalimumab in treating childhood refractory chronic uveitis when used as first biologic modifier drug: adalimumab as starting anti-TNF-alpha therapy in childhood chronic uveitis. Pediatr Rheumatol Online J 2013;11:16.
53. Verity DH, Wallace GR, Vaughan RW, et al. Behcet's disease: from Hippocrates to the third millennium. Br J Ophthalmol 2003;87(9):1175–83.
54. Atmaca L, Boyvat A, Yalcindag FN, et al. Behcet disease in children. Ocul Immunol Inflamm 2011;19(2):103–7.
55. Karincaoglu Y, Borlu M, Toker SC, et al. Demographic and clinical properties of juvenile-onset Behcet's disease: a controlled multicenter study. J Am Acad Dermatol 2008;58(4):579–84.
56. Tugal-Tutkun I, Urgancioglu M. Childhood-onset uveitis in Behcet disease: a descriptive study of 36 cases. Am J Ophthalmol 2003;136(6):1114–9.
57. Yazici H, Tuzun Y, Pazarli H, et al. Influence of age of onset and patient's sex on the prevalence and severity of manifestations of Behcet's syndrome. Ann Rheum Dis 1984;43(6):783–9.
58. Tugal-Tutkun I, Onal S, Altan-Yaycioglu R, et al. Uveitis in Behcet disease: an analysis of 880 patients. Am J Ophthalmol 2004;138(3):373–80.
59. Arevalo JF, Lasave AF, Al Jindan MY, et al. Uveitis in Behcet disease in a tertiary center over 25 years: the KKESH Uveitis Survey Study Group. Am J Ophthalmol 2015;159(1):177–84.e1-2.
60. Rose CD, Doyle TM, McIlvain-Simpson G, et al. Blau syndrome mutation of CARD15/NOD2 in sporadic early onset granulomatous arthritis. J Rheumatol 2005;32(2):373–5.
61. Caso F, Galozzi P, Costa L, et al. Autoinflammatory granulomatous diseases: from Blau syndrome and early-onset sarcoidosis to NOD2-mediated disease and Crohn's disease. RMD Open 2015;1(1):e000097.
62. Wouters CH, Maes A, Foley KP, et al. Blau syndrome, the prototypic autoinflammatory granulomatous disease. Pediatr Rheumatol Online J 2014;12:33.
63. Becker ML, Rose CD. Blau syndrome and related genetic disorders causing childhood arthritis. Curr Rheumatol Rep 2005;7(6):427–33.
64. Rose CD, Wouters CH, Meiorin S, et al. Pediatric granulomatous arthritis: an international registry. Arthritis Rheum 2006;54(10):3337–44.
65. Birnbaum AD, Oh FS, Chakrabarti A, et al. Clinical features and diagnostic evaluation of biopsy-proven ocular sarcoidosis. Arch Ophthalmol 2011;129(4):409–13.
66. Kawaguchi T, Hanada A, Horie S, et al. Evaluation of characteristic ocular signs and systemic investigations in ocular sarcoidosis patients. Jpn J Ophthalmol 2007;51(2):121–6.

67. Herbort CP, Rao NA, Mochizuki M, Members of Scientific Committee of First International Workshop on Ocular S. International criteria for the diagnosis of ocular sarcoidosis: results of the first International Workshop On Ocular Sarcoidosis (IWOS). Ocul Immunol Inflamm 2009;17(3):160–9.
68. Cunningham ET Jr, Rathinam SR, Tugal-Tutkun I, et al. Vogt-Koyanagi-Harada disease. Ocul Immunol Inflamm 2014;22(4):249–52.
69. O'Keefe GA, Rao NA. Vogt-Koyanagi-Harada disease. Surv Ophthalmol 2017; 62(1):1–25.
70. Rubsamen PE, Gass JD. Vogt-Koyanagi-Harada syndrome. Clinical course, therapy, and long-term visual outcome. Arch Ophthalmol 1991;109(5):682–7.
71. Moorthy RS, Inomata H, Rao NA. Vogt-Koyanagi-Harada syndrome. Surv Ophthalmol 1995;39(4):265–92.
72. Sakata VM, da Silva FT, Hirata CE, et al. Diagnosis and classification of Vogt-Koyanagi-Harada disease. Autoimmun Rev 2014;13(4–5):550–5.
73. Hamade IH, Al Shamsi HN, Al Dhibi H, et al. Uveitis survey in children. Br J Ophthalmol 2009;93(5):569–72.
74. Martin TD, Rathinam SR, Cunningham ET Jr. Prevalence, clinical characteristics, and causes of vision loss in children with Vogt-Koyanagi-Harada disease in South India. Retina 2010;30(7):1113–21.
75. Read RW, Holland GN, Rao NA, et al. Revised diagnostic criteria for Vogt-Koyanagi-Harada disease: report of an international committee on nomenclature. Am J Ophthalmol 2001;131(5):647–52.
76. Albaroudi N, Tijani M, Boutimzine N, et al. Clinical and therapeutic features of pediatric Vogt-Koyanagi-Harada disease. J Fr Ophtalmol 2020;43(5):427–32.
77. Goda C, Kotake S, Ichiishi A, et al. Clinical features in tubulointerstitial nephritis and uveitis (TINU) syndrome. Am J Ophthalmol 2005;140(4):637–41.
78. Mandeville JT, Levinson RD, Holland GN. The tubulointerstitial nephritis and uveitis syndrome. Surv Ophthalmol 2001;46(3):195–208.
79. Mackensen F, Smith JR, Rosenbaum JT. Enhanced recognition, treatment, and prognosis of tubulointerstitial nephritis and uveitis syndrome. Ophthalmology 2007;114(5):995–9.
80. Ferrara M, Eggenschwiler L, Stephenson A, et al. The challenge of pediatric uveitis: tertiary referral center experience in the United States. Ocul Immunol Inflamm 2019;27(3):410–7.
81. Rosenberg KD, Feuer WJ, Davis JL. Ocular complications of pediatric uveitis. Ophthalmology 2004;111(12):2299–306.
82. Souto FMS, Giampietro BV, Takiuti JT, et al. Clinical features of paediatric uveitis at a tertiary referral centre in Sao Paulo, SP, Brazil. Br J Ophthalmol 2018. https://doi.org/10.1136/bjophthalmol-2018-312313.
83. Makley TA, Long J, Suie T. Uveitis in children*: a follow-up study. J Pediatr Ophthalmol Strabismus 1969;6(3):136–9.
84. Soylu M, Ozdemir G, Anli A. Pediatric uveitis in southern Turkey. Ocul Immunol Inflamm 1997;5(3):197–202.
85. Paivonsalo-Hietanen T, Tuominen J, Saari KM. Uveitis in children: population-based study in Finland. Acta Ophthalmol Scand 2000;78(1):84–8.
86. Wang ZJ, Zhou M, Cao WJ, et al. Evaluation of the Goldmann-Witmer coefficient in the immunological diagnosis of ocular toxocariasis. Acta Trop 2016;158:20–3.
87. Lembo A, Pichi F, Santangelo E, et al. Two masquerade presentations of retinoblastoma. Int Ophthalmol 2016;36(2):275–9.
88. Heiligenhaus A, Klotsche J, Tappeiner C, et al. Predictive factors and biomarkers for the 2-year outcome of uveitis in juvenile idiopathic arthritis: data

from the Inception Cohort of Newly diagnosed patients with Juvenile Idiopathic Arthritis (ICON-JIA) study. Rheumatology (Oxford) 2019;58(6):975–86.

89. Skarin A, Elborgh R, Edlund E, et al. Long-term follow-up of patients with uveitis associated with juvenile idiopathic arthritis: a cohort study. Ocul Immunol Inflamm 2009;17(2):104–8.

90. Ophthalmology AAo. Basic and clinical science course 2020-2021. San Francisco, CA, USA: American Academy of Ophthalmology; 2020.

91. Henderson LA, Zurakowski D, Angeles-Han ST, et al. Medication use in juvenile uveitis patients enrolled in the Childhood Arthritis and Rheumatology Research Alliance Registry. Pediatr Rheumatol Online J 2016;14(1):9.

92. Sabri K, Saurenmann RK, Silverman ED, et al. Course, complications, and outcome of juvenile arthritis-related uveitis. J AAPOS 2008;12(6):539–45.

93. Gregory AC 2nd, Kempen JH, Daniel E, et al. Risk factors for loss of visual acuity among patients with uveitis associated with juvenile idiopathic arthritis: the systemic immunosuppressive therapy for eye diseases study. Ophthalmology 2013;120(1):186–92.

94. Acevedo S, Quinones K, Rao V, et al. Cataract surgery in children with juvenile idiopathic arthritis associated uveitis. Int Ophthalmol Clin 2008;48(2):1–7.

95. Grajewski RS, Zurek-Imhoff B, Roesel M, et al. Favourable outcome after cataract surgery with IOL implantation in uveitis associated with juvenile idiopathic arthritis. Acta Ophthalmol 2012;90(7):657–62.

96. Van Gelder RN, Leveque TK. Cataract surgery in the setting of uveitis. Curr Opin Ophthalmol 2009;20(1):42–5.

97. Akbarali S, Rahi JS, Dick AD, et al. Imaging-based uveitis surveillance in juvenile idiopathic arthritis: feasibility, acceptability, and diagnostic performance. Arthritis Rheumatol 2021;73(2):330–5.

98. Sharma S, Lowder CY, Vasanji A, et al. Automated analysis of anterior chamber inflammation by spectral-domain optical coherence tomography. Ophthalmology 2015;122(7):1464–70.

99. Qu Y, Zhao C, Pei M, et al. Anterior segment inflammation in pediatric uveitis is associated with reduced retinal vascular density as quantified by optical coherence tomography angiography. Ocul Immunol Inflamm 2020;1–5. https://doi.org/10.1080/09273948.2020.1803923.

100. Bou R, Adan A, Borras F, et al. Clinical management algorithm of uveitis associated with juvenile idiopathic arthritis: interdisciplinary panel consensus. Rheumatol Int 2015;35(5):777–85.

101. Heiligenhaus A, Michels H, Schumacher C, et al. Evidence-based, interdisciplinary guidelines for anti-inflammatory treatment of uveitis associated with juvenile idiopathic arthritis. Rheumatol Int 2012;32(5):1121–33.

102. Angeles-Han ST, Ringold S, Beukelman T, et al. 2019 American College of Rheumatology/Arthritis Foundation guideline for the screening, monitoring, and treatment of juvenile idiopathic arthritis-associated uveitis. Arthritis Care Res (Hoboken) 2019;71(6):703–16.

103. Eiger-Moscovich M, Tomkins-Netzer O, Amer R, et al. Visual and clinical outcome of macular edema complicating pediatric noninfectious uveitis. Am J Ophthalmol 2019;202:72–8.

104. Maccora I, Sen ES, Ramanan AV. Update on noninfectious uveitis in children and its treatment. Curr Opin Rheumatol 2020;32(5):395–402.

105. Thorne JE, Woreta FA, Dunn JP, et al. Risk of cataract development among children with juvenile idiopathic arthritis-related uveitis treated with topical corticosteroids. Ophthalmology 2010;117(7):1436–41.

106. Thorne JE, Sugar EA, Holbrook JT, et al. Periocular triamcinolone vs. intravitreal triamcinolone vs. intravitreal dexamethasone implant for the treatment of uveitic macular edema: the PeriOcular vs. INTravitreal corticosteroids for uveitic macular edema (POINT) Trial. Ophthalmology 2019;126(2):283–95.

107. Angeles-Han ST, Lo MS, Henderson LA, et al. Childhood arthritis and rheumatology research alliance consensus treatment plans for juvenile idiopathic arthritis-associated and idiopathic chronic anterior uveitis. Arthritis Care Res (Hoboken) 2019;71(4):482–91.

108. Weiss AH, Wallace CA, Sherry DD. Methotrexate for resistant chronic uveitis in children with juvenile rheumatoid arthritis. J Pediatr 1998;133(2):266–8.

109. Foeldvari I, Wierk A. Methotrexate is an effective treatment for chronic uveitis associated with juvenile idiopathic arthritis. J Rheumatol 2005;32(2):362–5.

110. Gangaputra S, Newcomb CW, Liesegang TL, et al. Methotrexate for ocular inflammatory diseases. Ophthalmology 2009;116(11):2188–98.e1.

111. Ramanan AV, Dick AD, Jones AP, et al. Adalimumab plus methotrexate for uveitis in juvenile idiopathic arthritis. N Engl J Med 2017;376(17):1637–46.

112. Quartier P, Baptiste A, Despert V, et al. ADJUVITE: a double-blind, randomised, placebo-controlled trial of adalimumab in early onset, chronic, juvenile idiopathic arthritis-associated anterior uveitis. Ann Rheum Dis 2018;77(7):1003–11.

113. Davies R, De Cock D, Kearsley-Fleet L, et al. The risk of uveitis in patients with JIA receiving etanercept: the challenges of analysing real-world data. Rheumatology (Oxford) 2020;59(6):1391–7.

114. Foeldvari I, Becker I, Horneff G. Uveitis events during adalimumab, etanercept, and methotrexate therapy in juvenile idiopathic arthritis: data from the biologics in pediatric rheumatology registry. Arthritis Care Res (Hoboken) 2015;67(11):1529–35.

115. Tynjala P, Lindahl P, Honkanen V, et al. Infliximab and etanercept in the treatment of chronic uveitis associated with refractory juvenile idiopathic arthritis. Ann Rheum Dis 2007;66(4):548–50.

116. Simonini G, Taddio A, Cattalini M, et al. Prevention of flare recurrences in childhood-refractory chronic uveitis: an open-label comparative study of adalimumab versus infliximab. Arthritis Care Res (Hoboken) 2011;63(4):612–8.

117. Cecchin V, Zannin ME, Ferrari D, et al. Longterm safety and efficacy of adalimumab and infliximab for uveitis associated with juvenile idiopathic arthritis. J Rheumatol 2018;45(8):1167–72.

118. Atienza-Mateo B, Martin-Varillas JL, Calvo-Rio V, et al. Comparative study of infliximab versus adalimumab in refractory uveitis due to Behcet's disease: National Multicenter Study of 177 cases. Arthritis Rheumatol 2019;71(12):2081–9.

119. Sukumaran S, Marzan K, Shaham B, et al. High dose infliximab in the treatment of refractory uveitis: does dose matter? ISRN Rheumatol 2012;2012:765380.

120. Sen ES, Ramanan AV. Juvenile idiopathic arthritis-associated uveitis. Best Pract Res Clin Rheumatol 2017;31(4):517–34.

121. Dipasquale V, Atteritano M, Fresta J, et al. Tocilizumab for refractory uveitis associated with juvenile idiopathic arthritis: a report of two cases. J Clin Pharm Ther 2019;44(3):482–5.

122. Maleki A, Manhapra A, Asgari S, et al. Tocilizumab employment in the treatment of resistant juvenile idiopathic arthritis associated uveitis. Ocul Immunol Inflamm 2020;1–7. https://doi.org/10.1080/09273948.2020.1817501.

123. Papo M, Bielefeld P, Vallet H, et al. Tocilizumab in severe and refractory noninfectious uveitis. Clin Exp Rheumatol 2014;32(4 Suppl 84):S75–9.

124. Ramanan AV, Dick AD, Guly C, et al. Tocilizumab in patients with anti-TNF refractory juvenile idiopathic arthritis-associated uveitis (APTITUDE): a multicentre, single-arm, phase 2 trial. Lancet Rheumatol 2020;2(3):e135–41.
125. Marrani E, Paganelli V, de Libero C, et al. Long-term efficacy of abatacept in pediatric patients with idiopathic uveitis: a case series. Graefes Arch Clin Exp Ophthalmol 2015;253(10):1813–6.
126. Zulian F, Balzarin M, Falcini F, et al. Abatacept for severe anti-tumor necrosis factor alpha refractory juvenile idiopathic arthritis-related uveitis. Arthritis Care Res (Hoboken) 2010;62(6):821–5.
127. Tappeiner C, Miserocchi E, Bodaghi B, et al. Abatacept in the treatment of severe, longstanding, and refractory uveitis associated with juvenile idiopathic arthritis. J Rheumatol 2015;42(4):706–11.
128. Birolo C, Zannin ME, Arsenyeva S, et al. Comparable efficacy of abatacept used as first-line or second-line biological agent for severe juvenile idiopathic arthritis-related uveitis. J Rheumatol 2016;43(11):2068–73.
129. Davatchi F, Shams H, Rezaipoor M, et al. Rituximab in intractable ocular lesions of Behcet's disease; randomized single-blind control study (pilot study). Int J Rheum Dis 2010;13(3):246–52.
130. Lasave AF, You C, Ma L, et al. Long-term outcomes of rituximab therapy in patients with noninfectious posterior uveitis refractory to conventional immunosuppressive therapy. Retina 2018;38(2):395–402.
131. Umran RMR, Shukur ZYH. Rituximab for sight-threatening refractory pediatric Vogt-Koyanagi-Harada disease. Mod Rheumatol 2018;28(1):197–9.
132. Miserocchi E, Modorati G, Berchicci L, et al. Long-term treatment with rituximab in severe juvenile idiopathic arthritis-associated uveitis. Br J Ophthalmol 2016; 100(6):782–6.
133. Miserocchi E, Giuffre C, Cornalba M, et al. JAK inhibitors in refractory juvenile idiopathic arthritis-associated uveitis. Clin Rheumatol 2020;39(3):847–51.
134. Bauermann P, Heiligenhaus A, Heinz C. Effect of Janus kinase inhibitor treatment on anterior uveitis and associated macular edema in an adult patient with juvenile idiopathic arthritis. Ocul Immunol Inflamm 2019;27(8):1232–4.
135. Henry PE, Sanacore KA. Relaxation methods in the control of essential hypertension. J N Y State Nurses Assoc 1987;18(2):18–32.
136. Yamada Y, Sugita S, Tanaka H, et al. Timing of recurrent uveitis in patients with Behcet's disease receiving infliximab treatment. Br J Ophthalmol 2011;95(2): 205–8.
137. Cai J, Qi L, Chen Y, et al. Evaluation of factors for predicting risk of uveitis recurrence in Behcet's disease patients. Braz J Med Biol Res 2020;53(6):e9118.
138. Reddy AK, John FT, Justin GA, et al. Vogt-Koyanagi-Harada disease in a native American population in Oklahoma. Int Ophthalmol 2021;41(3):915–22.
139. Diallo K, Revuz S, Clavel-Refregiers G, et al. Vogt-Koyanagi-Harada disease: a retrospective and multicentric study of 41 patients. BMC Ophthalmol 2020; 20(1):395.
140. Rathinam SR, Vijayalakshmi P, Namperumalsamy P, et al. Vogt-Koyanagi-Harada syndrome in children. Ocul Immunol Inflamm 1998;6(3):155–61.
141. Halyabar O, Mehta J, Ringold S, et al. Treatment withdrawal following remission in juvenile idiopathic arthritis: a systematic review of the literature. Paediatr Drugs 2019;21(6):469–92.
142. Acharya NR, Patel S, Homayounfar G, et al. Relapse of juvenile idiopathic arthritis-associated uveitis after discontinuation of immunomodulatory therapy. Ocul Immunol Inflamm 2019;27(4):686–92.

143. Saboo US, Metzinger JL, Radwan A, et al. Risk factors associated with the relapse of uveitis in patients with juvenile idiopathic arthritis: a preliminary report. J AAPOS 2013;17(5):460–4.

144. Simonini G, Bracaglia C, Cattalini M, et al. Predictors of relapse after discontinuing systemic treatment in childhood autoimmune chronic uveitis. J Rheumatol 2017;44(6):822–6.

145. Shakoor A, Esterberg E, Acharya NR. Recurrence of uveitis after discontinuation of infliximab. Ocul Immunol Inflamm 2014;22(2):96–101.

146. Lerman MA, Lewen MD, Kempen JH, et al. Uveitis reactivation in children treated with tumor necrosis factor alpha inhibitors. Am J Ophthalmol 2015; 160(1):193–200.e1.

147. Kalinina Ayuso V, van de Winkel EL, Rothova A, et al. Relapse rate of uveitis post-methotrexate treatment in juvenile idiopathic arthritis. Am J Ophthalmol 2011;151(2):217–22.

148. Foell D, Wulffraat N, Wedderburn LR, et al. Methotrexate withdrawal at 6 vs 12 months in juvenile idiopathic arthritis in remission: a randomized clinical trial. JAMA 2010;303(13):1266–73.

Pharmacosurveillance in Juvenile Idiopathic Arthritis

Natalie J. Shiff, MD, MHSc[a], Timothy Beukelman, MD, MSCE[b],*

KEYWORDS

- JIA • Pediatric rheumatology • Pharmacosurveillance • Biologics

KEY POINTS

- Safety monitoring of therapeutics in JIA is challenging, particularly for rare events and those with long latency periods.
- Traditional spontaneous reporting systems for adverse events form the backbone of pharmacosurveillance for adverse events.
- Pharmacoepidemiology using diverse data sources, such as electronic health records, administrative claims data, and single drug, multidrug, or disease-specific registries, is increasingly important to further assess safety signals, including those raised through spontaneous reporting systems.
- Assessing and controlling for confounding (eg, disease activity and severity, glucocorticoid use) is crucial to produce valid relative estimates of medication safety.
- Although each of these data sources has limitations that are important to recognize, they are critical to improve the understanding of the long-term risks of therapy in JIA.

INTRODUCTION

The advent of biologic disease-modifying antirheumatic drugs (bDMARDs) targeting specific cytokines or cell-cell interactions has dramatically changed the outlook of patients with juvenile idiopathic arthritis (JIA).[1] These therapies are now standard of care for JIA unresponsive to first-line agents or when poor prognostic factors are present.[2,3] However, safety concerns remain around the use of these targeted immunosuppressives. Foremost among these are the risks of serious infections and malignancy. Malignancies are rare events, and determining whether bDMARDs increase malignancy rates requires long-term follow-up of a large number of patients. Additionally, attribution of adverse events, such as the development of uveitis, psoriasis, and inflammatory bowel disease (IBD), is challenging because these could be

[a] Department of Community Health and Epidemiology, College of Medicine, University of Saskatchewan, Room 3250 – East Wing – Health Sciences Boulevard, 104 Clinic Place, Saskatoon, Saskatchewan S7N 2Z4, Canada; [b] Department of Pediatrics, Division of Rheumatology, University of Alabama at Birmingham, 1600 7th Avenue South, CPPN G10, Birmingham, AL 35233, USA
* Corresponding author.
E-mail address: tbeukelman@peds.uab.edu

Rheum Dis Clin N Am 47 (2021) 643–653
https://doi.org/10.1016/j.rdc.2021.07.012
0889-857X/21/© 2021 Elsevier Inc. All rights reserved.

caused by underlying disease or be potential adverse drug effects. This review provides an overview of methodologies for pharmacosurveillance in JIA and then briefly reviews the risks of infections and malignancies from various data sources.

PHARMACOSURVEILLANCE

Pharmacosurveillance deals with the study of adverse drug reactions (ADRs) and adverse drug events (ADEs), which the World Health Organization defines as "a response to a medicine which is noxious and unintended, and which occurs at doses normally used in man," and "any untoward medical occurrence that may present during treatment with a medicine but which does not necessarily have a causal relationship with this treatment," respectively. Serious ADEs include any events that are fatal, life threatening, permanently/significantly disabling, requiring or prolonging hospitalization, causes a congenial anomaly, or requires intervention to prevent permanent impairment or damage.[4,5]

Although the gold standard for evidence of efficacy, randomized controlled trials (RCTs) have limited ability to assess drug safety. The short duration of RCTs generally precludes identification of adverse events because of cumulative long-term use or with a long latency period, whereas rare events may not be detected because of the small sample size. RCTs generally have strict entry requirements, and often exclude patients with comorbidities or polypharmacy, which are common in the wider population for whom a drug is likely to be prescribed. Regulatory approval of bDMARDs in JIA is often based on one study of a small group of patients using a placebo withdrawal design, paired with extrapolation from adult studies where suitable.[6–10] In placebo withdrawal studies, all qualifying patients are treated with the drug of interest, making treatment-related ADRs particularly difficult to interpret because there is no comparator arm without any exposure to the drug of interest, and carryover-effect in the treatment withdrawal arm cannot be eliminated.[1]

Pharmacovigilance has dramatically changed since its formal beginnings in the early 1960s through the development of common definitions, infrastructure, regulatory processes, and international cooperation around drug safety monitoring and safety signal management throughout the life cycle of pharmaceuticals.[11] Pharmacosurveillance (postmarketing surveillance) describes the monitoring for ADRs after a medical product receives approval to be brought to market and is critical to ensure drug safety. It encompasses pharmacovigilance and pharmacoepidemiology.[12] Pharmacovigilance has been defined as detecting, assessing, and preventing adverse effects from medical products,[5] whereas pharmacoepidemiology describes population-level assessments of drug uses and related risks.[12] Pharmacovigilance relies on several reporting mechanisms for ongoing postmarketing monitoring of ADEs, including spontaneous reporting of suspected adverse events, mandated observational studies carried out by pharmaceutical companies after a drug receives regulatory approval (a type of phase IV clinical trial),[13,14] and more recently through the increasing use of "big data."

SPONTANEOUS REPORTING SYSTEMS

Spontaneous reporting of suspected ADRs to regulatory agencies by health care providers, patients, and pharmaceutical companies remains the most common source of postmarketing surveillance safety data routinely evaluated for safety signals.[11,12,15] In the United States, data from individual case safety reports are compiled and analyzed through the Food and Drug Administration (FDA) Adverse Event Reporting System, and in Europe through EudraVigilance, whereas globally national data from member countries is compiled through the World Health Organization Programme for International Drug Monitoring database (VigiBase).[11,12,15]

Spontaneous reporting is limited by underreporting, which can stem from lack of awareness of pharmacovigilance and spontaneous reporting systems, ADR reporting criteria, and how to report an ADR, difficulties attributing an adverse event to a particular drug, and the burden of reporting.[12,15,16] Safety signal assessments using spontaneous reporting systems are subject to biases, including the Weber effect, which describes the increase in ADR reporting in the first 2 years after a drug comes to market; protopathic bias, in which a drug is initiated to treat symptoms of an undiagnosed underlying condition, and the diagnosis is then attributed to the drug, thus overestimating risk; confounding by indication; notoriety bias, in which an adverse reaction is attributed to a drug known to cause that type of adverse reaction when a different drug is actually responsible; and duplicate reporting.[12,16] Clinical context is often missing in these reports, which is limiting. The lack of information about the size of the population exposed to the drug makes the choice of an appropriate denominator for risk assessment challenging, which can significantly alter the calculated risk of the adverse response.[16]

ADR safety signals generated by spontaneous reporting are validated and further assessed using pharmacoepidemiologic data from existing population-based "big data" (discussed next).[16–18] This is the purpose of the FDA Sentinel System, which consists of a National Data Network with large amounts of electronic health information from administrative claims and electronic health records (EHRs) that are housed at their home institutions in a common format, and infrastructure and analytical tools to use these data for pharmacosurveillance of FDA-approved medical products.[19]

BIG DATA

Now almost ubiquitous, big data describes large complex datasets that require specialized management tools and processes.[20,21] EHRs and administrative claims data are two examples of big data in health care that are not generated for research but provide population-level data that are analyzed to answer research questions. Registries may sometimes be considered alternate sources of big data, especially if linkages to external data sources are performed.

Ideally, validated case ascertainment algorithms are used to identify the study cohort and minimize patient misclassification. Exposures of interest are determined using prescriptions written or medications dispensed, and subsequent outcomes are typically identified using diagnosis codes. Limitations of big data include missing data; misclassification of exposures or outcomes; and loss to follow-up, particularly in US health insurance databases because patients often change insurance providers.[22] In a pharmacosurveillance setting, the readily available and large sample size in big data allows researchers to further assess potential safety signals noted through spontaneous reporting systems.

ELECTRONIC HEALTH RECORDS

EHRs are prospectively and systematically collected in real time, and their widespread availability, level of detail, and volume make EHRs attractive sources of data for research, particularly when studying rare diseases or rare outcomes.[17,22,23] However, EHRs often contain multiple versions of data of interest (clinic notes, diagnoses codes) entered by several providers that may conflict[16,23] or may risk double counting patients.[16] Medication records are often derived from prescriptions written and can have limited or inaccurate information about refills and discontinuation dates.

Additionally, some written prescriptions are never dispensed from the pharmacy. Providers who are not part of a given EHR system may care for patients, and therefore EHR information may not be complete and adverse events may be missed. EHR components within or across systems often are not easily combined, limiting data pooling.[16]

EHR data are structured (organized in a fixed way, such as laboratory values), or unstructured (eg, free text in clinic notes, scanned documents, radiology images).[21–23] Unstructured data need to be converted into analyzable elements through artificial intelligence techniques, such as natural language processing and machine learning.[21,23] Although a promising supplement to the underreporting seen in spontaneous reporting systems that could provide clinical context,[18,23] the need for processing of unstructured EHR data remains a barrier to their broad use for safety monitoring.

ADMINISTRATIVE CLAIMS DATA

Administrative claims are generated for billing and insurance purposes when a patient encounters the health care system. As such, they contain more limited information than EHRs, and generally do not contain structured results or unstructured clinical notes. Administrative claims do not capture nonprescription drugs and uninsured prescriptions, and the amount of information available for hospitalized patients (diagnoses, procedures, and medications) may vary. However, they do contain data about medications dispensed from the pharmacy. Although patient adherence cannot necessarily be assumed, medications that are regularly dispensed are likely to have been taken. These data capture all claims for a covered patient regardless of care provider, unlike EHRs; therefore, the likelihood of missing medical encounters is small.[24] Diagnosis codes submitted to insurers via administrative claims may be biased by reimbursement policies or habit and convenience, making them less reliable than clinical notes.[17]

REGISTRIES

The US Agency for Healthcare Research and Quality defines a patient registry as "an organized system that uses observational study methods to collect uniform data (clinical and other) to evaluate specified outcomes for a population defined by a particular disease, condition, or exposure, and that serves one or more stated scientific, clinical, or policy purposes."[25] Registry medication records are generally derived from the medical record but may be more accurate than relying on prescriptions written because additional information is derived from physician notes or other nonstructured components of the medical record enabling members of the registry team to focus specific attention to medication details. In pediatric rheumatology, real-world data from registries using each of these population definitions contribute important safety information for rare adverse events, or adverse events in rare diseases.

DRUG-SPECIFIC REGISTRIES

A drug-specific registry enrolls patients prescribed the drug of interest, providing real-world longitudinal data for longer periods and in a broader group of patients than most clinical trials required for product registration. These registries are therefore more likely to capture rare events or events with long latency periods, and may be mandated by regulatory agencies for postmarketing safety monitoring. The Dutch Arthritis and Biologicals in Children (ABC) Registry is an example of a drug-specific registry that followed all patients with JIA treated with etanercept in the Netherlands between 1999 and 2006.[26] At that time, a central board determined whether patients were eligible for etanercept treatment, and patients deemed eligible were automatically included in the registry. Unlike safety signals from spontaneous reporting systems, this type of open label single-drug study has a known denominator, facilitating the calculation of the risk of any adverse events that are observed. A key weakness of drug-specific registries is the lack of a comparator arm to assess relative safety, which is particularly important if patients are taking multiple medications that can cause adverse reactions or drug interactions, have comorbidities, or are at higher risk than the general population for certain adverse events. Alternatively, particularly when a medication is new, the potential for selection bias within the registry remains if providers are hesitant to prescribe the drug to individuals taking certain medications or with comorbidities.[27] Additional potential limitations of single-drug registries include difficulties recruiting and retaining patients, often leading to registries that are too small for the intended safety monitoring.[14] Sample size is of particular concern for pediatric rheumatic diseases because they affect small groups of patients, and the number of patients needed for multiple competing single-drug registries over time could exceed the number of existing patients.[7]

MULTIDRUG REGISTRIES

Multidrug registries, like single-drug registries, allow for long-term follow-up of a more varied and larger group of patients than a clinical trial. Their advantages over single-drug registries lie in the availability of comparator arms for risk assessment, because they contain information about patients prescribed a select group of drugs, and the potential to evaluate sequential therapies. The German BiKeR registry (Biologika in der Kinderrheumatologie), for example, follows most German patients with JIA treated with bDMARDs since 2001. Klein and colleagues[28] published safety data for 3873 patients with nonsystemic JIA enrolled as of September 2018. The multidrug nature of this registry allowed researchers to compare baseline characteristics and safety data for patients prescribed etanercept, adalimumab, infliximab, golimumab, tocilizumab, or abatacept. They found that baseline characteristics, time to bDMARDs, and ADRs differed by bDMARD, observations that would not be possible in a single-drug registry.

DISEASE-SPECIFIC REGISTRIES

Disease-specific registries provide numerous advantages for drug safety surveillance in addition to their larger size and longer-term follow-up compared with clinical trials.[29] For example, the Childhood Arthritis and Rheumatology Research Alliance (CARRA) Registry enrolls pediatric patients with rheumatic diseases including JIA. It will follow these patients for at least 10 years, with ongoing follow-up via a call center when patients leave pediatric care, further enhancing long-term safety follow-up. As of January 2021, 9840 of the 11,001 patients enrolled had JIA.[30] Entry into the registry is determined by diagnosis, not therapy, and therefore the full spectrum of disease severity is captured. Competition for patients among registries is eliminated, because multiple safety surveillance programs can occur concurrently along with outcomes assessments and other projects of interest. A selection of comparators is available, including an array of active treatments and patients with similar disease activity, comorbidities, or polypharmacy.[29] Real-world use of therapeutics and complex exposure patterns such as sequential medication use or combination therapy can be assessed in terms of safety and effectiveness.

ASSESSING MEDICATION SAFETY IN JUVENILE IDIOPATHIC ARTHRITIS

Studying bDMARDs in JIA is challenging, because pediatric rheumatic diseases affect small populations. Although in adults bDMARDs are studied and targeted to specific types of inflammatory arthritis, in children these arthritides are grouped together under the umbrella diagnosis of JIA. JIA encompasses seven different categories of chronic arthritis, and is considered the most common pediatric rheumatic disease. Although JIA itself may not be rare (depending on geographic location),[31] each category of JIA is rare disease.[7] Targeting therapies to specific categories of JIA with limited patient populations requires thoughtful nontraditional study designs.[7,10] Growth and development throughout childhood and adolescence are unique considerations in the pediatric population, potentially putting these patients at risk of disease complications and adverse drug responses not seen in adults. Different stages of growth and development may also differentially affect pharmacokinetics and pharmacodynamics, underlining the need for pediatric-specific information.[6,7] Transition to adult care also poses a challenge to long-term follow-up for adverse event monitoring, and is a type of loss to follow-up unique to the pediatric population.

INFECTIONS

As immunomodulatory agents, bDMARDs have the potential to increase the rate of severe infection in children with JIA. Serious infections were observed at low rates in the placebo withdrawal studies that led to their authorization[32–36]; however, since the authorization of tumor necrosis factor inhibitors (TNFi) conflicting results have been reported ([28,37–40], reviewed in[36,41]), a selection of which are shown in **Table 1**. Some of the

Table 1
Risk of serious infections in children with juvenile idiopathic arthritis treated with bDMARDs

Study, Ref.		Infection Rate per 100 Person-Years (95% CI)	Adjusted Relative Risk or Hazard Ratio (95% CI)	
Administrative Claims				
Beukelman et al,[37] 2012	MTX	3.3 (2.7–4.0)	TNFi vs MTX	1.2 (0.8–1.8)
	TNFi ± MTX	3.5 (2.6–4.5)		
Lee et al,[39] 2018	DMARDs	1.28 (0.76–2.02)	TNFi vs DMARDs	2.65 (1.06–6.65)
	TNFi	2.72 (1.36–4.86)		
			2 to <16 y of age[a]	2.53 (0.98–6.55)
			Excluding other rheumatic disease, IBD[a]	1.15 (0.28–4.17)
National Registers				
Dutch National Register[26]	ETN	1.3	Not provided	
Registries				
BiKeR Registry[28]	TNFi	1.15 (0.92–1.43)	MTX vs TNFi + abatacept + tocilizumab	0.56 (0.34–0.91)
BSPAR- ETN Cohort[38]	MTX	1.7 (0.9–3.0)	ETN ± MTX vs MTX	1.36 (0.60–3.07)
	ETN	2.2 (1.6–3.0)		

Examples are provided from administrative claims studies, The Dutch National Register, and registries.
Abbreviations: CI, confidence interval; ETN, etanercept; MTX, methotrexate.
[a] Sensitivity analyses.

discrepancies in results are explained by differing definitions of qualifying infections, and whether researchers controlled for potential confounders such as use of methotrexate and systemic glucocorticoids, prior treatment failures, and disease activity.[41] A large administrative claims–based study using Medicaid data for low-income children in the United States found that patients with JIA who were not being treated with methotrexate or a TNFi had almost twice the risk of a serious infection requiring hospitalization compared with children without JIA after adjusting for glucocorticoid treatment and patient characteristics (adjusted hazard ratio [HR], 2.0; 95% confidence interval [CI], 1.5–2.5), highlighting a potential increased risk of infection for children with JIA irrespective of treatment.[37] The risk was similar in patients treated with methotrexate and those treated with TNFi, but patients with JIA taking high-dose glucocorticoids ($\geq$10 mg/d of prednisone equivalents) had a three-fold increased risk of hospitalization for an infection (adjusted HR, 3.1; 95% CI, 2.0–4.7). In contrast, an administrative data–based study using a commercial database study showed an increased risk of serious infections with TNFi therapy compared with methotrexate, but results was no longer statistically significant when patients with other rheumatic diagnoses and IBD were excluded or age was limited to 2 years to less than 16 years old.[39]

Registry studies have generally reported low but increased risks of infections in patients treated with bDMARDs. The Dutch ABC Registry reported 4 serious infections in 312 patient-years of etanercept use; however, no comparator was available. The British Society for Pediatric and Adolescent Rheumatology Etanercept Cohort Study is a single-drug registry that includes methotrexate comparator patients in which there was an increased risk of medically significant infections (as determined by physician opinion) in patients treated with etanercept compared with methotrexate, but this difference disappeared when analysis was restricted to serious infections defined by traditional serious ADE criteria rather than physician opinion.[38] The BiKeR Registry reported an increased risk of serious infections in patients treated with TNFi (etanercept or adalimumab) compared with methotrexate alone. In this study, disease activity was significantly associated with an increased risk of serious infection, highlighting the need to control for disease activity as a potential confounder.[40] More recently, in patients with polyarticular JIA, this registry reported similar rates of medically important infections for etanercept, adalimumab, infliximab, abatacept, and tocilizumab, but a five-fold higher rate for golimumab, although the latter estimate had low patient numbers and years of exposure, high prior bDMARD failures, and concurrent treatment with methotrexate, potentially biasing the estimate. Patients treated with methotrexate alone had a lower relative risk of medically important infection compared with any of the bDMARDs (relative risk, 0.63; 95% CI, 0.41–0.98), but authors acknowledged that the methotrexate group had shorter disease duration and analyses were not adjusted for disease severity.[28]

MALIGNANCIES

One of the major concerns with using bDMARDs in pediatric patients with developing immune systems is the potential for an increased risk of malignancy. In 2008, the FDA first reported a safety signal based on spontaneous reporting indicating increased risk of malignancies in children treated with TNFi, particularly leukemias and lymphomas, the interpretation of which was limited by an unknown true population denominator and lack of a comparator arm of patients with JIA not treated with TNFi.[42] Subsequent registry and administrative claims data have not clearly supported a link between TNFi and malignancy, especially in JIA. Rather, growing evidence indicates that bDMARD-naive children with JIA likely have an increased malignancy rate compared with the general population.[43,44] Recent studies do not exclude an increased risk with TNFi but suggest if present, the risk is small in absolute terms.[28] Beukelman and colleagues[45] compared malignancy rates in patients with IBD, JIA, and psoriasis (the three most common indications for TNFi) with those in patients with attention-deficit/hyperactivity disorder (ADHD, a chronic noninflammatory condition) using US administrative claims data. In the 15,598 TNFi users identified, the standardized incidence ratios were 2.9 (1.6–4.9) for all patients who had been treated with TNFi; 2.1 (1.5–2.9) for patients with IBD, JIA, and psoriasis who had not used TNFi; and 0.97 (0.91–1.05) for patients with ADHD. TNFi were not associated with an increased risk of malignancy (although numbers of malignancies were small and therefore a small increased risk could not be excluded). The standardized incidence ratios for lymphoma were 1.05 (0.89–1.24) for patients with ADHD; 2.7 (1.2–5.2) for patients with JIA, IBD, and psoriasis without TNFi exposure; and 6.0 (2.4–14.5) for patients with TNFi exposure. Even in the absence of TNFi exposure, patients with these three diagnoses had approximately twice the number of lymphomas compared with those with ADHD. The HR for lymphoma for patients with these three diagnoses was 2.64 (95% CI, 0.93–7.51) for those with versus without TNFi exposure. A true association is therefore possible, although this study was also limited by a small number of lymphomas and inability to control for disease activity and severity, which could potentially affect lymphoma risk. In the BiKeR Registry, patients with JIA treated with etanercept had a higher rate of malignancies than reported in the German Childhood Cancer Registry, but a similar rate to patients with JIA treated with methotrexate.[46] Disease-based registries for JIA collecting longitudinal data and disease activity measures on a large group of patients will help to address these questions, as well as the role of sequential and concurrent therapies.

FUTURE CHALLENGES

The availability of bDMARDs and advent of other therapies, such as Janus kinase inhibitors, have changed the outlook for children with JIA yet questions remain about the long-term safety effects of these therapeutics. Ongoing pharmacosurveillance through registry-based studies, EHRs, and claims data are critical to answering these questions. As an increasing number of therapeutic agents receive authorization, a smaller number of inadequately controlled patients will be available for authorization and safety studies for each new drug. Long-term safety monitoring remains difficult, particularly when patients move from pediatric to adult care and are often lost to follow-up. Current registries, such as the CARRA Registry, are attempting to address this gap. Increased use of social media combined with rapidly evolving technology is leading to new potential sources of safety signals that could be digitally mined to enhance pharmacosurveillance,[47] and there are ongoing efforts to determine how best to make use of this wealth of publicly available information.

DISCLOSURE

N.J. Shiff is a stockowner of AbbVie, Gilead, Pfizer, Novartis, and Sanofi; and has previously received salary support from CARRA. T. Beukelman receives salary support from CARRA; and has received consulting fees from Novartis and UCB.

REFERENCES

1. Smith EMD, Foster HE, Beresford MW. The development and assessment of biological treatments for children. Br J Clin Pharmacol 2014;79(3):379–94.

2. Ringold S, Angeles-Han ST, Beukelman T, et al. 2019 American College of Rheumatology/Arthritis Foundation guideline for the treatment of juvenile idiopathic arthritis: therapeutic approaches for non-systemic polyarthritis, sacroiliitis, and enthesitis. Arthritis Care Res (Hoboken) 2019;71(6):717–34.

3. Ringold S, Weiss PF, Beukelman T, et al. 2013 update of the 2011 American College of Rheumatology recommendations for the treatment of juvenile idiopathic arthritis: recommendations for the medical therapy of children with systemic juvenile idiopathic arthritis and tuberculosis screening among children receiving biologic medications. Arthritis Rheum 2013;65(10):2499–512.

4. World Health Organization. Quality Assurance and Safety of Medicines Team. Safety of medicines: a guide to detecting and reporting adverse drug reactions: why health professionals need to take action. Geneva (Switzerland); 2002. Available at: https://apps.who.int/iris/handle/10665/67378. Accessed February 26, 2021.

5. World Health Organization. Quality Assurance and Safety of Medicines Team. The safety of medicines in public health programmes: pharmacovigilance, an essential tool. 2006. Available at: https://apps.who.int/iris/handle/10665/43384. Accessed February 26, 2021.

6. European Medicines Agency. Reflection paper on the use of extrapolation in the development of medicines for paediatrics (EMA/189724/2018. 2018. Available at: https://apps.who.int/iris/handle/10665/43384. Accessed February 27, 2021.

7. Schanberg LE, Ramanan AV, Benedetti F De, et al. Toward accelerated authorization and access to new medicines for juvenile idiopathic arthritis. Arthritis Rheumatol 2019;71(12):1976–84.

8. Ruperto N, Brunner HI, Lovell DJ, et al. Extrapolation or controlled trials in paediatrics: the current dilemma. Arch Dis Child 2017;102(10):949–51.

9. Stefanska AM, Distlerová D, Musaus J, et al. Extrapolation in the development of paediatric medicines: examples from approvals for biological treatments for paediatric chronic immune-mediated inflammatory diseases. Arch Dis Child 2017; 102:952–7.

10. Ruperto N, Giannini EH, Pistorio A, et al. Is it time to move to active comparator trials in juvenile idiopathic arthritis? A review of current study designs. Arthritis Rheum 2010;62(11):3131–9.

11. Beninger P. Pharmacovigilance: an overview. Clin Ther 2018;40(12):1991–2004.

12. Alomar M, Tawfiq AM, Hassan N, et al. Post marketing surveillance of suspected adverse drug reactions through spontaneous reporting: current status, challenges and the future. Ther Adv Drug Saf 2020;11. 2042098620938595.

13. Survana V. Phase IV of drug development. Perspect Clin Res 2010;1(2):57–60.

14. Zhang X, Zhang Y, Ye X, et al. Overview of phase IV clinical trials for postmarket drug safety surveillance: a status report from the ClinicalTrials.gov registry. BMJ Open 2016;6:e010643.

15. Guner M, Ekmekci PE. Healthcare professionals' pharmacovigilance knowledge and adverse drug reaction reporting behavior and factors determining the reporting rates. J Drug Assess 2019;8(1):13–20.

16. Moore N, Berdaï D, Blin P, et al. Pharmacovigilance: the next chapter. Therapies 2019;74(6):557–67.

17. Ventola CL. Big data and pharmacovigilance: data mining for adverse drug events and interactions. P T 2018;43(6):340–51.

18. Liu F, Jagannatha A, Yu H. Towards drug safety surveillance and pharmacovigilance: current progress in detecting medication and adverse drug events from electronic health records. Drug Saf 2019;42(1):95–7.

19. Ball R, Robb M, Anderson SA, et al. The FDA's sentinel initiative: a comprehensive approach to medical product surveillance. Clin Pharmacol Ther 2016;99(3): 265–8.

20. Halevi G, Moed HF. The evolution of big data as a research and scientific topic: overview of the literature. Research trends. Available at: https://www. researchtrends.com/issue-30-september-2012/the-evolution-of-big-data-as-a-research-and-scientific-topic-overview-of-the-literature/. Accessed February 11, 2021.

21. Zhou N, Corsini EM, Jin S, et al. Advanced data analytics for clinical research part i: what are the tools ? Innovations 2020;15(2):114–9.

22. Christensen ML, Davis RL. Identifying the "blip on the radar screen": leveraging big data in defining drug safety and efficacy in pediatric practice. J Clin Pharmacol 2018;58(S10):S86–93.

23. Kim E, Rubinstein SM, Nead KT, et al. The evolving use of electronic health records (EHR) for research. Semin Radiat Oncol 2019;29(4):354–61.

24. European Medicines Agency. Guideline on good pharmacovigilance practices (GVP) Module XVI Addendum II: methods for effectiveness evaluation. Draft for public consultation (EMA/419982/2019). February 1, 2021. Available at: https://www. ema.europa.eu/en/human-regulatory/post-authorisation/pharmacovigilance/good-pharmacovigilance-practices#public-consultations-section. Accessed February 26, 2021.

25. Gliklich R, Leavy M, Dreyer N Sr, editors. Registries for evaluating patient outcomes: a user's guide. 4th ed. Rockville, MD: Agency for Healthcare Research and Quality; 2020. p. 18 (Prepared by L&M Policy Research, LLC, under Contract No. 290-2014-00004-C with partners OM1 and IQVIA) AHRQ Publication No. 19(20)-EHC020. Available at: https://effectivehealthcare.ahrq.gov/products/registries-guide-4th-edition/users-guide. Accessed February 26, 2021.

26. Prince FHM, Twilt M, Cate R, et al. Long-term follow-up on effectiveness and safety of etanercept in juvenile idiopathic arthritis: the Dutch National Register. Ann Rheum Dis 2009;68:635–41.

27. Shahian DM, Jacobs JP, Badhwar V, et al. Risk aversion and public reporting. Part 1: observations from cardiac surgery and interventional cardiology. Ann Thorac Surg 2017;104(6):2093–101.

28. Klein A, Becker I, Minden K, et al. Biologic therapies in polyarticular juvenile idiopathic arthritis. Comparison of long-term safety data from the German BIKER registry. ACR Open Rheumatol 2020;2(1):37–47.

29. Lionetti G, Kimura Y, Schanberg LE, et al. Using registries to identify adverse events in rheumatic diseases abstract. Pediatrics 2013;132(5):e1384–94.

30. CARRA February Newsletter 20201 - Issue 1. Available at: https://carragroup.org/news/newsletters/archives/carra-february-newsletter-20201—issue-1. Accessed February 16, 2021.

31. Thierry S, Fautrel B, Lemelle I, et al. Prevalence and incidence of juvenile idiopathic arthritis: a systematic review. Jt Bone Spine 2014;81(2):112–7.

32. Lovell DJ, Giannini EH, Reiff A, et al. Etanercept in children with polyarticular juvenile rheumatoid arthritis. N Engl J Med 2000;342(11):763–9.

33. Ruperto N, Lovell DJ, Quartier P, et al. Abatacept in children with juvenile idiopathic arthritis: a randomised, double-blind, placebo-controlled withdrawal trial. Lancet 2008;372:383–91.

34. Lovell DJ, Ruperto N, Goodman S, et al. Adalimumab with or without methotrexate in juvenile rheumatoid arthritis. N Engl J Med 2008;359:810–20.

35. Brunner HI, Ruperto N, Zuber Z, et al. Efficacy and safety of tocilizumab in patients with polyarticular-course juvenile idiopathic arthritis: results from a phase 3, randomised, double-blind withdrawal trial. Ann Rheum Dis 2015;74:1110–7.

36. Horneff G. Safety of biologic therapies for the treatment of juvenile idiopathic arthritis. Expert Opin Drug Saf 2015;14(7):1111–26.

37. Beukelman T, Xie F, Chen L, et al. Rates of hospitalized bacterial infection associated with juvenile idiopathic arthritis and its treatment. Arthritis Rheum 2012; 64(8):2773–80.

38. Davies R, Southwood TR, Kearsley-Fleet L, et al, British Society for Paediatric and Adolescent Rheumatology Etanercept Cohort. Medically significant infections are increased in patients with juvenile idiopathic arthritis treated with etanercept: results from the British Society for Paediatric and Adolescent Rheumatology Etanercept Cohort Study. Arthritis Rheumatol 2015;67(9):2487–94.

39. Lee W, Lee TA, Suda KJ, et al. Risk of serious bacterial infection associated with tumour necrosis factor-alpha inhibitors in children with juvenile idiopathic arthritis. Rheumatol 2018;57:273–82.

40. Becker I, Horneff G. Risk of serious infection in juvenile idiopathic arthritis patients associated with tumor necrosis factor inhibitors and disease activity in the German Biologics in Pediatric Rheumatology Registry. Arthritis Care Res (Hoboken) 2017;69(4):552–60.

41. Marino A, Giani T, Cimaz R. Expert review of clinical immunology risks associated with use of TNF inhibitors in children with rheumatic diseases. Expert Rev Clin Immunol 2019;15(2):189–98.

42. AAP News. Updates boxed warning required for TNF blockers. 30(12). Available at: https://www.aappublications.org/content/30/12/11. Accessed February 25, 2021.

43. Simard J, Neovius M, Hagelberg S, et al. Juvenile idiopathic arthritis and risk of cancer a nationwide cohort study. Arthritis Rheum 2010;62(12):3776–82.

44. Horne A, Delcoigne B, Palmblad K, et al. Juvenile idiopathic arthritis and risk of cancer before and after the introduction of biological therapies. RMD Open 2019; 5:e001055.

45. Beukelman T, Xie F, Chen L, et al. Risk of malignancy associated with paediatric use of tumour necrosis factor inhibitors. Ann Rheum Dis 2018;77:1012–6.

46. Horneff G, Klein A, Oommen P, et al. Update on malignancies in children with juvenile idiopathic arthritis in the German BIKER Registry. Clin Exp Rheumatol 2016;1113–20.

47. Salathé M. Digital pharmacovigilance and disease surveillance: combining traditional and big-data systems for better. Public Health 2016;214(Suppl 4):399–403.

Outcome Measures in Pediatric Rheumatic Disease

Sarah Ringold, MD, MS[a],*, Alessandro Consolaro, MD, PhD[b], Stacy P. Ardoin, MD, MS[c]

KEYWORDS

- Outcome measure • Pediatrics • Juvenile idiopathic arthritis
- Juvenile dermatomyositis • Childhood-onset lupus • Vasculitis

KEY POINTS

- Outcome measures are essential to optimize clinical care and perform observational and interventional studies in pediatric rheumatic diseases.
- Largely developed by consensus methodology, disease activity, response, and damage outcome measures in juvenile idiopathic arthritis, juvenile dermatomyositis, childhood-onset systemic lupus erythematosus, and vasculitis are composite tools, which incorporate clinical and laboratory attributes.
- In recent years, the number and quality of outcome measures have increased rapidly and validation efforts are ongoing.

OUTCOME MEASURES IN PEDIATRIC RHEUMATIC DISEASE

Valid outcome measures that assess changes in disease activity, disease state, and disease damage accurately are of central importance in optimizing outcomes for pediatric rheumatic disease, improving the understanding of treatment efficacy and effectiveness in interventional and observational trials, and serving as treatment targets. Because no single variable can capture the multidimensional nature of disease activity in complex diseases like juvenile idiopathic arthritis (JIA), juvenile dermatomyositis (JDM), childhood-onset systemic lupus erythematosus (cSLE), and pediatric vasculitides adequately, assessment is based on composite measures, which incorporate multiple items and capture different manifestations of disease. Disease activity measures reflect reversible changes attributable to underlying disease whereas damage assessments measure cumulative organ damage after diagnosis. Patient-reported outcomes are central to monitoring the burden of rheumatic disease over time and are reviewed separately in this issue.

[a] Seattle Children's, 4800 Sand Point Way Northeast, Seattle, WA 98115, USA; [b] Rheumatology Unit, Istituto Giannina Gaslini, University of Genoa, Via Gerolamo Gaslini 5, 16147 Genoa, Italy; [c] Department of Pediatrics, Nationwide Children's Hospital, Ohio State University, 700 Children's Drive, Columbus, OH 43205, USA
* Corresponding author.
E-mail address: Sarah.Ringold@seattlechildrens.org

Rheum Dis Clin N Am 47 (2021) 655–668
https://doi.org/10.1016/j.rdc.2021.07.013

rheumatic.theclinics.com

OUTCOME MEASURES IN JUVENILE IDIOPATHIC ARTHRITIS

Dichotomous response measures were the first widely used measures of treatment response in JIA, and, more recently, continuous, composite measures of disease activity are available. Continuous composite measures currently are recommended for use in treat-to-target approaches for research and clinical care and are included in the recent American College of Rheumatology (ACR) JIA treatment guidelines.[1,2]

American College of Rheumatology Pediatric Criteria for Improvement and Flare

The ACR Pediatric response criteria, designed to distinguish between active treatment and placebo in efficacy trials of JIA,[1] measures response based on 6 consensus-derived response variables: (1) physician global assessment of overall disease activity (PGA), (2) parent or patient global assessment of overall well-being (PtGA), (3) functional ability, (4) number of joints with active arthritis, (5) number of joints with limited range of motion, and (6) acute-phase reactant. The ACR pediatric measures are dichotomous outcomes that assess percent improvement in disease activity relative to baseline, with the ACR Pedi 30 measure requiring 30% improvement in 3 of 6 variables and no more than 30% worsening in 1 variable (**Box 1**).[1] Although not formally validated, the ACR Pedi 20, ACR Pedi 50, ACR Pedi 70, ACR Pedi 90, and ACR Pedi 100 measures are used to report outcomes in pediatric trials and are defined as 20%, 50%, 70%, 90%, and 100% improvement, respectively. A preliminary definition of flare was proposed based on the same core set of variables (see **Box 1**).[3] Although development of the ACR Pedi response measures was a significant advance for pediatric rheumatology and remain standard for registration trials, utility of ACR Pedi measures is limited because they describe relative response (change in disease status relative to baseline), are dichotomous, and do not provide information regarding a patient's disease state. Due to these limitations, the ACR Pedi measures are not feasible for use in routine clinical care and do not allow for the description or

---

Box 1
Pediatric core set components, ACR pediatric juvenile idiopathic arthritis response criteria, and inactive disease definitions

Pediatric core set
1. PGA
2. PtGA
3. Functional ability
4. Number of joints with active arthritis
5. Number of joints with limited range of motion
6. ESR or CRP

ACR Pedi 30: a minimum of 30% improvement from baseline in a minimum of 3 out of 6 components, with no more than 1 component worsening by greater than 30%

Flare: a minimum of 40% worsening in a minimum of 2 out of 6 components, with no more than 1 component improving by greater than or equal to 30%

CID: no active synovitis; no fever, rash, splenomegaly or generalized lymphadenopathy attributable to JIA; no active uveitis; normal ESR and/or CRP; physician global assessment of disease activity indicating no active disease; morning stiffness duration less than or equal to 15 minutes

CR off medication: 12 months of sustained CID off of all JIA medications

CR on medication: 6 months of sustained CID while on JIA medications

comparison of patient disease status between cohorts, including among those enrolled in clinical trials.

Clinical Inactive Disease and Remission

The ACR provisional criteria for clinical inactive disease (CID) and remission in nonsystemic arthritis were the first definition of disease state in JIA (see **Box 1**), recognizing that CID and remission are important and achievable targets in JIA.[4] CID describes disease activity at a point in time, whereas definitions of remission reflect CID duration (see **Box 1**).[5] The CID definition was derived according to the ACR Quality of Care Committee guidance, using a combination of patient profiles and international consensus.[6] Subsequent validation was performed applying the criteria to other existing data sets, and CID was used as the primary outcome for the Trial of Early Aggressive Therapy in Polyarticular Juvenile Idiopathic Arthritis, which illustrated that CID was an achievable target in polyarticular JIA.[7] CID and remission, however, are dichotomous measures and do not provide additional information on disease state outside of CID or remission. In addition, although CID status is the goal of therapy, many children do not attain or maintain this level of disease control.[8–10] Alternate CID definitions have been developed using the Juvenile Arthritis Disease Activity Score (JADAS), and a recent report suggested that achievement of clinical JADAS based on 10 joints (cJADAS10) CID was more feasible and resulted in improved functional ability and psychosocial health compared with CID using the provisional ACR criteria.[11] Optimal definitions of JIA CID and remission require further exploration.

Continuous disease activity measures, such as the disease activity score (DAS), are widely used in adult rheumatoid arthritis clinical care and reasearch.[12] The JADAS met the need for a pediatric-specific continuous JIA measure that would be easy to use in routine clinical care and research. JADAS is a continuous, composite disease activity measure derived by consensus and subsequent factor analysis.[13] Different forms of the JADAS exist, based on different joint counts and presence or absence of acute-phase reactants. The JADAS-10 incorporates any combination of active joints to a maximum of 10, whereas JADAS-71 is based on a patient's total active joint count, and the JADAS-27 is derived from a count of 27 specific joints. Additionally, versions of the JADAS can be calculated incorporating an inflammatory marker (erythrocyte sedimentation rate [ESR] [JADAS-10/ESR or JADAS-71/ESR] or C-reactive protein [CRP] [JADAS-10/CRP; JADAS-71/CRP]) (**Box 2**).[13,14] Cutoff values are available for remission, minimal disease activity, and acceptable symptom state for various JADAS versions and were derived by performing receiver-operator curve analyses and

---

Box 2
Examples of the Juvenile Arthritis Disease Activity Score

- cJADAS = AJC + MDGA + PGH

- JADAS–ESR = AJC + MDGA + PGH + (ESR mm/h–20)/10

- JADAS–CRP = AJC + MDGA + PGH + (CRP mg/L–10)/10

AJC, active joint count; MDGA, physician global assessment of disease activity measured on a 0 to 10-cm numeric rating scale; PGH, parent or patient assessment of global health measured on a 0 to 10-cm numeric rating scale; ESR, ESR with all ESR values greater than 120 mm/h rounded to 120.

Different JADAS versions are available based on complete 71-joint AJC, 10-joint AJC (total AJC >10 capped at 10), and 27-AJC (restricted joint count).

measuring the range of JADAS values associated with different levels of disease activity and parent/child assessments of disease activity. New ACR-endorsed cutoffs are in preparation. The JADAS has yet to be utilized as a primary outcome in registration trials, due to lack of complete validation of JADAS cutoffs and determination of JADAS values associated with important changes in disease activity. JADAS is broadly accepted, however, as feasible for clinical care and has been incorporated into JIA treat to target strategies and the 2019 ACR JIA treatment guidelines.[2,15] Preliminary studies indicate that use of JADAS as a target for treatment can result in improved disease outcomes.[16,17] A JADAS recently was developed for systemic JIA that includes the PGA, PtGA, active joint count (maximum of 10), normalized ESR or CRP value, and a systemic manifestation score, which assigns points to extraarticular manifestations of sJIA (eg, fever, rash, and hepatosplenomegaly) generating a score between 0 and 10.[18] Similarly, the continuous Juvenile Spondylarthritis Disease Activity index has been developed to capture specific manifestations of juvenile spondyloarthropathies (eg, active entheses count, pain, uveitis, and clinical sacroiliitis).[19] Both measures are undergoing additional validation.

OUTCOME MEASURES IN JUVENILE DERMATOMYOSITIS

A lack of standardized and validated measures for assessing therapy response in JDM historically hampered a rational therapeutic approach to JDM. To address this gap, the International Myositis Assessment and Clinical Studies Group (IMACS) identified a core set of measures for the assessment of JDM patients.[20] The measures assess 5 domains: global activity (PGA and PtGA), muscle strength, physical function, laboratory assessment, and extraskeletal muscle disease. A collaboration between the Paediatric Rheumatology International Trials Organisation (PRINTO), the ACR, and the European League Against Rheumatism (EULAR) developed and validated a core set of outcome measures and definition of clinical improvement for measurement of treatment response.[21] The 6 domains include PGA, PtGA, muscle strength, a global JDM disease activity tool, functional ability, and health-related quality of life (**Box 3**). In 2017, an international group of researchers, using consensus methodology, identified 123 items collected in clinical practice to capture disease outcome and treatment

Box 3
Core set measures for disease activity for clinical studies and therapeutic trials in juvenile dermatomyositis and recommended measures by the International Myositis Assessment and Clinical Studies Group and Paediatric Rheumatology International Trials Organisation

Domain	Recommended Measure by the International Myositis Assessment and Clinical Studies Group	Recommended Measure by the Paediatric Rheumatology International Trials Organisation
Global activity	PGA, PtGA	PGA, PtGA
Muscle strength	MMT	CMAS
		MMT
Physical function	CMAS	Childhood Health Assessment Questionnaire
Laboratory assessment	At least 2 serum muscle-associated enzymes	Muscle enzymes
Extramuscle disease	MDAAT	MDAAT; DAS
Health-related quality of life		Child Health Questionnaire

response, facilitating patient care and translational research.[22] Three groups of items include those 3 groups: (1) measured only at first visit, (2) measured at every visit, and (3) measured at first visit and annually. A key difference from the JIA core sets is that the consensus data set does not propose specific tools to record disease activity but rather disaggregated items.

Both IMACS and PRINTO proposed a definition of improvement based on the percent change of the core set items.[23,24] To better understand the degree of improvement in JDM, a 2016 EULAR/ACR joint effort proposed a new definition of response in which the sum of improvement in each of the 6 core measures generates a total improvement score (ranging from 0 to 100).[25] These response criteria provide categorical outcomes of minimal improvement, moderate improvement, and major improvement. Criteria for CID in JDM, established using a data-driven approach by PRINTO, have evidence-based cutoffs for muscle strength/endurance, muscle enzymes, and physical global evaluation of disease activity.[26]

Muscle Strength and Physical Function Measures

Muscle strength assessment is crucial in the evaluation of JDM. The most widely adopted tool is the manual muscle test (MMT),[27] available in several versions, differing in the number of muscle groups tested and the methods of scoring. The MMT-8, in which 8 proximal, distal, and axial muscle groups are tested unilaterally (patient's dominant side), is an important outcome measure in clinical trials and clinical care. Each muscle group examined is scored on a 0 to 10 scale (0 = extreme weakness; 10 = normal strength).[28] Muscle groups are assessed based on strength opposing gravity or pressure applied by the examiner. More recently, versions of the MMT-8 were developed evaluating strength in fewer muscle groups (6 or 4).[29] A limitation of MMT is the lack of inclusion of the abdominal muscles.

The PRINTO/ACR/EULAR JDM core set includes the Childhood Myositis Assessment Scale (CMAS), which assesses the capacity of the patient to perform 14 maneuvers or the duration of performance of tasks. The CMAS is a measure of muscle strength and endurance as well as physical function. It is a comprehensive and reliable tool,[30] but its scoring not always is feasible in a busy clinical setting.

In order to obtain a measure of muscle strength more complete than the MMT-8 but more feasible than the CMAS, Varnier and colleagues[31] developed and preliminarily validated the hybrid MMT-CMAS, which adds the assessment of abdominal muscle strength, time of head lift, and floor rise derived from the CMAS to the MMT-8 items. Handheld dynamometry may be useful in muscle strength evaluation,[32] but currently no studies in pediatric patients are available.

Other Disease Activity Measures

The DAS was devised to evaluate physical function, weakness, skin involvement, and the presence of vasculitis in JDM.[33] Most items are dichotomous, whereas physical function and skin involvement are rated as continuous measures according to the level of activity (total score range 0–20).

The Myositis Disease Activity Assessment Tool (MDAAT) is a comprehensive tool that assesses muscular and extramuscular disease activity in adult myositis and pediatric myositis.[34] It is composed of the Myositis Disease Activity Assessment Visual Analogue Scale (MYOACT) and the Myositis Intention-to-Treat Activities Index (MITAX). The MYOACT includes several 0 to 10 visual analog scales (VASs) for organ system–specific disease activity. The MITAX assesses specific manifestations in 7 organs/systems and is based on an intention-to-treat approach, derived from the British Isles Lupus Assessment Group (BILAG) approach to assess disease activity in SLE.[35]

A recently developed tool for the assessment of global disease activity, the Juvenile Dermatomyositis Activity Index (JDMAI) incorporates scores for muscle and skin activity, PGA, and PtGA and awaits further validation.[36]

Skin disease activity

Few tools exist for the quantification of skin involvement. The DAS has a section devoted to skin involvement[33] that assesses severity of skin erythema and Gottron papules, distribution, and the presence of erythema and telangiectasias of the eyelid, periungual region, and palate. The Cutaneous Assessment Tool (CAT)[37] was designed to assess JDM skin disease; shortened versions, the CAT-Binary Method and abbreviated CAT (aCAT), currently are preferred over the original version.[38] The aCAT tool includes 21 items, yielding an activity and damage score. The Cutaneous Dermatomyositis Disease Area and Severity Index captures the extent of skin disease in 15 anatomic locations with 3 activity measures and 2 damage measures. The resulting activity and damage scores range from 0 to 100 and 0 to 32, respectively.[39,40]

Damage Measures

The myositis damage index (MDI)[41] is endorsed by IMACS and is the preferred damage measure in the PRINTO/ACR/EULAR JDM core set and assesses the extent of damage in muscle, skeletal, cutaneous, gastrointestinal, pulmonary, cardiac, peripheral vascular, endocrine, ocular, infectious, malignancy, and other organ/systems. Three versions of the MDI are available to assess damage in children (35 items), adolescents (37 items), and adults (38 items).

OUTCOME MEASURES IN CHILDHOOD-ONSET LUPUS

Many lupus disease measures developed for use in adults with SLE have been validated in cSLE populations. Recently, pediatric-specific tools examining lupus flare and treatment response are available.

Systemic Lupus Erythematosus Disease Activity Measures

Lupus disease activity measures (**Box 4**) are composite tools that incorporate clinical and laboratory findings. No consensus exists regarding an optimal measure of cSLE disease activity. Available tools cover similar domains with differing definitions and item weighting, and each has its own advantages and disadvantages. For example, the BILAG is comprehensive but time consuming whereas the Systemic Lupus Erythematosus Disease Activity Index (SLEDAI) is less comprehensive but is easy to complete quickly. Unless otherwise indicated, validation results in cSLE populations are available for all measures discussed later.

The SLEDAI[42] is a weighted index that includes attributes across 9 organ systems and reflects disease activity in the past 10 days or 30 days, with a score ranging from 0 to 105.[43] The SLEDAI is used and iterations include the Safety of Estrogens in Lupus Erythematosus: National Assessment (SELENA)-SLEDAI[44] and SLEDAI 2000 (SLEDAI-2K).[45] SLEDAI-2K added ongoing disease activity, and SELENA-SLEDAI incorporated a PGA (ranging from 0 to 3) and flare index. For the SLEDAI and all other clinician reported disease activity measures discussed subsequently, a thorough physical examination is required with attention to mucocutaneous, cardiovascular, musculoskeletal, and neurologic cSLE manifestations. Urinalysis, complete blood cell count; C3 and C4 levels; and anti–double-stranded DNA levels are necessary to complete the SLEDAI.

Additional disease activity measures, the BILAG[35] and subsequent BILAG-2004,[46] measure disease activity over the preceding 4 weeks with separate scores for each

---

Box 4
Outcome measures proposed for childhood-onset systemic lupus erythematosus

Global disease
  Disease activity
    SLEDAI
    BILAG
    ECLAM
    SLAM
  PRINTO/PCRSG disease activity core set
    PGA (10-cm VAS)
    PGA/PtGA (10-cm VAS)
    Proteinuria (grams over 24 h)
    Global disease activity tool (ECLAM, SLEDAI, or SLAM)
    Health-related quality-of-life assessment (Child Health Questionnaire physical health
    summary score)
  Disease flare and response measures
    PRINTO/ACR provisional criteria for the evaluation of response to therapy
    ID
    Complete remission
    SRI
    ACR provisional criteria for global flare
    CHILI
  Disease status
    ID
    Complete remission
    LLDAS
  Disease damage
    SDI

Specific organ manifestations
  Cutaneous lupus
    CLASI
  Lupus nephritis
    CARRA core renal parameters and definitions for renal flare and response
  Neuropsychiatric SLE–cognitive impairment
    ACR neurocognitive battery
    Pediatric Automated Neuropsychological Assessment Metrics

---

organ system and categorization of disease activity (grades A–E) and incorporate an intent-to-treat approach. Grade A reflects highly active disease requiring therapeutic intervention; grade B, moderate disease; grade C, mild and stable disease; grade D; no current disease activity in previously impacted domain(s); and grade E, no current or prior disease activity in domain. The BILAG-2004 eliminated the vasculitis domain and added ophthalmic and gastrointestinal sections. To complete the BILAG, additional data are needed, including measurement of blood pressure, serum creatinine, lupus anticoagulant, Coombs test, and renal biopsy results (if performed in past 3 months). The BILAG is convertible to a continuous, numerical score.[47]

The European Consensus Lupus Activity Measurements (ECLAM) includes 33 items organized into 12 domains, and the score ranges from 0 to 10. The period of observation is unspecified although preceding month typically is used and required laboratory data are as in SLEDAI. ECLAM includes concepts of evolving disease manifestations and hypocomplementemia. In cSLE, the ECLAM has slightly higher sensitivity to change compared to the SLEDAI but is not as widely adopted as the SLEDAI.[48]

The Systemic Lupus Activity Measure (SLAM)[49] and SLAM-Revised (SLAM-R)[50] assess disease activity over prior 4 weeks; scores range 0 to 86 for SLAM and 0 to 81 for SLAM-R. Providers grade each attribute on a 1 to 3 Likert scale. In SLAM-R, revisions included definitions and weighting, and removal of pneumonitis, and "other" categories. In cSLE, SLAM has comparable sensitivity to change as SLEDAI and BILAG. Like BILAG, SLAM includes blood pressure and serum creatinine measurement.[51]

Systemic Lupus Erythematosus Disease Activity Core Set, Response Measures, and Disease State Measures

A collaborative effort between PRINTO and the Pediatric Rheumatology Collaborative Study Group proposed[21] and subsequently validated[52] a cSLE disease activity core set, which includes PGA (0–10 cm VAS), PtGA (0–10 cm VAS), ECLAM score (can substitute SLEDAI or SLAM), proteinuria (grams/24 h), and the Child Health Questionnaire physical health summary score. Subsequently, using this core set, ACR/PRINTO proposed a definition of meaningful improvement as greater than or equal to 50% improvement in any 2 of the 5 core set variables, with less than or equal to 1 variable worsening by 30% or more.[53]

Another international consensus exercise proposed preliminary definitions of inactive disease (ID), which represents a single time point, and clinical remission (CR), which requires 6-month duration of ID.[54] ID requires a normal physical examination but tolerates some laboratory abnormalities (eg, low C4 and stable proteinuria) and symptoms (eg, fatigue and arthralgia). Furthermore, the group described remission as occurring on medications, on preventive medication, or off medication. The group also described minimally active lupus.[52]

The SLE Responder Index (SRI) incorporates changes in PGA (0–3 cm VAS) and SELENA-SLEDAI scores to measure global activity and the BILAG domain scores to assure no significant organ system worsening.[55] A pediatric validation study of the SRI showed modest sensitivity for measuring cSLE improvement.[55] The SRI served as primary outcome measure, and PRINTO/ACR provisional criteria as secondary outcome measure, in the first randomized clinical trial leading to Food and Drug Administration approval for a drug (belimumab) to treat cSLE.[56]

Recently, the ACR provisionally endorsed the Childhood Lupus Improvement Index (CHILI) as a tool to measure clinically meaningful improvement in cSLE. Developed to improve on the PRINTO/ACR Provisional Response to Therapy and the SRI, particularly in its capacity to measure minor and moderate improvements in cSLE, CHILI is a composite of SLEDAI-2K, PGA, urine protein/creatinine ratio (random or timed), and PtGA. Total scores range from 0 to 100 with defined cutoffs for minor, moderate, and major improvement.[57]

Recognizing that low disease activity is a more realistic target than remission in SLE, the Lupus Low Disease Activity State (LLDAS) was developed for adults requiring SLEDAI-2K score less than or equal to 4 with no activity in major organ systems, no new lupus activity compared with previous assessment, SELENA-SLEDAI PGA less than or equal to 1, prednisone dose less than or equal to 7.5 mg/d, and standard immunosuppressive drug maintenance therapy.[58] LLDAS shows promise in predicting lower disease damage in adult cohorts[58] but awaits further evaluation in cSLE.

Disease Flare Definition in Childhood Systemic Lupus Erythematosus

The ACR provisionally endorsed Criteria for Global Flares in cSLE, which include an SLEDAI or BILAG numeric score, PGA, urine protein/creatinine ratio (random or timed) and ESR with specific cutoffs for minor, moderate and major flares.[59] Other approaches to measure SLE flares, not specifically validated in cSLE, include the SELENA-SLEDAI categorization of mild, moderate, or severe flare[44] and the BILAG flare tool.[60]

Systemic Lupus Erythematosus Disease Damage Measurement

The Systemic Lupus International Collaborating Clinics/ACR Damage Index (SDI) is a universally used measure[61] but has received criticism for not adequately capturing pediatric-specific concerns, such as growth and cognitive development.[62] On the other hand, having separate adult and pediatric damage measures limits opportunities to compare populations or to track damage across the life span. A proposed pediatric version lacks extensive validation and has not achieved universal adoption.[62]

Measures for Specific Organ Involvement

The Cutaneous Lupus Erythematosus Disease Area and Severity Index (CLASI), validated in cSLE and in isolated cutaneous lupus, captures both disease activity and damage across several anatomic sites.[63]

For measuring outcomes in lupus nephritis, the Childhood Arthritis and Rheumatology Research Alliance (CARRA) proposed use of core renal parameters (proteinuria, creatinine clearance or serum creatinine, urine white blood cells, red blood cells, and casts) and provided definitions for renal response (substantial response/complete remission, moderate, mild, and no response), and renal flare (proteinuric/nephrotic flare and nonproteinuric/nephritic flare).[64] Alternate renal outcome measures include renal components of SLEDAI or BILAG.[65]

For measuring cognitive outcomes in neuropsychiatric lupus, the ACR endorsed a neurocognitive battery in cSLE[66] and the computer-based, pediatric version of Automated Neuropsychological Assessment Metrics also has been used.[67]

OUTCOME MEASURES IN VASCULITIS

The Birmingham Vasculitis Activity Score (BVAS) assesses disease activity in patients with a broad spectrum of vasculitides and subsequently has been updated in BVAS for Granulomatosis and Polyangiitis[68] and BVAS version 3.[69] Scored items represent 9 organ systems. The BVAS version 3, validated in a pediatric cohort with ANCA-associated vasculitis, has lower correlation with PGA compared with use in adults.[70] A pediatric modification of the BVAS, the Pediatric Vasculitis Activity Score (PVAS), includes 56 items in 9 organ systems and categorizes new/worsening or persistent disease manifestations. The PVAS demonstrated validity in a pediatric cohort with systemic vasculitides, including polyarteritis nodosa, granulomatosis with polyangiitis and Takayasu arteritis.[71]

Developed for adult populations, the Vasculitis Damage Index assesses 64 items of damage across 11 organ systems and is used widely in studies of various vasculitides.[72] A proposed Pediatric Vasculitis Damage Index inventories 72 items across 10 systems and includes a separate assessment of days of missed school since last evaluation; validation studies have yet to be published.[73]

FUTURE DIRECTIONS

Disease activity and damage assessments in JIA, JDM, SLE, and vasculitis have evolved rapidly. The development of continuous measures is an important advance, with significant potential to improve disease activity assessment in routine care and research. Use of these measures will continue to become more common, particularly as measure validation continues. Primarily clinical measures of disease activity, however, may not be sensitive enough to detect subclinical disease, and work is ongoing to standardize more sensitive outcome measures, including magnetic resonance imaging and ultrasound protocols, for use in JIA and JDM. As understanding of disease pathogenesis evolves, development of serum, urine, and tissue biomarkers hopefully will follow, allowing improved detection of subclinical disease and assessment of early response to medications. These additional disease activity outcomes, incorporated into existing disease activity and damage assessment measures, will enhance the ability to answer key questions about response to treatment and long-term outcomes.

CLINICS CARE POINTS

- Valid outcome measures that evaluate changes in disease activity, disease state and disease damage are important to study and optimize outcomes for children with rheumatic disease.

- Outcome measures in pediatric rheumatic disease are typically composite outcome measures, reflecting the multidimensional nature of the diseases, and they commonly include elements of the physical examination, lab results, and patient-reported outcomes.

- Validated outcome measures for JIA, JDM and childhood onset SLE and are available for use for research and for clinical assessment of disease status.

DISCLOSURE

Stacy Ardoin: Consulting for Aurinia Pharmaceuticals. Consolaro: Research grants from Pfizer and AlfaSigma.

REFERENCES

1. Giannini EH, Ruperto N, Ravelli A, et al. Preliminary definition of improvement in juvenile arthritis. Arthritis Rheum 1997;40(7):1202–9.
2. Ringold S, Angeles-Han ST, Beukelman T, et al. 2019 American College of Rheumatology/Arthritis Foundation Guideline for the Treatment of Juvenile Idiopathic Arthritis: Therapeutic approaches for non-systemic polyarthritis, sacroiliitis, and enthesitis. Arthritis Rheumatol 2019;71(6):846–63.
3. Brunner HI, Lovell DJ, Finck BK, et al. Preliminary definition of disease flare in juvenile rheumatoid arthritis. J Rheumatol 2002;29(5):1058–64.
4. Wallace CA, Giannini EH, Huang B, et al. American College of Rheumatology provisional criteria for defining clinical inactive disease in select categories of juvenile idiopathic arthritis. Arthritis Care Res (Hoboken) 2011;63(7):929–36.
5. Wallace CA, Ravelli A, Huang B, et al. Preliminary validation of clinical remission criteria using the OMERACT filter for select categories of juvenile idiopathic arthritis. J Rheumatol 2006;33(4):789–95.
6. Singh JA, Solomon DH, Dougados M, et al. Development of classification and response criteria for rheumatic diseases. Arthritis Rheum 2006;55(3):348–52.
7. Wallace CA, Giannini EH, Spalding SJ, et al. Trial of early aggressive therapy in polyarticular juvenile idiopathic arthritis. Arthritis Rheum 2012;64(6):2012–21.
8. Wallace CA, Huang B, Bandeira M, et al. Patterns of clinical remission in select categories of juvenile idiopathic arthritis. Arthritis Rheum 2005;52(11):3554–62.
9. Ringold S, Seidel KD, Koepsell TD, et al. Inactive disease in polyarticular juvenile idiopathic arthritis: current patterns and associations. Rheumatology (Oxford) 2009;48(8):972–7.
10. Shoop-Worrall SJW, Kearsley-Fleet L, Thomson W, et al. How common is remission in juvenile idiopathic arthritis: a systematic review. Semin Arthritis Rheum 2017;47(3):331–7.

11. Shoop-Worrall SJW, Verstappen SMM, McDonagh JE, et al. Long-term outcomes following achievement of clinically inactive disease in juvenile idiopathic arthritis: the importance of definition. Arthritis Rheumatol 2018;70(9):1519-29.

12. van der Heijde DM, van 't Hof M, van Riel PL, et al. Development of a disease activity score based on judgment in clinical practice by rheumatologists. J Rheumatol 1993;20(3):579-81.

13. Consolaro A, Ruperto N, Bazso A, et al. Development and validation of a composite disease activity score for juvenile idiopathic arthritis. Arthritis Rheum 2009;61(5):658-66.

14. Nordal EB, Zak M, Aalto K, et al. Validity and predictive ability of the juvenile arthritis disease activity score based on CRP versus ESR in a Nordic population-based setting. Ann Rheum Dis 2012;71(7):1122-7.

15. Ravelli A, Consolaro A, Horneff G, et al. Treating juvenile idiopathic arthritis to target: recommendations of an international task force. Ann Rheum Dis 2018; 77(6):819-28.

16. Klein A, Minden K, Hospach A, et al. Treat-to-target study for improved outcome in polyarticular juvenile idiopathic arthritis. Ann Rheum Dis 2020;79(7):969-74.

17. Swart JF, van Dijkhuizen EHP, Wulffraat NM, et al. Clinical Juvenile Arthritis Disease Activity Score proves to be a useful tool in treat-to-target therapy in juvenile idiopathic arthritis. Ann Rheum Dis 2018;77(3):336-42.

18. Tibaldi J, Pistorio A, Aldera E, et al. Development and initial validation of a composite disease activity score for systemic juvenile idiopathic arthritis. Rheumatology (Oxford) 2020;59(11):3505-14.

19. Weiss PF, Colbert RA, Xiao R, et al. Development and retrospective validation of the juvenile spondyloarthritis disease activity index. Arthritis Care Res (Hoboken) 2014;66(12):1775-82.

20. Miller FW, Rider LG, Chung YL, et al. Proposed preliminary core set measures for disease outcome assessment in adult and juvenile idiopathic inflammatory myopathies. Rheumatology (Oxford) 2001;40(11):1262-73.

21. Ruperto N, Ravelli A, Murray KJ, et al. Preliminary core sets of measures for disease activity and damage assessment in juvenile systemic lupus erythematosus and juvenile dermatomyositis. Rheumatology (Oxford) 2003;42(12):1452-9.

22. McCann LJ, Pilkington CA, Huber AM, et al. Development of a consensus core dataset in juvenile dermatomyositis for clinical use to inform research. Ann Rheum Dis 2018;77(2):241-50.

23. Rider LG, Giannini EH, Brunner HI, et al. International consensus on preliminary definitions of improvement in adult and juvenile myositis. Arthritis Rheum 2004;50(7):2281-90.

24. Ruperto N, Pistorio A, Ravelli A, et al. The Paediatric Rheumatology International Trials Organisation provisional criteria for the evaluation of response to therapy in juvenile dermatomyositis. Arthritis Rheum 2010;62(11):1533-41.

25. Rider LG, Aggarwal R, Pistorio A, et al. 2016 American College of Rheumatology/European League Against Rheumatism Criteria for Minimal, Moderate, and Major Clinical Response in Juvenile Dermatomyositis: An International Myositis Assessment and Clinical Studies Group/Paediatric Rheumatology International Trials Organisation Collaborative Initiative. Ann Rheum Dis 2017;76(5):782-91.

26. Lazarevic D, Pistorio A, Palmisani E, et al. The PRINTO criteria for clinically inactive disease in juvenile dermatomyositis. Ann Rheum Dis 2013;72(5):686-93.

27. Rider LG, Werth VP, Huber AM, et al. Measures of adult and juvenile dermatomyositis, polymyositis, and inclusion body myositis: Physician and Patient/Parent Global Activity, Manual Muscle Testing (MMT), Health Assessment Questionnaire (HAQ)/Childhood Health Assessment Questionnaire (C-HAQ), Childhood Myositis Assessment Scale (CMAS), Myositis Disease ActivAssessment Tool

(MDAAT), Disease Activity Score (DAS), Short Form 36 (SF-36), Child Health Questionnaire (CHQ), physician global damage, Myositis Damage Index (MDI), Quantitative Muscle Testing (QMT), Myositis Functional Index-2 (FI-2), Myositis Activities Profile (MAP), Inclusion Body Myositis Functional Rating Scale (IBMFRS), Cutaneous Dermatomyositis Disease Area and Severity Index (CDASI), Cutaneous Assessment Tool (CAT), Dermatomyositis Skin Severity Index (DSSI), Skindex, and Dermatology Life Quality Index (DLQI). Arthritis Rheum 2011;63(Suppl 11):S118–57.

28. Kendall FP, Mcreary EK, Provance PG. Muscles: testing and function. Baltimore (MD): Williams and Wilkins; 1993.

29. Rosina S, Varnier GC, Pistorio A, et al. Development and testing of reduced versions of the MMT-8 in juvenile dermatomyositis. J Rheum 2021;48(6):898–906.

30. Lovell DJ, Lindsley CB, Rennebohm RM, et al. Development of validated disease activity and damage indices for the juvenile idiopathic inflammatory myopathies. II. The Childhood Myositis Assessment Scale (CMAS): a quantitative tool for the evaluation of muscle function. The Juvenile Dermatomyositis Disease Activity Collaborative Study Group. Arthritis Rheum 1999;42(10):2213–9.

31. Varnier GC, Rosina S, Ferrari C, et al. Development and testing of a hybrid measure of muscle strength in juvenile dermatomyositis for use in routine care. Arthritis Rheum 2018;70(9):1312–9.

32. Saygin D, Oddis CV, Moghadam-Kia S, et al. Hand-held dynamometry for assessment of muscle strength in patients with inflammatory myopathies. Oxford, England: Rheumatology; 2020.

33. Bode RK, Klein-Gitelman MS, Miller ML, et al. Disease activity score for children with juvenile dermatomyositis: reliability and validity evidence. Arthritis Rheum 2003;49(1):7–15.

34. Sultan SM, Allen E, Cooper RG, et al. Interrater reliability and aspects of validity of the myositis damage index. Ann Rheum Dis 2011;70(7):1272–6.

35. Hay EM, Bacon PA, Gordon C, et al. The BILAG index: a reliable and valid instrument for measuring clinical disease activity in systemic lupus erythematosus. Q J Med 1993;86(7):447–58.

36. Rosina S, Consolaro A, van Dijkhuizen P, et al. Development and validation of a composite disease activity score for measurement of muscle and skin involvement in juvenile dermatomyositis. Rheumatology (Oxford) 2019;58(7):1196–205.

37. Huber AM, Dugan EM, Lachenbruch PA, et al. The Cutaneous Assessment Tool: development and reliability in juvenile idiopathic inflammatory myopathy. Rheumatology (Oxford) 2007;46(10):1606–11.

38. Huber AM, Dugan EM, Lachenbruch PA, et al. Preliminary validation and clinical meaning of the Cutaneous Assessment Tool in juvenile dermatomyositis. Arthritis Rheum 2008;59(2):214–21.

39. Tiao J, Feng R, Berger EM, et al. Evaluation of the reliability of the Cutaneous Dermatomyositis Disease Area and Severity Index and the Cutaneous Assessment Tool-Binary Method in juvenile dermatomyositis among paediatric dermatologists, rheumatologists and neurologists. Br J Dermatol 2017;177(4):1086–92.

40. Anyanwu CO, Fiorentino DF, Chung L, et al. Validation of the Cutaneous Dermatomyositis Disease Area and Severity Index: characterizing disease severity and assessing responsiveness to clinical change. Br J Dermatol 2015;173(4):969–74.

41. Isenberg DA, Allen E, Farewell V, et al. International consensus outcome measures for patients with idiopathic inflammatory myopathies. Development and initial validation of myositis activity and damage indices in patients with adult onset disease. Rheumatology (Oxford) 2004;43(1):49–54.

42. Bombardier C, Gladman DD, Urowitz MB, et al. Derivation of the SLEDAI. A disease activity index for lupus patients. The Committee on Prognosis Studies in SLE. Arthritis Rheum 1992;35(6):630–40.

43. Touma Z, Urowitz MB, Ibañez D, et al. SLEDAI-2K 10 days versus SLEDAI-2K 30 days in a longitudinal evaluation. Lupus 2011;20(1):67–70.

44. Petri M, Kim MY, Kalunian KC, et al. Combined oral contraceptives in women with systemic lupus erythematosus. N Engl J Med 2005;353(24):2550–8.

45. Gladman DD, Ibañez D, Urowitz MB. Systemic lupus erythematosus disease activity index 2000. J Rheumatol 2002;29(2):288–91.

46. Isenberg DA, Rahman A, Allen E, et al. BILAG 2004. Development and initial validation of an updated version of the British Isles Lupus Assessment Group's disease activity index for patients with systemic lupus erythematosus. Rheumatology (Oxford) 2005;44(7):902–6.

47. Cresswell L, Yee CS, Farewell V, et al. Numerical scoring for the Classic BILAG index. Rheumatology (Oxford) 2009;48(12):1548–52.

48. Brunner HI, Silverman ED, Bombardier C, et al. European Consensus Lupus Activity Measurement is sensitive to change in disease activity in childhood-onset systemic lupus erythematosus. Arthritis Rheum 2003;49(3):335–41.

49. Liang MH, Socher SA, Larson MG, et al. Reliability and validity of six systems for the clinical assessment of disease activity in systemic lupus erythematosus. Arthritis Rheum 1989;32(9):1107–18.

50. Bae SC, Koh HK, Chang DK, et al. Reliability and validity of systemic lupus activity measure-revised (SLAM-R) for measuring clinical disease activity in systemic lupus erythematosus. Lupus 2001;10(6):405–9.

51. Brunner HI, Feldman BM, Bombardier C, et al. Sensitivity of the Systemic Lupus Erythematosus Disease Activity Index, British Isles Lupus Assessment Group Index, and Systemic Lupus Activity Measure in the evaluation of clinical change in childhood-onset systemic lupus erythematosus. Arthritis Rheum 1999;42(7):1354–60.

52. Ruperto N, Ravelli A, Cuttica R, et al. The Pediatric Rheumatology International Trials Organization criteria for the evaluation of response to therapy in juvenile systemic lupus erythematosus: prospective validation of the disease activity core set. Arthritis Rheum 2005;52(9):2854–64.

53. Ruperto N, Ravelli A, Oliveira S, et al. The Pediatric Rheumatology International Trials Organization/American College of Rheumatology provisional criteria for the evaluation of response to therapy in juvenile systemic lupus erythematosus: prospective validation of the definition of improvement. Arthritis Rheum 2006; 55(3):355–63.

54. Mina R, Klien-Gitelman MS, Ravelli A. Inactive disease and remission in childhood-onset systemic lupus erythematosus. Arthritis Care Res 2012;64(5):683–93.

55. Mina R, Klein-Gitelman MS, Nelson S, et al. Validation of the systemic lupus erythematosus responder index for use in juvenile-onset systemic lupus erythematosus. Ann Rheum Dis 2014;73(2):401–6.

56. Brunner HI, Abud-Mendoza C, Viola DO, et al. Safety and efficacy of intravenous belimumab in children with systemic lupus erythematosus: results from a randomised, placebo-controlled trial. Ann Rheum Dis 2020;79(10):1340–8.

57. Brunner HI, Holland MJ, Beresford MW, et al. American College of Rheumatology Provisional Criteria for Clinically Relevant Improvement in Children and Adolescents With Childhood-Onset Systemic Lupus Erythematosus. Arthritis Care Res (Hoboken) 2019;71(5):579–90.

58. Ugarte-Gil MF, Wojdyla D, Pons-Estel GJ, et al. Remission and Low Disease Activity Status (LDAS) protect lupus patients from damage occurrence: data from a

multiethnic, multinational Latin American Lupus Cohort (GLADEL). Ann Rheum Dis 2017;76(12):2071–4.

59. Brunner HI, Holland M, Beresford MW, et al. American College of Rheumatology Provisional Criteria for Global Flares in Childhood-Onset Systemic Lupus Erythematosus. Arthritis Care Res (Hoboken) 2018;70(6):813–22.

60. Isenberg D, Sturgess J, Allen E, et al. Study of Flare Assessment in Systemic Lupus Erythematosus Based on Paper Patients. Arthritis Care Res (Hoboken) 2018;70(1):98–103.

61. Gladman D, Ginzler E, Goldsmith C, et al. The development and initial validation of the Systemic Lupus International Collaborating Clinics/American College of Rheumatology damage index for systemic lupus erythematosus. Arthritis Rheum 1996;39(3):363–9.

62. Holland MJ, Beresford MW, Feldman BM, et al. Measuring disease damage and its severity in childhood-onset systemic lupus erythematosus. Arthritis Care Res (Hoboken) 2018;70(11):1621–9.

63. AIE'ed A, Aydin POA, Al Mutairi N, et al. Validation of the Cutaneous Lupus Erythematosus Disease Area and Severity Index and pSkindex27 for use in childhood-onset systemic lupus erythematosus. Lupus Sci Med 2018;5(1):e000275.

64. Mina R, von Scheven E, Ardoin SP, et al. Consensus treatment plans for induction therapy of newly diagnosed proliferative lupus nephritis in juvenile systemic lupus erythematosus. Arthritis Care Res (Hoboken) 2012;64(3):375–83.

65. Mina R, Abulaban K, Klein-Gitelman MS, et al. Validation of the lupus nephritis clinical indices in childhood-onset systemic lupus erythematosus. Arthritis Care Res (Hoboken) 2016;68(2):195–202.

66. Mikdashi JA, Esdaile JM, Alarcón GS, et al. Proposed response criteria for neurocognitive impairment in systemic lupus erythematosus clinical trials. Lupus 2007; 16(6):418–25.

67. Brunner HI, Ruth NM, German A, et al. Initial validation of the Pediatric Automated Neuropsychological Assessment Metrics for childhood-onset systemic lupus erythematosus. Arthritis Rheum 2007;57(7):1174–82.

68. Stone JH, Hoffman GS, Merkel PA, et al. A disease-specific activity index for Wegener's granulomatosis: modification of the Birmingham Vasculitis Activity Score. International Network for the Study of the Systemic Vasculitides (INSSYS). Arthritis Rheum 2001;44(4):912–20.

69. Mukhtyar C, Lee R, Brown D, et al. Modification and validation of the Birmingham Vasculitis Activity Score (version 3). Ann Rheum Dis 2009;68(12):1827–32.

70. Morishita K, Li SC, Muscal E, et al. Assessing the performance of the Birmingham Vasculitis Activity Score at diagnosis for children with antineutrophil cytoplasmic antibody-associated vasculitis in A Registry for Childhood Vasculitis (ARChiVe). J Rheumatol 2012;39(5):1088–94.

71. Dolezalova P, Price-Kuehne FE, Özen S, et al. Disease activity assessment in childhood vasculitis: development and preliminary validation of the Paediatric Vasculitis Activity Score (PVAS). Ann Rheum Dis 2013;72(10):1628–33.

72. Exley AR, Bacon PA, Luqmani RA, et al. Development and initial validation of the Vasculitis Damage Index for the standardized clinical assessment of damage in the systemic vasculitides. Arthritis Rheum 1997;40(2):371–80.

73. Dolezalova P, Wilkinson N, Brogan PA, et al. Paediatric Vasculitis Damage Index: a new tool for standardised disease assessment. Ann Rheum Dis 2014;73:696–7.

Updates on Juvenile Dermatomyositis from the Last Decade: Classification to Outcomes

Hanna Kim, MS, MD[a],*, Adam M. Huber, MSc, MD[b], Susan Kim, MD, MMSc[c]

KEYWORDS

- Juvenile myositis (JM) • Juvenile dermatomyositis (JDM)
- Myositis-specific autoantibodies (MSA) • Pathogenesis • Treatment
- Biologic therapies • Outcomes

KEY POINTS

- New classification criteria for juvenile dermatomyositis (JDM) have been developed, but their role remains unclear. New serologic classifications that define distinct subgroups within juvenile myositis may be more useful in practice.
- There are many validated assessment tools available to assess disease activity in JDM. Future studies will optimize these tools and improve feasibility in clinical and research contexts.
- Genetic and environmental risk factors, causes of perifascicular atrophy in muscle, and vascular dysfunction provide new insights into the pathogenesis of JDM. Biomarkers related to endothelial function, interferon, and immune cells also have shown correlation to disease activity.
- Outcomes of children with JDM have improved with immunomodulatory therapies but many patients have persistent disease sequelae.
- An expanding repertoire of medications is helpful in subsets of JDM patients, but additional investigation to identify optimal individualized treatment regimens is essential to improve future outcomes in JDM

[a] Juvenile Myositis Pathogenesis and Therapeutics Unit, National Institute of Arthritis Musculoskeletal and Skin Diseases, National Institutes of Health, 10 Center Drive, Building 10, 12N-240, Bethesda, MD 20892, USA; [b] IWK Health Centre and Dalhousie University, Division of Pediatric Rheumatology, 5850 University Avenue, Halifax, Nova Scotia B3K 6R8, Canada; [c] University of California, San Francisco, 550 16th Street, San Francisco, CA 94158, USA
* Corresponding author.
E-mail address: Hanna.kim@nih.gov

Rheum Dis Clin N Am 47 (2021) 669–690
https://doi.org/10.1016/j.rdc.2021.07.003
0889-857X/21/Published by Elsevier Inc.

rheumatic.theclinics.com

INTRODUCTION

Juvenile dermatomyositis (JDM) is a rare heterogeneous immune-medicated condition with characteristic skin rashes, muscle weakness, vasculopathy, and other organ involvement. Myositis-specific autoantibodies (MSAs) help define clinical associations within subgroups of JDM.[1,2] The authors present key updates from the past 10 years on the classification, pathogenesis, MSA groups, assessment, and treatment of JDM.[3]

CLASSIFICATION

Historically, classification criteria for JDM have been limited to those of Bohan and Peter from 1975.[4] These were not originally intended to be used, however, for JDM. Lundberg and colleagues[5] recently conducted a large, international, consensus-based effort to develop new classification criteria for inflammatory myositis in both adults and children. The criteria assign scores to a variety of characteristics, such as presence of classic rash, age, or biopsy features, giving a total score, which can be used to determine the likelihood that a patient has an idiopathic inflammatory myopathy. Additional validation of the criteria in JDM suggest excellent sensitivity but specificity that is lower than previous criteria.[6] The role of the new criteria for clinical research or diagnosis remains to be determined.

SEROLOGIC CLASSIFICATION OF JUVENILE DERMATOMYOSITIS

MSAs are found in 50% to 70% of juvenile myositis and have multiple clinical associations.[1,2] MSAs are present exclusively in patients with myositis, as summarized in **Table 1**. Myositis-associated autoantibodies (MAAs) are present in patients with myositis as well as in patients with other autoimmune diseases but have clinical associations in myositis.

Myositis-specific Autoantibodies

In the past decade, several studies assessing clinical associations of MSAs have shown generally consistent findings. Anti-transcriptional intermediary factor 1 (TIF1) is the most common MSA, distinct from adult myositis in which anti-synthetase autoantibody is most common. The largest cohorts are based in North America (n = 365–454)[1,7–9] and the United Kingdom (n = 285–380),[2,10,11] with smaller cohorts from India[12,13] and Japan.[14,15] MSA-related clinical phenotype subgroups have been defined based on not only clinical features but also demographics and disease course (**Table 1**). Other distinctions are highlighted.

Environmental associations were also identified. Anti-p155/140 or TIF1 has an association with higher UV indices,[16] consistent with the clinical association of anti-TIF1 with photosensitivity.[1,2,9,14] Higher UV index also was associated with lower odds of antinuclear matrix protein 2 (NXP2), also known as anti-MJ.[16]

In one study, the IFN score of anti-TIF1 autoantibody-positive JDM patients had higher correlation with skin activity than in JDM generally or other disease activity measures, even though anti-TIF1 patients did not have significantly higher skin disease activity.[17] This suggests that biomarkers may have distinct associations by MSA group, which may point to differences in pathogenic mechanisms, but this needs further evaluation.

JDM patients with anti-Mi2 were less likely to remain on treatment despite more severe muscle biopsy findings, indicating they may be more responsive to treatment.[18] Thus, although muscle biopsy general indicates disease severity, MSA group also should be considered when considering disease course and treatment.

Table 1
Myositis-specific autoantibodies in juvenile myositis

MSA Group	Alias(es)	Frequency (%)	Cohort Sizes	Associations	References
Anti-TIF1	p155/140, TIF1-gamma	17.9–35.0	21–380	Associated with photosensitivity, Gottron papules, malar rash, V-, and shawl-sign rash, cuticular overgrowth, cutaneous ulceration, and chronic or polycyclic disease course	[1,2,9,12,14]
Anti-NXP2	MJ	15.1–23.8	21–380	Associated with muscle cramps, more weakness, dysphonia, calcinosis, hospitalization, younger age of onset, and less remission at 2 years	[1,2,11,14]
Anti-MDA5	CADM-140	6.1–23.8	13–453	Associated with oral and skin ulceration, amyopathic disease, ILD (sometimes RP-ILD), arthralgia/arthritis, fever, weight loss, adenopathy, and older age of diagnosis	[2,7,10,12,14,15]
Anti-synthetase	Jo-1, PL-7, PL-12, other aminoacyl-tRNA synthetases	0.0–5.1	21–380	Associated with ILD, arthralgia, less weakness, mechanic's hands, lipoatrophy, and older age of onset	[1,2,12–14]
Anti–Mi-2	NuRD	0.0–3.9	21–380	Associated with malar rash, more muscle weakness including pharyngeal weakness, edema, less ILD, lower mortality, and more common in Hispanic patients	[1,2,12–14]
Anti-SRP		0.0–1.8	22–380	Associated with polymyositis (without rash), severe onset, more weakness including distal weakness, falling episodes, necrosis on muscle biopsy, Raynaud phenomenon, cardiac involvement, cutaneous ulceration, high CK, frequent hospitalization, wheelchair use, poor response to treatment, chronic disease course, and more common in African American patients.	[1,2,12,13]

(continued on next page)

Table 1
(continued)

MSA Group	Alias(es)	Frequency (%)	Cohort Sizes	Associations	References
Anti-HMGCR		1.1	380–440	Associated with severe proximal and distal weakness, necrosis on muscle biopsy, muscle atrophy, joint contractures, arthralgias, dysphagia, high CK, HLA DRB1*0701, poor response to medication, and chronic course. No previous statin medication exposure.	2,8
Anti-SAE		0.3–9.1	11–380	Too few cases with in juvenile myositis for any clear clinical associations	1,2,19

Abbreviations: CK, creatine kinase; NuRD, nucleosome remodeling deacetylase complex; RP-ILD, rapidly progressive ILD.

For the anti–melanoma differentiation-associated gene 5 (MDA5) MSA group, there are notable differences in cohorts based on geography. In general, the anti-MDA5 MSA group has less weakness with more joint symptoms (arthritis and arthralgia), skin ulcerations, and systemic features (eg, fever). In Japanese JDM cohorts, however, anti-MDA5 antibody was more frequent (23.8%–38.5%)[14,15] and associated with rapidly progressive interstitial lung disease (ILD).[15] In other cohorts, anti-MDA5 was less common (6.1%–7.7%), associated with ILD, but not associated with rapidly progressive ILD.[2,7,10,12]

Necrotizing myopathy includes anti–signal recognition particle (SRP), which is associated with juvenile polymyositis (JPM) (without skin findings) and the recently described anti-3-hydroxy-3-methylglutaryl-coenzyme A reductase (anti-HMGCR). Anti-HMGCR recently was detected in 1.1% cases of JDM, JPM, and necrotizing myositis of both North American and UK-based cohorts.[2,8] Distinct from adults, it has not been associated with previous statin exposure and has a different HLA-type association (DRB1*0701) compared with adult myositis.[8]

Anti–small ubiquitin-like modifier activating enzyme (anti-SAE) is another rare MSA in juvenile myositis. There is limited information on the few cases from 3 cohorts (1/374 North American cohort, 3/380 UK cohort, and 1/11 Japanese cohort), which is too limited to establish clear clinical correlations.[1,2,19]

There can be differences in testing sensitivity and specificity by MSA testing method, so care should be taken when interpreting results.[20] This is an important area of continued study.

Myositis-associated Autoantibodies Updates

Anti-NT5C1A, a more recently identified MAA, was identified in adults with inclusion body myositis. Of 380 US-based juvenile myositis patients, 27% were found to have anti-NT5C1A with greater pulmonary symptoms at diagnosis, more frequent hospitalizations, and required more medication.[21] Also, anti-Ro52 MAA was assessed in juvenile myositis (14% in North American cohort of 698) to be more frequent with anti-synthetase and anti-MDA5 MSA groups. In general, it was associated with ILD, chronic disease course, less remission, and more medications.[22]

ASSESSMENT

Assessment of children with JDM for the purposes of clinical care or research is challenging due to the complexity of the illness. Consideration needs to be given to various aspects of muscle involvement, a wide range of skin manifestations, and involvement of multiple organ systems as well as other aspects of disease impact, including quality of life (QoL). Measurement tools in JDM are reviewed by Rider and colleagues.[23] New or updated/modified assessments discussed in this article are listed in **Table 2**. A key development in the understanding of the assessment of JDM was the advent of core sets, consensus-derived groups of outcome measures, which attempt to assess the full spectrum of disease manifestations. The core sets were developed independently by the International Myositis Assessment and Clinical Studies Group (IMACS)[24] and Pediatric Rheumatology International Trials Organization (PRINTO) groups[25] and are summarized in **Table 3**. Although this approach acknowledged the multidimensional nature of JDM, completion of all recommended core set measures is a time-consuming, challenging process that is difficult to use in a clinical context.

Consensus Core Data Set in Juvenile Dermatomyositis

To facilitate collaboration and standardization of data collection across international centers, McCann and colleagues[26] developed a consensus core data set. They developed a preliminary minimal data set using consensus methods. Subsequently, this

Table 2
New and updated/modified juvenile dermatomyositis assessment tools discussed in this article

Measure	What is Assessed?	Author (Reference)
IMACS core set	Disease Activity	Miller et al,[24] 2001
PRINTO core set	Disease Activity	Ruperto et al,[25] 2003
Consensus core set	Comprehensive assessment	McCann et al,[26] 2014; McCann et al,[27] 2015; McCann et al,[28] 2014
Hybrid MMT-8/CMAS	Muscle strength/function	Varnier et al,[29] 2018
JDMAI	Muscle strength/function	Rosina et al,[30] 2019
Abbreviated MMT-8	Muscle strength	Rosina et al,[31] 2020
Whole-body MRI score	MRI muscle inflammation	Malattia et al,[33] 2014
Pelvic girdle MRI score	MRI muscle inflammation	Thyoka et al,[34] 2018
Muscle biopsy score	Muscle biopsy assessment	Wedderburn et al,[36] 2007; Varsani et al,[37] 2015
CAT	Skin disease activity	Huber et al,[38] 2008
CDASI	Skin disease activity	Klein et al,[39] 2008
DSSI	Skin disease activity	Klein et al,[39] 2008
DAS	Skin disease activity	Bode et al,[40] 2003
Inactive disease	Inactive disease	Lazarevic et al,[47] 2013; Almeida et al,[48] 2015
Definition of improvement	Response/improvement	Ruperto et al,[49] 2010
Response to therapy	Response/improvement	Rider et al,[50–52] 2017

Table 3 Juvenile myositis disease activity core set measures	
IMACS Core Set variables[59]	PRINTO Core Set variables[60]
Physician global disease activity (VAS or Likert)	Physician global disease activity (VAS or Likert)
Parent/Patient Global Disease Activity (VAS or Likert)	Parent/patient assessment of overall well-being (VAS or Likert)
CHAQ and CMAS	CHAQ
MMT	CMAS and MMT
Muscle enzymes (at least 2)	Muscle enzymes
Extraskeletal muscle disease activity (to be developed)	Global JDM disease activity tool

data set was reviewed and refined through an international email-based Delphi survey, including both medical specialists and patients/parents, followed by a smaller consensus meeting of JDM experts using nominal group technique.[27] The resulting data set included 123 items and was renamed a "core" rather than "minimal" data set.[28] Several organizations, including the Childhood Arthritis and Rheumatology Research Alliance (CARRA), have adopted the core data set. Collecting a common data set in both clinical and research contexts will facilitate future collaboration between sites and research networks.

Changes to Core Set Tools

Recent work seeks to streamline the assessment process. Varnier and colleagues[29] published preliminary validation work of a hybrid tool, which combines the manual muscle test 8 (MMT 8) with 3 items from the Childhood Myositis Assessment Scale (CMAS) to give a score from 0 to 100. Their work supported face and content validity, construct validity, reliability, internal consistency, responsiveness and discriminant validity, while reducing completion time. Rosina and colleagues[30] reported on the development of a composite measure of disease activity in JDM, called the Juvenile DermatoMyositis Activity Index (JDMAI). The JDMAI incorporates physician and parent/patient global scales, an assessment of muscle strength and an assessment of skin disease activity. All 6 versions of the JDMAI demonstrated face and content validity, construct validity, internal consistency, responsiveness, and the ability to discriminate between disease states and parental satisfaction. Future validation work will allow selection of a final version. Rosina and colleagues' group also has reported on the measurement properties of shortened versions of the MMT-8.[31] Rather than testing 8 muscle groups, they studied versions using 6 and 4 muscle groups, documenting similar construct validity, internal consistency, discriminant validity and somewhat better responsiveness to the original tool. Together, these publications demonstrate ongoing attempts to improve assessment of children with JDM, maintaining validity while facilitating use in clinical settings.

Magnetic Resonance Imaging

The use of magnetic resonance imaging (MRI) to assess and document muscle involvement in children with JDM has become common, even though MRI is not included in any diagnostic criteria. For example, in the CARRA Legacy Registry, which included 483 children with JDM, 90% had MRI as part of their evaluation.[32] Malattia and colleagues[33] reported on the use of whole-body MRI in 41 JDM patients and controls. They developed and validated a whole-body MRI score, demonstrating reliability, construct validity, and responsiveness, and showed the presence of muscle inflammation in muscles not clinically affected. More recently, Thyoka and colleagues[34] refined a previous MRI scoring tool for children with JDM, using pelvic girdle MRI,[35] demonstrating good inter-rater and intra-rater reliability. Unfortunately, MRI results from this study were not linked to weakness or disease activity, limiting further assessment of the clinical utility of the score.

Muscle Biopsy

The use of muscle biopsy in the assessment of JDM has declined, largely due to its invasiveness and replacement by other methods that document muscle involvement. Many experts, however, continue to advocate for its routine use. Wedderburn and colleagues[36] described a consensus-derived scoring tool for comprehensive assessment of muscle biopsies. A subsequent update and validation showed good intra-rater and inter-rater reliability and strong correlations with clinical measures of disease activity.[37] Its use allows standardization of muscle biopsy assessment in clinical and research contexts. Deakin and colleagues[18] showed that muscle biopsy combined with myositis specific autoantibodies predicted clinically relevant outcomes, including future treatment status, suggesting that muscle biopsy could be part of an assessment to tailor therapy for individual patients.

Assessment of Skin Disease in Juvenile Dermatomyositis

The assessment of skin disease in JDM is complicated by the use of multiple tools, including the Cutaneous Assessment Tool (CAT),[38] the Cutaneous Dermatomyositis Disease Activity and Severity Index (CDASI),[39] the Dermatomyositis Skin Severity Index (DSSI),[39] and the Disease Activity Score (DAS),[40] with little consensus about which tool is optimal. Given the number of patients with persistent skin disease long after resolution of muscle disease, the lack of consensus on assessment negatively affects the study of effective therapies. Several recent studies have attempted to address this lack of consensus.

Tiao and colleagues[41] compared the CDASI and the CAT when used by pediatric dermatologists, rheumatologists, and neurologists in children with JDM. They found that both tools had good inter-rater reliability and correlations with other measures of activity and damage when used by dermatologists and rheumatologists, although performance was worse when used by neurologists. Both tools also were compared in adults with dermatomyositis (DM), with demonstration of good inter-rater and intra-rater reliability, construct validity, and responsiveness.[42] In the adult study, including 10 dermatologists, the CDASI was preferred. A review of the CDASI, primarily in adults with DM, recently has been published.[43] Determination of the optimal tool to assess skin disease in children remains an area in need of consensus.

Quality of Life and Other Measures

There is increased recognition of the impact of JDM beyond physical manifestations like skin and muscle disease. Apaz and colleagues[44] reported on QoL, as assessed by the Child Health Questionnaire, in an international cohort of children with JDM. They found that QoL was impaired in children with JDM, particularly in the physical domain, compared with healthy controls, with baseline disability and disease duration predicting lower scores 6 months later. Tory and colleagues[45] surveyed health care providers and families of children with JDM to identify the most important components of high-quality care. They found that although patients and families generally gave higher scores than physicians, there was consensus on the 5 most important items: QoL, timely diagnosis, access to rheumatology care, normalization of function/strength, and ability for self-care. In another publication, Tory and colleagues[46] studied discordance between physician and patient/family global visual analog scales (VASs). They found that nearly 40% of the global VAS scores in a large registry were discordant, defined as a difference of greater than or equal to 2 points on a 10-point scale. More work is needed to understand the reasons for discordance between physician and patient/family global assessments and the impact on patient care.

Inactive Disease

Achieving inactive disease, either on or off medications, is an important goal in the management of JDM. Lazarevic and colleagues[47] used a large, international cohort of 275 children with JDM to develop and validate a data-driven definition (meeting at least 3 of 4 criteria: creatine phosphokinase (CPK) less than or equal to 150, CMAS greater than or equal to 48, MMT8 greater than or equal to 78, and physician global VAS less than or equal to 0.2). The definition, however, may overemphasize the importance of muscle disease, because a patient with marked persistent skin involvement or other active extramuscular disease would meet the definition of inactive disease if they had normal strength and normal muscle enzymes.[48] Almeida and colleagues[48] proposed an amendment whereby the physician global VAS is an essential criterion. Further work is needed to develop a more acceptable definition.

Definition of Improvement/Clinical Response in Juvenile Dermatomyositis

Defining improvement or response to therapy is critical to conducting clinical trials. Ruperto and colleagues[49] initially reported provisional response criteria for JDM. Using previously established core set variables for JDM, the criteria defined permitted percentages of improvement and worsening for a patient to be "improved." More recently, an international effort developed new criteria for response to therapy in JDM.[50–52] The criteria generate a continuous total improvement score, based on points assigned for the absolute percent change of each of the core set variables. This approach allows for the definition of minimal, moderate, and major improvement, permitting quantification of the degree of response. The response calculator can be found online at https://www.niehs.nih.gov/research/resources/imacs/response_criteria/index.cfm.

PATHOGENESIS
Genetics

Although the etiology of JDM is not fully understood, genetic and environmental risk factors are key contributors. One study found that approximately half of JDM families had at least 1 other family member with autoimmune disease, most commonly type 1 diabetes mellitus or systemic lupus erythematosus.[53] Genome-wide association studies of single-nucleotide polymorphisms (SNPs) comparing adult DM and JDM to controls found multiple major histocompatibility complex (MHC) region signals, strongest at HLA 8.1 ancestral haplotype, with HLA DRB1*03:01 strongest in adult and JDM. Three SNPs also were more common from *PLCL1*, *BLK*, and *CCL21*, as has been seen in other autoimmune diseases.[54,55] Lower C4a gene copy number (deficiency) is more common in JDM than controls, particularly among those with an HLA DR3-positive background.[56] Genetic changes have been validated as an important component in JDM, identifying variants associated with immune response, particularly MHC class II, B cell signaling, and C4.

Environment

Because photosensitivity is a common manifestation of disease and flares often occur after sun exposure, UV radiation is considered an environmental trigger of JDM.[57] Higher UV index was associated more strongly with JDM and more prominently among those positive for anti-TIF1 MSA compared with juvenile myositis without skin involvement (JPM).[16] Higher UV index in the month prior to symptom onset was associated with increased odds of developing calcinosis in non–African Americans with JDM.[58] When matched to healthy control mothers, maternal exposures to school chalk dust, gasoline vapor, smoking, and carbon monoxide during the third trimester were significant risk factors for having a child with JDM.[59] Direct UV exposure and maternal toxic exposures (chalk dust, gasoline vapor, smoking, and carbon monoxide) are environmental triggers associated with JDM.

Muscle Pathology

Perifascicular atrophy (PFA) is a characteristic finding on muscle biopsy in DM, with or without clinical myopathy.[60] In early DM without PFA, there already is focal capillary depletion found on biopsy.[61] In chronic DM, biopsies show a combination of chronic ischemia with replacement of normal capillaries by abnormal lumens and thickened walls as well as neoangiogenesis.[60] *RIG-I*, an IFN-response gene part of innate immune system response, is overexpressed in areas of PFA. With hypoxia, *RIG-I* expression and type I IFN increase, indicating a connection between hypoxia, IFN, and PFA.[62] When compared with adult myositis biopsies, JDM biopsies show predominantly hypoxia-driven pathology in perifascicular areas with atrophy, regional loss of capillaries, and less IFN-inducible gene expression.[63] Decreased vascular density, ischemia, cell death, neoangiogenesis, and IFN expression all contribute to PFA, a characteristic finding of JDM muscle biopsies.

Interferon

An increased interferon (IFN) regulated signature is present in JDM.[64] Human myogenic precursor cells from JDM patients' muscle biopsies show an angiogenic gene expression signature recapitulated with type I IFN treatment, indicating JDM's proangiogenic features may be type I IFN driven.[65] Galectin-9 and CXCL10, IFN-stimulated proteins, were validated as reliable biomarkers for disease activity in multiple JDM cohorts, showing elevated or rising levels prior to flare in longitudinal analysis.[66] Weakness and joint disease activity were the best predictors of a high IFN score from blood in JDM.[17] Untreated JDM muscle biopsies had higher type I and type II IFN scores, both associated with muscle biopsy pathology and higher disease activity, whereas only type II IFN scores correlated with longer time to clinically inactive disease.[67] A UK group found MxA (myxovirus-resistance protein A) staining of JDM muscle biopsies by immunohistochemistry correlated inversely with muscle strength measurements.[68] Type I and type II IFN signatures are high in untreated JDM blood and muscle, correlating with disease activity and angiogenic changes.

Endothelial Markers

Endothelial dysfunction and vasculopathy are prominent in JDM. Low soluble intercellular adhesion molecule 1 (ICAM-1) and high endoglin levels are associated with increased vasculopathy assessed by nailfold capillary end-row loop scoring.[69] Endothelial injury markers (von Willebrand factor (vWF) antigen and circulating endothelial cells) correlate with extramuscular activity, whereas circulating endothelial progenitor cells negatively correlate with muscle activity.[70] Endothelial activation with elevated vascular cell adhesion molecule (VCAM)-1 was higher with shorter duration of un-treated JDM (early in disease) in JDM muscle biopsy.[71] Peripherally, endothelial acti-vation (VCAM-1) and inhibition of angiogenesis (angiopoietin-2, soluble vascular endothelial growth factor receptor 1 (VEGFR-1)) also relate to JDM disease activity.[72] As described previously, vasculopathy is a prominent feature of JDM with multiple endothelial markers that correlate to disease activity.

Immune Cells

Immature transitional B cells are expanded in pretreatment baseline JDM peripheral blood correlating with disease activity.[73] Genes related to B-cell survival, including BAFF, correlate with disease activity.[74] Increased plasmablasts correlate with some T-helper subsets and disease activity in JDM.[75] Although peripheral T-regulatory cells were found in the same proportion as controls, those cells from active JDM patients were found to be functionally impaired.[76] There are multiple immune cell subset changes in JDM, including B-cell and T-cell differences in level or function, which correlate with disease activity.

TREATMENT

There are few clinical trials to inform optimal treatment of JDM; therefore, treatment is largely based on empiric and expert opinion. Consensus recommendations and key clinical trial results are summarized.

Consensus Recommendations

Over the past decade, CARRA,[77–79] Single Hub and Access point for paediatric Rheu-matology in Europe (SHARE),[80] the JDM working group of the Society for Pediatric Rheumatology[81] and others have published standardized treatment approaches. Initial therapy for the average patient presenting with JDM typically includes a combi-nation of steroids and methotrexate, with escalation or modification of therapy for resistant disease. See **Figs. 1 and 2** for summaries of the CARRA and SHARE treat-ment recommendations.

Clinical Trials

The Rituximab Therapy in Refractory Adult and Juvenile Idiopathic Inflammatory Myopathy Trial was a randomized, double blind, placebo-phase trial[82] for treatment of refractory myositis, which included 48 children. Although the study did not meet the primary outcome and definition of improvement, post hoc analyses suggest pre-dictors of rituximab response included anti–Jo-1 and anti–Mi-2 or other antibodies compared with autoantibody negative patients.[83] The findings suggest a role for B-cell–depleting therapy for subsets of patients with JDM.

The PRINTO Network completed an international, multicenter, randomized, open-label superiority trial using steroids with or without methotrexate or cyclosporine,[84] enrolling 139 newly diagnosed JDM patients from 54 centers and 22 countries. The study confirmed the combination treatment with steroids and either methotrexate or cyclosporine to be superior to steroid monotherapy and methotrexate was more effec-tive with less adverse events compared with cyclosporine.

Other Immunomodulatory Therapies

Intravenous immunoglobulin (IVIG) commonly is used as adjunctive treatment of JDM, but its efficacy is not well studied. A retrospective inception cohort of 78 Canadian JDM patients was assessed[85] to determine whether IVIG-treated patients had less

---

MODERATE JDM

Plan 1
Methotrexate[a] 15 mg/m^2 or 1 mg/kg weekly
AND
Prednisone[b] 2 mg/kg/d for 4 wk then decrease by 20%

Plan 2
Plan 1 AND
IV methylprednisolone 30 mg/kg for 3 d, then weekly[c]

Plan 3
Plan 2 AND
IVIG 2 g/kg[d] q2wk X 3 doses then monthly

SKIN PREDOMINANT JDM

Plan 1
Hydroxychloroquine 5 mg/kg/d[e]

Plan 2
Plan 1 AND
Methotrexate[a] 15 mg/m^2 or 1 mg/kg weekly

Plan 3
Plan 2 AND
Prednisone[b] 2 mg/kg/d for 4 wk then decrease by 20%

SKIN RESISTANT JDM

Plan 1
IVIG 2 g/kg[d] q2wks X 3 doses then monthly

Plan 2
Plan 1 AND
Mycophenolate mofetil[f] BID 10 mg/kg/dose OR 600 mg/m^2

Plan 3
Cyclosporine 3 mg/kg[g]

Fig. 1. Recommended consensus treatment plans from CARRA, for JDM patients with moderate, skin-predominant, and skin-resistant disease. IV, intravenous; IG, immunoglobulin. [a] Lesser of 15 mg/m^2 or 1 mg/kg (max 40 mg), [b]max 60mg, [c]optional, [d]max 70 grams, [e]max 400mg, [f]max 1500mg bid, [g]higher doses based on toxicity, efficacy.

disease activity and achieved inactive disease sooner than patients not treated with IVIG. Marginal structural modeling showed IVIG-treated patients started with greater disease activity compared with patients not treated with IVIG. After controlling for confounding, IVIG-treated patients maintained similar or lower disease activity compared with controls.

Mycophenolate mofetil is used to treat JDM patients with resistant and refractory disease. A small case series of 8 patients published in 2012[86] suggested mycophenolate mofetil was safe and efficacious with improvement in strength and the ability to wean steroids.

Cyclophosphamide typically is reserved for severe or resistant disease, with limited published efficacy data. Cyclophosphamide was used to treat 19 steroid-resistant JDM patients from a single Japanese hospital[87] and considered effective, including 4 patients whose interstitial pneumonitis resolved with treatment. However, 8 patients with calcinosis progressed without improvement. 56 patients from a UK JDM cohort received cyclophosphamide and showed improvement in global, skin, and muscle disease activity, with the greatest benefit in skin disease and global disease activity at 12 months.[88]

The use of biologic agents to treat refractory JDM is evolving. Two small studies suggested that etanercept was not beneficial and could cause worsening of

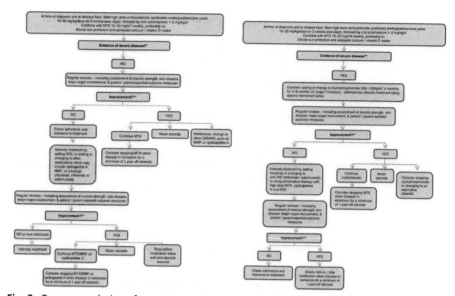

Fig. 2. Recommendations from SHARE, for treatment of JDM, ranging from mild to severe disease.* such as major organ involvement / extensive ulcerative skin disease; ** improvement based on clinical opinion. DMARD, disease modifying antirheumatic drug; MMF, mycophenolate mofetil; MTX, methotrexate.

disease.[89,90] Other anti-TNF therapies, however, show promise for resistant disease. A retrospective analysis of 60 JDM patients treated with adalimumab or infliximab in the United Kingdom demonstrated benefit,[91] including improvement of calcinosis. Smaller case reports and series also suggest anti-TNF therapies may be useful in resistant cases.[92,93]

Single case reports of the benefit of abatacept in the treatment of JDM with associated calcinosis have been reported[44,94] and a larger pilot trial is under way (NCT02594735).

The use of Janus kinase inhibitors (JAKinibs) to treat JDM is increasing.[95–98] In a 2020 case series, of 25 refractory JDM patients treated with JAKinibs, 96% (24/25) reported improvement and 66.7% (16/24) had complete resolution of rash.[99,100] Kim and colleagues[95] reported 4 patients with chronically active JDM in a compassionate use study of baricitinib, which also supported JAKinibs efficacy, according to physician, patient, and extramuscular VAS, as well as skin scoring measures, biomarker response, and MRI.

Exercise

JDM patients may have long-term issues with exercise intolerance, muscle weakness, and fatigue, despite aggressive treatment and apparent clinical remission.[101,102] A growing body of evidence suggests a role for exercise training as an important non-pharmacologic adjunct treatment of JDM,[103–107] without causing flares in disease.

LONG-TERM OUTCOMES

Long-term outcomes reported from several international JDM cohorts[108–116] over the past decade continue to show suboptimal outcomes and long-term morbidity. These patient cohorts, followed for 3.7 to nearly 17 years, have chronic or polycyclic disease course in up to two-thirds of patients, suggesting that monocyclic disease course and remission are uncommon.

Although 60% of PRINTO's 490 patient cohort had no impairment (Childhood Health Assessment Questionnaire [CHAQ] score = 0) after a mean disease duration of 7.7 years (range 2–25.2 y), approximately 7% had severe functional impairment (CHAQ score >1.5).[108] Adult JDM patients from 2 US adult referral subspecialty centers (n = 49)[109] had mild to moderate disability (median American College of Rheumatology [ACR] functional class 2, Health Assessment Questionnaire 0.4). More than half of JDM patients have reduced endurance and ongoing weakness,[108,113] with up to 10% reporting severe impairment[113] at long-term follow-up, after a median of at least 6 years disease duration (range 2–25.2 y)[108,113] in 2 cohorts. These findings suggest that although some JDM patients have good functional outcomes, a subset of patients continue to have significant impairment due to JDM.

Cumulative damage at long-term follow-up, after a median of at least 6 years (range 2–25.2 years) disease duration,[108,113] is common, reported in up to 69% of patients.[108,113] Cutaneous damage also is frequent in these published JDM cohorts, including calcinosis and lipodystrophy, reported in up to 2% to 60% and 10% to 33% of patient, respectively.[108,109,113,114] Long-term musculoskeletal damage based on MRI findings is present in up to 52% of patients[110] and joint contractures in 18% to 63%.[108,109] There also is long-term growth delay in 8% to 40% of long-term cohorts followed for a median of at least 6 years (range 2–25 years).[108,109,114,115] In summary, the long-term damage described in JDM patients likely is related to many factors, including disease activity as well as medication toxicity from corticosteroids. The high frequency of damage in these cohorts point to the urgent need for better JDM treatments.

Although mortality rates for JDM have improved since the 1960s, when it was reported in one-third of patients,[117] current rates remain unacceptably high. The JDM specific mortality rate from the National Institutes of Health natural history questionnaire–based protocols administered between 1989 and 2011 was estimated at 2.4%, most commonly attributed to ILD.[118] In other cohorts, death was attributed to severe JDM manifestations, including cutaneous ulceration with infections, gastrointestinal vasculitis, and lung disease, including ILD and respiratory failure.[114–116,118] The dramatic differences in mortality ranging from 2[118] to 11%,[114–116] suggest not only differences in patient populations, but disparities in access to care and treatment.

Risk factors for worse outcomes

The trajectory of disease is variable in JDM and it is challenging to predict long-term patient outcomes. Predicting treatment resistance or poor outcomes earlier in the course of disease could help guide treatment decisions to improve long-term prognosis.

There are inconsistent reports of age-based risk for worse outcomes in several cohorts that suggest possible regional or environmental differences contributing to worse outcome, and additional study is necessary.[109,112,118,119]

Longer disease duration, including chronic or continuous disease course, predicted long-term damage and worse outcomes, including functional impairment and death, in several cohorts.[108,109,112,113,118] Similarly, calcinosis is reported to be less common in patients with a monocyclic course.[115] High disease activity, according to muscle and total DAS scores, 1 year after diagnosis predicted poor outcomes in a Norwegian cohort.[110] Worse baseline ACR functional class and baseline skin disease and severity (including erythroderma, heliotrope rash, and shawl sign) also were found to predict damage and risk for mortality in JDM.[109,118] These findings suggest that patients with delayed or severe disease at diagnosis or persistent disease activity at 1 year may benefit from proactive, aggressive treatment to achieve rapid disease control and remission that may help limit unsatisfactory outcomes.

Ravelli and colleagues[108] reported female patients had more long-term functional impairment and worse health-related QoL. The JDM CARRA Registry found that higher mean UV radiation exposure 1 month prior to disease onset increased calcinosis risk and varied by race.[58] Decreased end row loops (ERLs) in nail fold capillaries at JDM diagnosis was associated with longer untreated disease and more active skin disease compared with children with normal ERLs.[120] The UK Juvenile Dermatomyositis Cohort and Biomarker Study found differences in muscle biopsy scores when comparing MSA subgroups and increased severity of the histopathologic features predictive of longer treatment duration.[18] Weight loss was found an early illness feature associated with mortality.[118] These findings suggest that the clinical history, physical examination at onset, and diagnostic work-up may be useful to inform treatment recommendations and help to improve future long-term outcomes.

Earlier prognostication with modifications in therapy tailored to each patients' risk for worse outcome may be possible if the current wide-ranging predictors are validated in future studies. Additional research is needed to identify more effective treatment approaches targeted toward these patients at risk for worse outcomes.

SUMMARY

JDM is a heterogeneous disease with new classification criteria and updates in MSA and MAA groups, helping define clinical subgroups. There are many validated assessment tools for assessing disease activity in JDM. Future studies will optimize the tools, improving feasibility of use in clinical and research contexts. Genetic and environmental risk factors, mechanisms of muscle pathology, role of IFN, vascular markers, and changes in immune cells provide insights to JDM pathogenesis. Outcomes have improved, but chronic disease activity, damage, and mortality highlight the need for improved predictors of outcome and treatment efficacy. Increased international collaboration of patients, clinicians, scientists, and other key stakeholders in patient registries and biorepositories as well as clinical trials may overcome current barriers that exist for improving research, treatment, and outcomes for this rare condition.

CLINICS CARE POINTS

- Validated tools should be used for the clinical assessment of children with JDM.
- Identification of specific JDM phenotypes using MSA and clinical features may help to predict course and outcome and influence treatment decisions.
- Prompt diagnosis and treatment are needed to improve long-term outcomes in JDM.
- Guidelines and recommendations developed through expert opinion and consensus should be used to treat JDM patients.

DISCLOSURE

This research was support in part by the Intramural Research Program of the National Institutes of Health (NIH), National Institute of Arthritis and Musculoskeletal and Skin diseases (NIAMS). H.K. has been part of a clinical study at NIAMS that received grant support for under a government CRADA from Eli Lilly. The authors have no other disclosures.

REFERENCES

1. Rider LG, Shah M, Mamyrova G, et al. The myositis autoantibody phenotypes of the juvenile idiopathic inflammatory myopathies. Medicine (Baltimore) 2013; 92(4):223–43.
2. Tansley SL, Simou S, Shaddick G, et al. Autoantibodies in juvenile-onset myositis: their diagnostic value and associated clinical phenotype in a large UK cohort. J Autoimmun 2017;84:55–64.
3. Rider LG, Katz JD, Jones OY. Developments in the classification and treatment of the juvenile idiopathic inflammatory myopathies. Rheum Dis Clin North Am 2013;39(4):877–904.
4. Bohan A, Peter JB. Polymyositis and dermatomyositis (second of two parts). N Engl J Med 1975;292(8):403–7.
5. Lundberg IE, Tjarnlund A, Bottai M, et al. 2017 European League Against Rheumatism/American College of Rheumatology classification criteria for adult and juvenile idiopathic inflammatory myopathies and their major subgroups. Ann Rheum Dis 2017;76(12):1955–64.
6. Sag E, Demir S, Bilginer Y, et al. Validation of the EULAR/ACR 2017 idiopathic inflammatory myopathy classification criteria in juvenile dermatomyositis patients. Clin Exp Rheumatol 2021 May-Jun;39(3):688–94.
7. Mamyrova G, Kishi T, Shi M, et al. Childhood Myositis Heterogeneity Collaborative Study Group. Anti-MDA5 autoantibodies associated with juvenile dermatomyositis constitute a distinct phenotype in North America. Rheumatology (Oxford) 2021 Apr 6;60(4):1839–49.
8. Kishi T, Rider LG, Pak K, et al. Association of Anti-3-Hydroxy-3-Methylglutaryl-coenzyme a reductase autoantibodies with DRB1*07:01 and severe myositis in juvenile myositis patients. Arthritis Care Res (Hoboken) 2017;69(7):1088–94.
9. Habers GE, Huber AM, Mamyrova G, et al. Brief report: association of myositis autoantibodies, clinical features, and environmental exposures at illness onset with disease course in juvenile myositis. Arthritis Rheumatol 2016;68(3):761–8.
10. Tansley SL, Betteridge ZE, Gunawardena H, et al. Anti-MDA5 autoantibodies in juvenile dermatomyositis identify a distinct clinical phenotype: a prospective cohort study. Arthritis Res Ther 2014;16(4):R138.
11. Tansley SL, Betteridge ZE, Shaddick G, et al. Calcinosis in juvenile dermatomyositis is influenced by both anti-NXP2 autoantibody status and age at disease onset. Rheumatology (Oxford) 2014;53(12):2204–8.
12. Hussain A, Rawat A, Jindal AK, et al. Autoantibodies in children with juvenile dermatomyositis: a single centre experience from North-West India. Rheumatol Int 2017;37(5):807–12.
13. Srivastava P, Dwivedi S, Misra R. Myositis-specific and myositis-associated autoantibodies in Indian patients with inflammatory myositis. Rheumatol Int 2016; 36(7):935–43.
14. Iwata N, Nakaseko H, Kohagura T, et al. Clinical subsets of juvenile dermatomyositis classified by myositis-specific autoantibodies: experience at a single center in Japan. Mod Rheumatol 2019;29(5):802–7.
15. Kobayashi I, Okura Y, Yamada M, et al. Anti-melanoma differentiation-associated gene 5 antibody is a diagnostic and predictive marker for interstitial

lung diseases associated with juvenile dermatomyositis. J Pediatr 2011;158(4): 675–7.

16. Shah M, Targoff IN, Rice MM, et al. Childhood Myositis Heterogeneity Collaborative Study G. Brief report: ultraviolet radiation exposure is associated with clinical and autoantibody phenotypes in juvenile myositis. Arthritis Rheum 2013; 65(7):1934–41.

17. Kim H, Gunter-Rahman F, McGrath JA, et al. Expression of interferon-regulated genes in juvenile dermatomyositis versus Mendelian autoinflammatory interferonopathies. Arthritis Res Ther 2020;22(1):69.

18. Deakin CT, Yasin SA, Simou S, et al. Muscle biopsy findings in combination with myositis-specific autoantibodies aid prediction of outcomes in juvenile dermatomyositis. Arthritis Rheumatol 2016;68(11):2806–16.

19. Fujimoto M, Matsushita T, Hamaguchi Y, et al. Autoantibodies to small ubiquitin-like modifier activating enzymes in Japanese patients with dermatomyositis: comparison with a UK Caucasian cohort. Ann Rheum Dis 2013;72(1):151–3.

20. Tansley SL, Li D, Betteridge ZE, et al. The reliability of immunoassays to detect autoantibodies in patients with myositis is dependent on autoantibody specificity. Rheumatology (Oxford) 2020;59(8):2109–14.

21. Yeker RM, Pinal-Fernandez I, Kishi T, et al. Anti-NT5C1A autoantibodies are associated with more severe disease in patients with juvenile myositis. Ann Rheum Dis 2018;77(5):714–9.

22. Sabbagh S, Pinal-Fernandez I, Kishi T, et al. Anti-Ro52 autoantibodies are associated with interstitial lung disease and more severe disease in patients with juvenile myositis. Ann Rheum Dis 2019;78(7):988–95.

23. Rider LG, Werth VP, Huber AM, et al. Measures of adult and juvenile dermatomyositis, polymyositis, and inclusion body myositis: physician and Patient/Parent Global Activity, Manual Muscle Testing (MMT), Health Assessment Questionnaire (HAQ)/Childhood Health Assessment Questionnaire (C-HAQ), Childhood Myositis Assessment Scale (CMAS), Myositis Disease Activity Assessment Tool (MDAAT), Disease Activity Score (DAS), Short Form 36 (SF-36), Child Health Questionnaire (CHQ), physician global damage, Myositis Damage Index (MDI), Quantitative Muscle Testing (QMT), Myositis Functional Index-2 (FI-2), Myositis Activities Profile (MAP), Inclusion Body Myositis Functional Rating Scale (IBMFRS), Cutaneous Dermatomyositis Disease Area and Severity Index (CDASI), Cutaneous Assessment Tool (CAT), Dermatomyositis Skin Severity Index (DSSI), Skindex, and Dermatology Life Quality Index (DLQI). Arthritis Care Res (Hoboken) 2011;63(Suppl 11):S118–57.

24. Miller FW, Rider LG, Chung YL, et al. Proposed preliminary core set measures for disease outcome assessment in adult and juvenile idiopathic inflammatory myopathies. Rheumatology (Oxford) 2001;40(11):1262–73.

25. Ruperto N, Ravelli A, Murray KJ, et al. Preliminary core sets of measures for disease activity and damage assessment in juvenile systemic lupus erythematosus and juvenile dermatomyositis. Rheumatology (Oxford) 2003;42(12):1452–9.

26. McCann LJ, Arnold K, Pilkington CA, et al. Developing a provisional, international minimal dataset for Juvenile Dermatomyositis: for use in clinical practice to inform research. Pediatr Rheumatol Online J 2014;12:31.

27. McCann LJ, Kirkham JJ, Wedderburn LR, et al. Development of an internationally agreed minimal dataset for juvenile dermatomyositis (JDM) for clinical and research use. Trials 2015;16:268.

28. McCann LJ, Pilkington CA, Huber AM, et al. Development of a consensus core dataset in juvenile dermatomyositis for clinical use to inform research. Ann Rheum Dis 2018;77(2):241–50.
29. Varnier GC, Rosina S, Ferrari C, et al. Development and testing of a hybrid measure of muscle strength in juvenile dermatomyositis for use in routine care. Arthritis Care Res (Hoboken) 2018;70(9):1312–9.
30. Rosina S, Consolaro A, van Dijkhuizen P, et al. Development and validation of a composite disease activity score for measurement of muscle and skin involvement in juvenile dermatomyositis. Rheumatology (Oxford) 2019;58(7):1196–205.
31. Rosina S, Varnier GC, Pistorio A, et al. Pediatric Rheumatology International Trials Organization (PRINTO). Development and Testing of Reduced Versions of the Manual Muscle Test-8 in Juvenile Dermatomyositis. J Rheumatol 2021 Jun; 48(6):898–906.
32. Robinson AB, Hoeltzel MF, Wahezi DM, et al. Clinical characteristics of children with juvenile dermatomyositis: the Childhood Arthritis and Rheumatology Research Alliance Registry. Arthritis Care Res (Hoboken) 2014;66(3):404–10.
33. Malattia C, Damasio MB, Madeo A, et al. Whole-body MRI in the assessment of disease activity in juvenile dermatomyositis. Ann Rheum Dis 2014;73(6): 1083–90.
34. Thyoka M, Adekunle O, Pilkington C, et al. Introduction of a novel magnetic resonance imaging-based scoring system for assessing disease activity in children with juvenile dermatomyositis. Rheumatology (Oxford) 2018;57(9):1661–8.
35. Davis WR, Halls JE, Offiah AC, et al. Assessment of active inflammation in juvenile dermatomyositis: a novel magnetic resonance imaging-based scoring system. Rheumatology (Oxford) 2011;50(12):2237–44.
36. Wedderburn LR, Varsani H, Li CK, et al. International consensus on a proposed score system for muscle biopsy evaluation in patients with juvenile dermatomyositis: a tool for potential use in clinical trials. Arthritis Rheum 2007;57(7): 1192–201.
37. Varsani H, Charman SC, Li CK, et al. Validation of a score tool for measurement of histological severity in juvenile dermatomyositis and association with clinical severity of disease. Ann Rheum Dis 2015;74(1):204–10.
38. Huber AM, Dugan EM, Lachenbruch PA, et al. Preliminary validation and clinical meaning of the Cutaneous Assessment Tool in juvenile dermatomyositis. Arthritis Rheum 2008;59(2):214–21.
39. Klein RQ, Bangert CA, Costner M, et al. Comparison of the reliability and validity of outcome instruments for cutaneous dermatomyositis. Br J Dermatol 2008; 159(4):887–94.
40. Bode RK, Klein-Gitelman MS, Miller ML, et al. Disease activity score for children with juvenile dermatomyositis: reliability and validity evidence. Arthritis Rheum 2003;49(1):7–15.
41. Tiao J, Feng R, Berger EM, et al. Evaluation of the reliability of the Cutaneous Dermatomyositis Disease Area and Severity Index and the Cutaneous Assessment Tool-Binary Method in juvenile dermatomyositis among paediatric dermatologists, rheumatologists and neurologists. Br J Dermatol 2017;177(4): 1086–92.
42. Goreshi R, Okawa J, Rose M, et al. Evaluation of reliability, validity, and responsiveness of the CDASI and the CAT-BM. J Invest Dermatol 2012;132(4):1117–24.
43. Ahmed S, Chen KL, Werth VP. The validity and utility of the Cutaneous Disease Area and Severity Index (CDASI) as a clinical outcome instrument in dermatomyositis: a comprehensive review. Semin Arthritis Rheum 2020;50(3):458–62.

44. Apaz MT, Saad-Magalhaes C, Pistorio A, et al. Health-related quality of life of patients with juvenile dermatomyositis: results from the Pediatric Rheumatology International Trials Organisation multinational quality of life cohort study. Arthritis Rheum 2009;61(4):501–17.

45. Tory HO, Carrasco R, Griffin T, et al. Comparing the importance of quality measurement themes in juvenile idiopathic inflammatory myositis between patients and families and healthcare professionals. Pediatr Rheumatol Online J 2018; 16(1):28.

46. Tory H, Zurakowski D, Kim S, et al. Patient and physician discordance of global disease assessment in juvenile dermatomyositis: findings from the Childhood Arthritis & Rheumatology Research Alliance Legacy Registry. Pediatr Rheumatol Online J 2020;18(1):5.

47. Lazarevic D, Pistorio A, Palmisani E, et al. The PRINTO criteria for clinically inactive disease in juvenile dermatomyositis. Ann Rheum Dis 2013;72(5):686–93.

48. Almeida B, Campanilho-Marques R, Arnold K, et al. Analysis of published criteria for clinically inactive disease in a large juvenile dermatomyositis cohort shows that skin disease is underestimated. Arthritis Rheumatol 2015;67(9): 2495–502.

49. Ruperto N, Pistorio A, Ravelli A, et al. The Paediatric Rheumatology International Trials Organisation provisional criteria for the evaluation of response to therapy in juvenile dermatomyositis. Arthritis Care Res (Hoboken) 2010;62(11):1533–41.

50. Rider LG, Aggarwal R, Pistorio A, et al. 2016 American College of Rheumatology/European League Against Rheumatism Criteria for Minimal, Moderate, and Major Clinical Response in Juvenile Dermatomyositis: An International Myositis Assessment and Clinical Studies Group/Paediatric Rheumatology International Trials Organisation Collaborative Initiative. Arthritis Rheumatol 2017; 69(5):911–23.

51. Rider LG, Aggarwal R, Pistorio A, et al. 2016 American College of Rheumatology/European League Against Rheumatism Criteria for Minimal, Moderate, and Major Clinical Response in Juvenile Dermatomyositis: An International Myositis Assessment and Clinical Studies Group/Paediatric Rheumatology International Trials Organisation Collaborative Initiative. Ann Rheum Dis 2017;76(5): 782–91.

52. Rider LG, Ruperto N, Pistorio A, et al. 2016 ACR-EULAR adult dermatomyositis and polymyositis and juvenile dermatomyositis response criteria-methodological aspects. Rheumatology (Oxford) 2017;56(11):1884–93.

53. Niewold TB, Wu SC, Smith M, et al. Familial aggregation of autoimmune disease in juvenile dermatomyositis. Pediatrics 2011;127(5):e1239–46.

54. Miller FW, Chen W, O'Hanlon TP, et al. Genome-wide association study identifies HLA 8.1 ancestral haplotype alleles as major genetic risk factors for myositis phenotypes. Genes Immun 2015;16(7):470–80.

55. Miller FW, Cooper RG, Vencovsky J, et al. Genome-wide association study of dermatomyositis reveals genetic overlap with other autoimmune disorders. Arthritis Rheum 2013;65(12):3239–47.

56. Lintner KE, Patwardhan A, Rider LG, et al. Gene copy-number variations (CNVs) of complement C4 and C4A deficiency in genetic risk and pathogenesis of juvenile dermatomyositis. Ann Rheum Dis 2016;75(9):1599–606.

57. Mamyrova G, Rider LG, Ehrlich A, et al. Environmental factors associated with disease flare in juvenile and adult dermatomyositis. Rheumatology (Oxford) 2017;56(8):1342–7.

58. Neely J, Long CS, Sturrock H, et al. Association of short-term ultraviolet radiation exposure and disease severity in juvenile dermatomyositis: results from the childhood arthritis and rheumatology research alliance legacy registry. Arthritis Care Res 2019;71(12):1600–5.

59. Orione MA, Silva CA, Sallum AM, et al. Risk factors for juvenile dermatomyositis: exposure to tobacco and air pollutants during pregnancy. Arthritis Care Res (Hoboken) 2014;66(10):1571–5.

60. Gitiaux C, Kostallari E, Lafuste P, et al. Whole microvascular unit deletions in dermatomyositis. Ann Rheum Dis 2013;72(3):445–52.

61. Emslie-Smith AM, Engel AG. Microvascular changes in early and advanced dermatomyositis: a quantitative study. Ann Neurol 1990;27(4):343–56.

62. De Luna N, Suarez-Calvet X, Lleixa C, et al. Hypoxia triggers IFN-I production in muscle: Implications in dermatomyositis. Sci Rep 2017;7(1):8595.

63. Preusse C, Allenbach Y, Hoffmann O, et al. Differential roles of hypoxia and innate immunity in juvenile and adult dermatomyositis. Acta Neuropathol Commun 2016;4(1):45.

64. Reed AM, Peterson E, Bilgic H, et al. Changes in novel biomarkers of disease activity in juvenile and adult dermatomyositis are sensitive biomarkers of disease course. Arthritis Rheum 2012;64(12):4078–86.

65. Gitiaux C, Latroche C, Weiss-Gayet M, et al. Myogenic progenitor cells exhibit Type I interferon-driven proangiogenic properties and molecular signature during juvenile dermatomyositis. Arthritis Rheumatol 2018;70(1):134–45.

66. Wienke J, Bellutti Enders F, Lim J, et al. Galectin-9 and CXCL10 as biomarkers for disease activity in juvenile dermatomyositis: a longitudinal cohort study and multicohort validation. Arthritis Rheumatol 2019;71(8):1377–90.

67. Moneta GM, Pires Marafon D, Marasco E, et al. Muscle expression of Type I and Type II interferons is increased in juvenile dermatomyositis and related to clinical and histologic features. Arthritis Rheumatol 2019;71(6):1011–21.

68. Soponkanaporn S, Deakin CT, Schutz PW, et al. Expression of myxovirus-resistance protein A: a possible marker of muscle disease activity and autoantibody specificities in juvenile dermatomyositis. Neuropathol Appl Neurobiol 2019;45(4):410–20.

69. Wienke J, Pachman LM, Morgan GA, et al. Endothelial and inflammation biomarker profiles at diagnosis reflecting clinical heterogeneity and serving as a prognostic tool for treatment response in two independent cohorts of patients with juvenile dermatomyositis. Arthritis Rheumatol 2020;72(7):1214–26.

70. Kishi T, Chipman J, Evereklian M, et al. Endothelial activation markers as disease activity and damage measures in juvenile dermatomyositis. J Rheumatol 2020;47(7):1011–8.

71. Kim E, Cook-Mills J, Morgan G, et al. Increased expression of vascular cell adhesion molecule 1 in muscle biopsy samples from juvenile dermatomyositis patients with short duration of untreated disease is regulated by miR-126. Arthritis Rheum 2012;64(11):3809–17.

72. Wienke J, Mertens JS, Garcia S, et al. Biomarker profiles of endothelial activation and dysfunction in rare systemic autoimmune diseases: implications for cardiovascular risk. Rheumatology (Oxford) 2021 Feb 1;60(2):785–801.

73. Piper CJM, Wilkinson MGL, Deakin CT, et al. CD19(+)CD24(hi)CD38(hi) B cells are expanded in juvenile dermatomyositis and exhibit a pro-inflammatory phenotype after activation through toll-like receptor 7 and interferon-alpha. Front Immunol 2018;9:1372.

74. Lopez De Padilla CM, McNallan KT, Crowson CS, et al. BAFF expression correlates with idiopathic inflammatory myopathy disease activity measures and autoantibodies. J Rheumatol 2013;40(3):294–302.

75. Morita R, Schmitt N, Bentebibel SE, et al. Human blood CXCR5(+)CD4(+) T cells are counterparts of T follicular cells and contain specific subsets that differentially support antibody secretion. Immunity 2011;34(1):108–21.

76. Vercoulen Y, Bellutti Enders F, Meerding J, et al. Increased presence of FOXP3+ regulatory T cells in inflamed muscle of patients with active juvenile dermatomyositis compared to peripheral blood. PLoS One 2014;9(8):e105353.

77. Huber AM, Kim S, Reed AM, et al. Childhood arthritis and rheumatology research alliance consensus clinical treatment plans for juvenile dermatomyositis with persistent skin rash. J Rheumatol 2017;44(1):110–6.

78. Kim S, Kahn P, Robinson AB, et al. Childhood Arthritis and Rheumatology Research Alliance consensus clinical treatment plans for juvenile dermatomyositis with skin predominant disease. Pediatr Rheumatol Online J 2017;15(1):1.

79. Huber AM, Giannini EH, Bowyer SL, et al. Protocols for the initial treatment of moderately severe juvenile dermatomyositis: results of a Children's Arthritis and Rheumatology Research Alliance Consensus Conference. Arthritis Care Res (Hoboken) 2010;62(2):219–25.

80. Bellutti Enders F, Bader-Meunier B, Baildam E, et al. Consensus-based recommendations for the management of juvenile dermatomyositis. Ann Rheum Dis 2017;76(2):329–40.

81. Hinze CH, Oommen PT, Dressler F, et al. Development of practice and consensus-based strategies including a treat-to-target approach for the management of moderate and severe juvenile dermatomyositis in Germany and Austria. Pediatr Rheumatol Online J 2018;16(1):40.

82. Oddis CV, Reed AM, Aggarwal R, et al. Rituximab in the treatment of refractory adult and juvenile dermatomyositis and adult polymyositis: a randomized, placebo-phase trial. Arthritis Rheum 2013;65(2):314–24.

83. Aggarwal R, Bandos A, Reed AM, et al. Predictors of clinical improvement in rituximab-treated refractory adult and juvenile Dermatomyositis and adult polymyositis. Arthritis Rheumatol 2014;66(3):740–9.

84. Ruperto N, Pistorio A, Oliveira S, et al. Prednisone versus prednisone plus ciclosporin versus prednisone plus methotrexate in new-onset juvenile dermatomyositis: a randomised trial. The Lancet 2016;387(10019):671–8.

85. Lam CG, Manlhiot C, Pullenayegum EM, et al. Efficacy of intravenous Ig therapy in juvenile dermatomyositis. Ann Rheum Dis 2011;70(12):2089–94.

86. Dagher R, Desjonquères M, Duquesne A, et al. Mycophenolate mofetil in juvenile dermatomyositis: a case series. Rheumatol Int 2012;32(3):711–6.

87. Kishi T, Miyamae T, Hara R, et al. Clinical analysis of 50 children with juvenile dermatomyositis. Mod Rheumatol 2013;23(2):311–7.

88. Deakin C, Campanilho-Marques R, Simou S, et al. Efficacy and safety of cyclophosphamide treatment in severe juvenile dermatomyositis shown by marginal structural modeling. Arthritis Rheumatol 2018;70(5):785–93.

89. Rouster-Stevens KA, Ferguson L, Morgan G, et al. Pilot study of etanercept in patients with refractory juvenile dermatomyositis. Arthritis Care Res (Hoboken) 2014 May;66(5):783–7.

90. Liu SW, Velez NF, Lam C, et al. Dermatomyositis induced by anti-tumor necrosis factor in a patient with juvenile idiopathic arthritis. JAMA Dermatol 2013 Oct; 149(10):1204–8.

91. Campanilho-Marques R, Deakin CT, Simou S, et al. Retrospective analysis of infliximab and adalimumab treatment in a large cohort of juvenile dermatomyositis patients. Arthritis Res Ther 2020;22(1):79.

92. Boulter EL, Beard L, Ryder C, et al. Effectiveness of anti-TNF-α agents in the treatment of refractory juvenile dermatomyositis. Pediatr Rheumatol 9, O29 2011.

93. Riley P, McCann LJ, Maillard SM, et al. Effectiveness of infliximab in the treatment of refractory juvenile dermatomyositis with calcinosis. Rheumatology (Oxford) 2008 Jun;47(6):877–80.

94. Sukumaran S, Vijayan V. Abatacept in the Treatment of juvenile dermatomyositis-associated calcifications in a 16-year-old girl. Case Rep Rheumatol 2020; 2020:1–4.

95. Kim H, Dill S, O'Brien M, et al. Janus kinase (JAK) inhibition with baricitinib in refractory juvenile dermatomyositis Annals of the Rheumatic Diseases 2021;80:406–8.

96. Papadopoulou C, Hong Y, Omoyinmi E, et al. Janus kinase 1/2 inhibition with baricitinib in the treatment of juvenile dermatomyositis. Brain 2019 Mar 1; 142(3):e8.

97. Aeschlimann FA, Frémond ML, Duffy D, et al. A child with severe juvenile dermatomyositis treated with ruxolitinib. Brain 2018 Nov 1;141(11):e80.

98. Yu Z, Wang L, Quan M, et al. Successful management with Janus kinase inhibitor tofacitinib in refractory juvenile dermatomyositis: a pilot study and literature review. Rheumatology (Oxford) 2021 Apr 6;60(4):1700–7.

99. Ding Y, Huang B, Wang Y, et al. Janus kinase inhibitor significantly improved rash and muscle strength in juvenile dermatomyositis. Ann Rheum Dis 2020 Oct 28;80(4):543–5. https://doi.org/10.1136/annrheumdis-2020-218582.

100. Levy DM, Bingham CA, Kahn PJ, et al. Favorable outcome of juvenile dermatomyositis treated without systemic corticosteroids. J Pediatr 2010;156(2):302–7.

101. Mathiesen PR, Ørngreen MC, Vissing J, et al. Aerobic fitness after JDM–a long-term follow-up study. Rheumatology (Oxford) 2013 Feb;52(2):287–95.

102. Berntsen KS, Tollisen A, Schwartz T, et al. Submaximal exercise capacity in juvenile dermatomyositis after longterm disease: the contribution of muscle, lung, and heart involvement. J Rheumatol 2017;44(6):827–34.

103. Omori C, Prado DML, Gualano B, et al. Responsiveness to exercise training in juvenile dermatomyositis: a twin case study. BMC Musculoskelet Disord 2010; 11:270.

104. Omori CH, Silva CAA, Sallum AME, et al. Exercise training in juvenile dermatomyositis. Arthritis Care Res (Hoboken) 2012 Aug;64(8):1186–94.

105. Riisager M, Mathiesen PR, Vissing J, et al. Aerobic training in persons who have recovered from juvenile dermatomyositis. Neuromuscul Disord 2013 Dec; 23(12):962–8.

106. Samhan A, Mohamed N, Elnaggar R, et al. Assessment of the clinical effects of aquatic-based exercises in the treatment of children with juvenile dermatomyositis: a 2×2 controlled-crossover trial. Arch Rheumatol 2020;35(1):97–106.

107. Habers EA, Van Brussel M, Langbroek-Amersfoort AC, et al. Design of the muscles in motion study: a randomized controlled trial to evaluate the efficacy and feasibility of an individually tailored home-based exercise training program for children and adolescents with juvenile dermatomyositis. BMC Musculoskelet Disord 2012;13:108.

108. Ravelli A, Trail L, Ferrari C, et al. Long-term outcome and prognostic factors of juvenile dermatomyositis: a multinational, multicenter study of 490 patients. Arthritis Care Res 2010;62(1):63–72.
109. Tsaltskan V, Aldous A, Serafi S, et al. Long-term outcomes in Juvenile Myositis patients. Semin Arthritis Rheum 2020;50(1):149–55.
110. Sanner H, Kirkhus E, Merckoll E, et al. Long-term muscular outcome and predisposing and prognostic factors in juvenile dermatomyositis: a case-control study. Arthritis Care Res 2010;62(8):1103–11.
111. Sanner H, Sjaastad I, Flatø B. Disease activity and prognostic factors in juvenile dermatomyositis: a long-term follow-up study applying the Paediatric Rheumatology International Trials Organization criteria for inactive disease and the myositis disease activity assessment tool. Rheumatology (United Kingdom) 2014;53(9):1578–85.
112. Mathiesen PR, Zak M, Herlin T, et al. Clinical features and outcome in a Danish cohort of juvenile dermatomyositis patients. Clin Exp Rheumatol 2010;28(5): 782–9.
113. Sharma A, Gupta A, Rawat A, et al. Long-term outcome in children with juvenile dermatomyositis: a single-center study from north India. Int J Rheum Dis 2020; 23(3):392–6.
114. Okong'o LO, Esser M, Wilmshurst J, et al. Characteristics and outcome of children with juvenile dermatomyositis in Cape Town: a cross-sectional study. Pediatr Rheumatol 2016;14(1):60.
115. Malek A, Raeeskarami SR, Ziaee V, et al. Clinical course and outcomes of Iranian children with juvenile dermatomyositis and polymyositis. Clin Rheumatol 2014;33(8):1113–8.
116. Singh S, Suri D, Aulakh R, et al. Mortality in children with juvenile dermatomyositis: two decades of experience from a single tertiary care centre in North India. Clin Rheumatol 2014;33(11):1675–9.
117. Bitnum S, Daeschner CW Jr, Travis LB, et al. Dermatomyositis. J Pediatr 1964; 64:101–31.
118. Huber AM, Mamyrova G, Lachenbruch PA, et al. Early illness features associated with mortality in the juvenile idiopathic inflammatory myopathies. Arthritis Care Res (Hoboken) 2014;66(5):732–40.
119. Patwardhan A, Rennebohm R, Dvorchik I, et al. Is juvenile dermatomyositis a different disease in children up to three years of age at onset than in children above three years at onset? A retrospective review of 23 years of a single center's experience. Pediatr Rheumatol 2012;10(1):34.
120. Ostrowski RA, Sullivan CL, Seshadri R, et al. Association of normal nailfold end row loop numbers with a shorter duration of untreated disease in children with juvenile dermatomyositis. Arthritis Rheum 2010;62(5):1533–8.

Chronic Nonbacterial Osteomyelitis

Insights into Pathogenesis, Assessment, and Treatment

Farzana Nuruzzaman, MD[a],*, Yongdong Zhao, MD, PHD[b],
Polly J. Ferguson, MD[c]

KEYWORDS

- Chronic nonbacterial osteomyelitis • Chronic recurrent multifocal osteomyelitis
- Autoinflammatory bone disease

KEY POINTS

- CNO is an autoinflammatory bone disorder that primarily occurs in childhood, but may persist into adulthood.
- CNO is a diagnosis of exclusion and symptoms often mimic other conditions including infectious osteomyelitis and malignancies.
- MRI is the imaging modality of choice because of sensitivity detecting lesions and distinguishing inflammation from normal physis in children.
- NSAIDs are first-line therapy. However, second-line treatments, such as DMARDs, biologic medications, and bisphosphonates, should be considered in children with severe disease.
- Inadequately treated CNO may lead to complications, such as pathologic fractures and limb-length discrepancy.

OVERVIEW

Chronic nonbacterial osteomyelitis (CNO) is an autoinflammatory bone disorder, which results from aberrant activation of the innate immune system.[1] CNO causes sterile skeletal inflammation characterized by bone pain and/or swelling that primarily

[a] Pediatric Rheumatology, Stony Brook Children's Hospital, Renaissance School of Medicine at Stony Brook University, 101 Nicolls Road, Health Sciences Tower T11-060, Stony Brook, NY 11794, USA; [b] Pediatric Rheumatology, Seattle Children's Hospital, University of Washington, 4800 Sand Point Way NE, MA.7.110 - Rheumatology, Seattle, WA 98105, USA; [c] Pediatrics - Rheumatology, Allergy and Immunology, University of Iowa Carver College of Medicine, Med Labs, 25 South Grand, Iowa City, IA 52242, USA
* Corresponding author.
E-mail address: farzana.nuruzzaman@stonybrookmedicine.edu

Rheum Dis Clin N Am 47 (2021) 691–705
https://doi.org/10.1016/j.rdc.2021.06.005
0889-857X/21/© 2021 Elsevier Inc. All rights reserved.

affects children. CNO was first described by Giedion and coworkers[2] in 1972. The term "chronic recurrent multifocal osteomyelitis," suggested by Probst and colleagues,[3] emphasized the recurrent nature of the disorder in its most severe form. However, patients with the disorder do not always have multiple bone lesions nor relapsing disease, so the term CNO is preferred as the umbrella term for all clinical presentations. This review focuses on recent insights into the pathogenesis of CNO and outlines recent advances and ongoing research contributing to the diagnosis, assessment of disease activity, and treatment.

EPIDEMIOLOGY

CNO is considered a rare disorder, although the exact prevalence and incidence is unknown; diagnostic delays are common, suggesting it is underrecognized.[4,5] Estimated incidences range from 0.4 to 2 per 100,000 children.[6,7] Disease onset of CNO typically occurs between 7 and 12 years of age, affecting girls approximately two times more frequently than boys.[8] Reports of CNO in the literature suggest that it affects multiple races and ethnicities.[9–11]

ETIOLOGY AND PATHOGENESIS

Although the exact cause of CNO remains unclear, there have been several recent developments leading to a clearer understanding of pathogenesis suggesting a multifactorial origin including cytokine dysregulation, osteoclastic activation, and genetic predisposition. Lack of sustained disease remission in patients with CNO treated with prolonged antibiotics supports a noninfectious cause.[12,13] Previous reports of the efficacy of azithromycin in CNO was likely related to the drug's anti-inflammatory rather than antimicrobial effects.[14] However, whether initial nonpathogenic infection leads to immune dysregulation and subsequent sterile osteomyelitis remains controversial. The common presence of *Cutibacterium acnes* within bone biopsy samples in adult patients classified with synovitis, acne, pustulosis, hyperostosis, osteitis (SAPHO) syndrome, thought to be a subgroup of CNO occurring mostly in adults, suggested that it may be associated with disease.[15] Although there are a few reports of *C acnes* in bone biopsies from pediatric patients, Girschick and colleagues[16] reported no evidence of a bacterial signature by molecular biology assays. The indirect role of microorganisms in the development of disease has not been well explored in CNO. Epigenetic factors may contribute to the development of disease in genetically predisposed individuals. Evidence showing the role of the microbiome in the alteration of immune homeostasis and development of inflammatory disease is expanding. Zeus and colleagues[17] reported that patients with CNO treated with nonsteroidal anti-inflammatory drugs (NSAIDs) had changes to the oral microbiome, although the causal relationship between perturbed microbiome and active CNO has not been established.

Cytokine Dysregulation

The pathogenesis of CNO seems to be related to a cytokine imbalance. Peripheral blood monocytes of patients with CNO usually have cytokine profiles characterized by overproduction of proinflammatory cytokines (interleukin [IL]-6, tumor necrosis factor [TNF], IL-1ß) and chemokines (IL-8, IP-10, membrane cofactor protein-1, macrophage inflammatory protein-1α and -1ß), and failure to produce immune regulatory cytokine IL-10 (and its homologue IL-19) in response to stimulation with lipopolysaccharide or toll-like receptor 4.[18–21] Decreased production of IL-10 (and IL-19) rises from decreased activation of the mitogen-activated protein kinase/extracellular signal regulated kinase pathway leading to reduced phosphorylation of signaling protein-1 and impaired recruitment to regulatory components within the IL-10 cytokine complex and the IL-10 gene promoters, and reduced phosphorylation of histone 3 at serine position 10 (H3S10). Less H3S10P phosphorylation results in epigenetic "closure" of the *IL10* promoter, which, in context with reduced availability of signaling protein-1, translates to decreased IL-10 expression.[22] Reduced expression of IL-10 and IL-19 contributes to enhanced NLRP3 inflammasome assembly and activation of caspase 1, leading to increased IL-1β release.[23,24] Proinflammatory cytokines TNF, IL-6, IL-20, and IL-1β increase the interaction of membrane-bound RANK receptors with their soluble ligand RANKL on osteoclast precursor cells leading to osteoclast differentiation and activation causing bone destruction.

Genetics

Evidence supporting a genetic component to CNO susceptibility is growing. The association of CNO with either a personal or family history of inflammatory disorders of skin (psoriasis) and intestine (inflammatory bowel disease) or inflammatory arthritis suggests a genetic predisposition to a spectrum of autoinflammatory conditions.[6]

Mutations in the filamin-binding LIM protein (FBLIM) 1 gene have been implicated in disease pathogenesis. Normally, FBLIM1 protein is anti-inflammatory and controls bone remodeling through inhibiting RANKL. In affected patients, mutated FBLIM1 protein results in a loss of function, leading to increased activation of RANKL and imbalanced bone remodeling.[25] Susceptibility genes for chronic recurrent multifocal osteomyelitis also include FGR, a member of the Src family tyrosine kinases (SRKS). A gain of function missense mutation in the C-terminal region of this protooncogene causes reduced negative regulatory phosphorylation of FGR leading to sterile osteomyelitis and systemic reduced bone mineral density.[26] Another gene, human mixed lineage kinase domain-like (MLKL), which is involved in a form of programmed lytic cell death called necroptosis, has been implicated as a human CNO susceptibility gene. Compound heterozygosity (both alleles have a different genetic variant) in the brace region of human MLKL gene was found at up to 12 times the frequency in European patients with CNO compared with matched control subjects.[27]

CLINICAL MANIFESTATIONS

Clinical features of CNO are nonspecific, often presenting with insidious onset of localized bone pain. Nocturnal bone pain may be misconstrued as "growing pains." The pain is often chronic and intermittent. Tenderness, swelling, or warmth overlying affected bone may be present, although physical examinations are often normal (**Fig. 1**). Fatigue is frequently reported. However, patients may also present with sequelae of bone lesions (ie, compression fractures of vertebral bodies) without preceding clinical symptoms.[28,29] Significant pain, fatigue, and physical limitations related to CNO and negative family and peer relationships cause challenges in performance and function at school and work demonstrating an unmet need for psychosocial and socioeconomic support for patients and families with this chronic disease.[30]

Although almost any bone can be affected, classic sites of CNO involvement are the clavicle, mandible, metaphysis of lower extremity long bones, vertebrae, and pelvis. Multiple bony lesions occur in up to 98% of cases[31] and are symmetric in 25% to 40% of individuals.[6] Underestimation of lesion number and underidentification of certain lesion locations may result from lack of assessment using whole-body MRI (WBMRI). As the use of WBMRI increases at diagnosis, correlation with clinical symptoms of affected anatomic sites may be determined. Andronikou and colleagues[32] identified two patterns of bony lesion involvement based on WBMRI in a cohort of

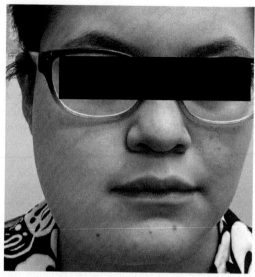

Fig. 1. A 15-year-old girl diagnosed with CNO of right mandible after 3 years of intermittent right facial swelling and pain.

37 children: "tibioappendicular multifocal patterns" (54%) in which lesions were located in the tibia without clavicular involvement; and "claviculospinal paucifocal pattern" (24%) with lesions in the clavicle, no tibial lesions, and a few more lesions mainly of spine. Further analysis of larger cohorts is needed to identify all patterns of CNO lesions and whether the patterns predict disease prognosis and outcomes.

CNO is associated with other inflammatory conditions affecting various organs including severe acne, pyoderma gangrenosum, palmoplantar pustulosis, inflammatory bowel disease, and spondyloarthritis affecting between 6% and 18% of patients with CNO in several reported cohorts.[6,8,9,33]

LABORATORY STUDIES

Traditional markers of inflammation are not uniformly elevated in CNO. Mild elevations of C-reactive protein (CRP) and erythrocyte sedimentation rate (ESR) were reported in frequencies ranging from 40% to 80% of patients in large cohorts of patients with CNO.[6,11] Levels of ESR and CRP were not associated with specific clinical manifestations or treatment response in a recent international study.[11] Highly elevated CRP and ESR greater than three times the upper limit of normal should raise suspicion of an alternative diagnosis.[30] Only a subset of children with CNO had elevated titers of antinuclear antibodies (8%–38%) and were positive for HLA-B27 antigen (2%–25%).[5,6,8,9,11,33]

As a bone resorption marker, urine N-terminal telopeptide was proposed as a biomarker of disease flare in patients with CNO treated with bisphosphonates.[34,35] However, it did not distinguish children with active CNO from healthy control subjects or correlate with disease activity when children were treated with medications other than bisphosphonates.[36]

DIAGNOSTIC IMAGING

Radiologic studies are helpful in establishing the diagnosis of CNO, as illustrated by its inclusion in all proposed diagnostic criteria.[4,6]

Radiographs

Plain radiographs are often the first step in evaluation of patients presenting with bone pain, although it only identified 13% of lesions detected by MRI.[37] One of the most common radiologic findings of CNO on plain radiographs is mixed osteolytic and sclerotic lesions, affecting primarily the metaphyses of long bones.[3,38,39] Rarely, when the epiphysis is involved, premature epiphyseal closure can occur. Diaphyseal lesions usually occur in conjunction with metaphyseal lesions. Other radiographic findings include periosteal reaction (new bone formation), cortical bone thickening, sclerosis, and hyperostosis (bony expansion) (**Fig. 2**).[40] Vertebral spine lesions range from reduced intervertebral spaces, erosion of vertebral plates, to frank pathologic vertebral collapse and compression fracture.[41–43] However, in early stages of disease, plain radiographs may be entirely normal. Therefore, relying on radiographs can delay diagnosis.

Bone Scintigraphy

Bone scintigraphy was previously used for whole-body imaging in CNO to identify asymptomatic lesions as it had been historically used for evaluation of bone tumors and metabolic bone disease. Typical patterns of bone involvement on bone scan may show abnormal radiotracer uptake at metaphyses of long bones, especially tibia, femur, and clavicle, but may miss symmetric metaphyseal disease.[44] Although useful in demonstrating abnormalities, greater radiation exposure and decreased sensitivity in identification of CNO lesions[45] make bone scintigraphy less desirable than MRI. Therefore, where available, WBMRI is used for initial work-up or disease monitoring.

Computed Tomography

Similarly, the use of computed tomography in the diagnosis of CNO is limited, because of its radiation burden in children and its limited ability to distinguish active from inactive lesions. Computed tomography findings of CNO lesions are specific to certain locations (eg, anterior chest wall, spine, and mandible) and include cortical erosion, sclerosis, and paravertebral bony bridging.[46]

MRI

MRI is the preferred imaging modality for CNO. Research has shown that MRI is superior to radiograph in the identification of CNO lesions[12] because of greater sensitivity,[45] particularly in early disease when plain radiographs are often entirely normal.[47–51] Early MRI findings of CNO include T2 signal hyperintensity suggesting bony edema and T1 signal hypointensity and altered diffusion capacity on diffusion-weighted imaging. Other MRI sequences useful in the diagnostic work-up of CNO are strongly T2-weighted sequences (turbo inversion recovery measurement) or short

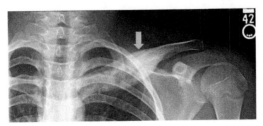

Fig. 2. Radiograph showing cortical thickening of medial two-thirds of left clavicle with mixed areas of sclerosis and lucency with adjacent periosteal reaction (*yellow arrow*).

tau inversion recovery images, which show signal hyperintensity. Additional MRI findings in active CNO inflammatory lesions include soft tissue inflammation, periosteal reaction, hyperostosis, and CNO-related damage including vertebral body compression and growth plate damage (**Figs. 3–7**).[40,45,52]

WBMRI should be performed at diagnosis to help exclude alternative diagnoses, to provide further diagnostic support if multifocal lesions are present, and help identify unexpected/clinically silent lesions particularly of the spinal column, which may necessitate more aggressive therapy to prevent long-term damage.[50] One-third of patients with CNO have asymptomatic lesions only detected by WBMRI[4,53] and clinical remission does not necessarily equate with radiologic remission.[51,54] Escalation of therapy for asymptomatic nonspinal MRI lesions remains controversial. However, total lesion counts detected by MRI is used commonly to determine response to treatment.[50,55,56]

Novel Imaging Techniques

A pilot study by Zhao and colleagues[57] explored the use of infrared thermal imaging as a rapid and inexpensive imaging tool to detect active bone lesions in the extremities of 30 children with CNO. Children with active CNO lesions in the distal tibia/fibula exhibited higher regional temperatures on average than unaffected extremities,[57] although this work needs validation.

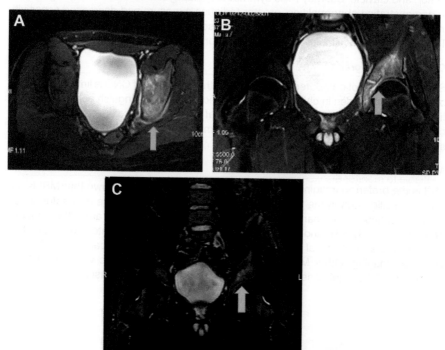

Fig. 3. (*A*) Axial fat saturation T2 images through the pelvis demonstrating extensive marrow edema at the left acetabulum with surrounding linear periosseous edema (*yellow arrow*). (*B*) Coronal fat saturation T2 images through the pelvis demonstrating extensive marrow edema at the left acetabulum with surrounding linear periosseous edema (*yellow arrow*). (*C*) Coronal short tau inversion recovery (STIR) images through the pelvis demonstrating interval decreased marrow edema at the left acetabulum and resolution of the periosseous edema after treatment (*yellow arrow*).

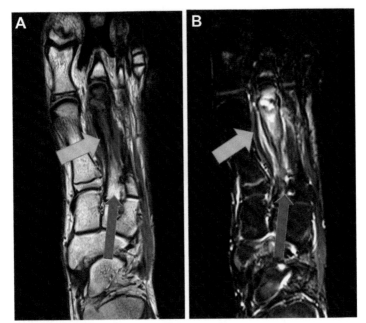

Fig. 4. Long axis T1 (*A*) and STIR (*B*) images through the left foot show extensive marrow edema at the second metatarsal (*yellow arrow*) with cystic changes distally at the metaphysis (*red arrow*) with exuberant periosseous edema.

MONITORING DISEASE ACTIVITY

Assessment of disease activity in CNO is challenging. Clinical examination may be normal. Pain assessments are prone to individual patient variability and may reflect potential comorbidities, such as pain amplification syndrome, rather than CNO disease activity. Because of the lack of specific disease markers, no laboratory tests are reliable to monitor disease activity in CNO. Instead, imaging is used to monitor disease activity.

Most pediatric rheumatologists caring for patients with CNO reported using new lesions on radiographic imaging as a marker of disease activity.[7,58] Indeed, a disease activity score (PedsCNO score) developed by Beck and colleagues[49] included the

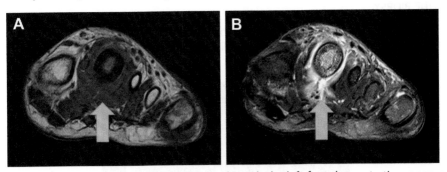

Fig. 5. Short axis T1 (*A*) and STIR (*B*) images through the left foot demonstrating marrow edema at the second metatarsal and the circumferential periosseous edema and adjacent soft tissue edema (*yellow arrow*).

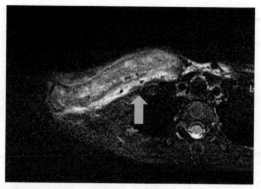

Fig. 6. Axial T2 fat saturation image of the right clavicle demonstrating marked deformity with expansion of the clavicle. There is extensive marrow edema throughout the right clavicle with interval focal areas increasing high T2 signal and surrounding periosseous edema(*yellow arrow*).

number of radiologic lesions. Prior studies proposed various methods of scoring MRIs to assess disease activity in CNO.[55,59,60] The proposed radiologic index for nonbacterial osteitis (RINBO) and the ChRonic nonbacterial Osteomyelitis MRI Scoring (CROMRIS) use similar parameters of bone edema or signal hyperintensity, extramedullary inflammation (soft tissue edema and periosteal reaction), hyperostosis, and presence of spinal lesions and vertebral body deformities to assess clinically active disease and chronic damage. Size of lesions are described in relative as opposed to absolute measurement of various body and bone sizes in the latter scoring tool, which was shown to have excellent interrater reliability. Recent studies by Capponi and colleagues[61] used the scoring tool to create a radiologic activity index that showed correlation with clinical disease activity, although findings are yet to be validated.

Core domain sets for outcome measurements in CNO need to be further developed enlisting all stakeholders (especially patient research partners) following established methodology, such as Outcome Measures in Rheumatology (OMERACT).[62] Domains including pathophysiology, life impact, and health outcomes will be considered for consensus by the CNO OMERACT Working Group, an independent initiative of international stakeholders interested in outcome measurement.

BONE BIOPSY

Because CNO is a diagnosis of exclusion, bone biopsy is often useful to rule out alternative diagnoses, such as infections, malignancy, Langerhans cell histiocytosis, or

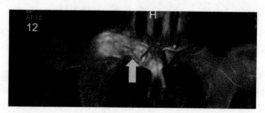

Fig. 7. Coronal fat saturation T2 image through the right clavicle demonstrating extensive marrow edema, expansion, and adjacent soft tissue edema (*yellow arrow*).

fibrous dysplasia, and is performed in most patients (60%–80%) reported in available literature.[4–6] Jansson and colleagues proposed a scoring system to determine whether to perform a bone biopsy in a child based on the presence of multiple clinical symptoms, laboratory findings, and imaging factors.[4,63] Histologically, samples from CNO lesions may vary drastically. Within early stage CNO lesions, neutrophil and monocyte predominate; whereas in later-stage lesions, lymphocytes and plasma cells with variable degrees of sclerosis and fibrosis are most common.[6] Monocytes and macrophages are seen in all phases.[23] The coexistence of innate and adaptive infiltrates may reflect relapsing disease with flares and remissions. In pediatric CNO, the biopsy is generally negative for bacterial, fungal, and mycobacterial cultures.

DIAGNOSTIC CRITERIA

Three groups have proposed diagnostic or classification criteria, none of which are prospectively validated,[4,6,50] and CNO remains a diagnosis of exclusion. Each of the suggested criteria include generally well-appearing children, with long-standing disease (>6 months), and the presence of multiple "typical" bone lesions on imaging or unifocal lesion without evidence of infection or malignancy. Certain clinical features may help distinguish mimics from CNO as described in a multinational case-control study,[64] although findings are still preliminary (**Fig. 8**).

TREATMENT

NSAIDs are generally considered first-line therapy for patients with nonspinal CNO.[49] About half of reported patients achieved remission on NSAIDs in several case series.[9,53,65] The Childhood Arthritis & Rheumatology Research Alliance has recently proposed consensus treatment plans for patients with NSAID-refractory disease or vertebral column lesions.[50] The three regimens are (1) methotrexate or sulfasalazine, (2) TNF inhibitor with optional methotrexate, and (3) bisphosphonates. Short courses of glucocorticoids and continuation of NSAIDs are included for all scenarios.

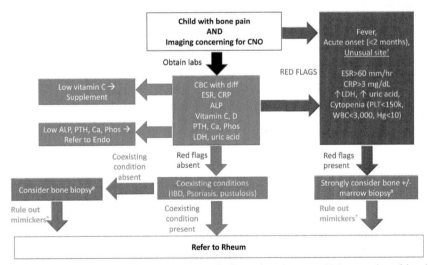

Fig. 8. Diagnostic algorithm for CNO. ALP, alkaline phosphatase; CBC, complete blood count; IBD, inflammatory bowel disease; LDH, lactate dehydrogenase; PLT, platelets; WBC, white blood cell count; Phos, phosphorus; PTH, parathyroid hormone.

Traditional nonbiologic disease-modifying agents (DMARDs), namely methotrexate and sulfasalazine, are effective in some patients as evidenced by case series reports.[9,66] Remission rates on methotrexate are lower than other DMARDs, ranging from 20% to 44%.[9,65,66] Concomitant arthritis increases the likelihood of remission with methotrexate in CNO.[65]

TNF inhibitors have been shown to induce remission in 46% to 73% of patients with CNO.[65,66] In patients with associated conditions, in which TNF inhibition is Food and Drug Administration approved, such as juvenile idiopathic arthritis, psoriasis, psoriatic arthritis, and inflammatory bowel disease, anti-TNF agents may be most beneficial.

Bisphosphonates are thought to be helpful in the treatment of CNO by inhibiting osteoclastic activity, thereby decreasing bone damage,[67] reducing pain, and decreasing inflammation.[34,52] Infusions of pamidronate (initial dose 0.5mg/kg/dose [with max 30mg/dose] and subsequent doses 1 mg/kg/dose [with max 60 mg/dose] for 3 consecutive days every 3 months or monthly for a total of 9– 12 months) have been reported.[34,68–70] Aggressive combination therapy with zoledronic acid and infliximab has been effective in a small cohort of patients with primary spinal involvement.[55] Remission rates for patients with CNO treated with bisphosphonates ranged from 51% in the EuroFever registry to 88.8% in several single-center studies.[53,65] Use of bisphosphonates in these studies was primarily in patients with spinal involvement.

Despite the critical role of IL-1 in the pathogenesis of CNO, evidence supporting the role of IL-1 inhibitors in CNO treatment is sparse. In a small case series, nine patients who had failed NSAIDs and/or bisphosphonates reported improvement after 6 months treatment with anakinra using a five-point scoring system (inactive, minimal, mild, moderate, severe disease) based on fever, number of active bone lesions detected by bone scintigraphy, inflammatory markers, and presence of pain and functional impairment. The decrease in disease activity was maintained after a median follow-up of 1.7 years.[71] Similarly, IL-17 blockers have not been tested for efficacy in large cohorts of patients with CNO, despite Food and Drug Administration approval for use in patients with overlapping features, such as psoriasis and spondyloarthritis, but may be a promising therapeutic option.[72]

Various individual patient factors may play a role in determining appropriate therapeutic choices in CNO, such as lesion location. In a recent retrospective review of 22 patients with CNO with mandibular involvement at a single US center, anti-TNF and pamidronate seemed superior to NSAIDs alone in treating mandibular CNO. Patients receiving pamidronate responded faster than those receiving anti-TNF therapies.[73]

Optimal duration of treatment to minimize disease recurrence is unknown and needs to be investigated prospectively, such as could be done through EuroFever or CHronic nonbacterial Osteomyelitis International Registry (CHOIR).[9] Because of the chronic nature of CNO, therapy is typically prolonged and for some, may be needed into adulthood.

OUTCOME AND PROGNOSIS

Delayed diagnosis is still common in CNO. Children experience an average diagnostic delay of 2 years,[9,30,33] leading to significant morbidity. Up to a quarter of children with CNO may have limitations in function, limp, and pathologic fractures even at initial presentation.[10,53] Complications of CNO in children include vertebral fractures, resulting in spine scoliosis and kyphosis.[10,74] Overall remission rates are favorable in long-term cohorts ranging from 50% to 80% based on composite scores that include clinical and imaging criteria.[33,53] More than half of children continue to have CNO flares within the first year of diagnosis[9,33] and after reaching adulthood.[51]

SUMMARY

CNO is an autoinflammatory bone disorder where the innate immune system is dysregulated. It often presents as insidious bone pain in children with or without systemic signs of inflammation. CNO is currently a diagnosis of exclusion with mimickers, such as infectious osteomyelitis and malignancy. Clinical manifestations range from a single episode of unifocal disease to multifocal, relapsing disease that primarily occurs in childhood, but may persist into adulthood. CNO typically affects the clavicle, mandible, metaphysis of lower extremity long bones, spine, and pelvis. Radiologic imaging, specifically MRI, increasingly aids diagnosis and long-term monitoring of patients with suspected and known CNO because of its sensitivity in identifying lesions. Treatments aim to decrease inflammation and include NSAIDs as first-line, with conventional and/or biologic DMARDs and bisphosphonates for more severe disease. Timely diagnosis and appropriate therapy are necessary in growing children with CNO to prevent long-standing complications, such as pathologic fractures and limb-length discrepancy.

CLINICS CARE POINTS

- The diagnosis of CNO can be challenging due to mimicking conditions including infectious osteomyelitis and malignancies.
- Whole body MR imaging is helpful in distinguishing CNO from alternative diagnoses.
- More severe disease may warrant escalation of therapy from NSAIDs to advanced therapies including DMARDs, biologic medications, and bisphosphonates to prevent poor outcomes.

DISCLOSURE

F. Nuruzzaman has nothing to disclose. Y. Zhao - Consultant for Novartis. P.J. Ferguson - Consultant for Novartis.

REFERENCES

1. Masters SL, Simon A, Aksentijevich I, et al. Horror autoinflammaticus: the molecular pathophysiology of autoinflammatory disease (*). Annu Rev Immunol 2009; 27:621–68.
2. Giedion A, Holthusen W, Masel LF, et al. [Subacute and chronic "symmetrical" osteomyelitis]. Ann Radiol (Paris) 1972;15(3):329–42.
3. Probst FP, Bjorksten B, Gustavson KH. Radiological aspect of chronic recurrent multifocal osteomyelitis. Ann Radiol (Paris) 1978;21(2–3):115–25.
4. Roderick MR, Shah R, Rogers V, et al. Chronic recurrent multifocal osteomyelitis (CRMO) - advancing the diagnosis. Pediatr Rheumatol Online J 2016;14(1):47.
5. Schnabel A, Range U, Hahn G, et al. Unexpectedly high incidences of chronic non-bacterial as compared to bacterial osteomyelitis in children. Rheumatol Int 2016;36(12):1737–45.
6. Jansson A, Renner ED, Ramser J, et al. Classification of non-bacterial osteitis: retrospective study of clinical, immunological and genetic aspects in 89 patients. Rheumatology (Oxford) 2007;46(1):154–60.
7. Grote V, Silier CC, Voit AM, et al. Bacterial Osteomyelitis or Nonbacterial Osteitis in Children: A Study Involving the German Surveillance Unit for Rare Diseases in Childhood. Pediatr Infect Dis J 2017;36(5):451–6.

8. Wipff J, Costantino F, Lemelle I, et al. A large national cohort of French patients with chronic recurrent multifocal osteitis. Arthritis Rheumatol 2015;67(4):1128–37.

9. Girschick H, Finetti M, Orlando F, et al. The multifaceted presentation of chronic recurrent multifocal osteomyelitis: a series of 486 cases from the Eurofever international registry. Rheumatology (Oxford) 2018;57(8):1504.

10. Concha S, Hernandez-Ojeda A, Contreras O, et al. Chronic nonbacterial osteomyelitis in children: a multicenter case series. Rheumatol Int 2020;40(1):115–20.

11. Gamalero L, Belot A, Zajc Avramovic M, et al. Chronic non-bacterial osteomyelitis: a retrospective international study on clinical manifestations and response to treatment. Clin Exp Rheumatol 2020;38(6):1255–62.

12. Schultz C, Holterhus PM, Seidel A, et al. Chronic recurrent multifocal osteomyelitis in children. Pediatr Infect Dis J 1999;18(11):1008–13.

13. Huber AM, Lam PY, Duffy CM, et al. Chronic recurrent multifocal osteomyelitis: clinical outcomes after more than five years of follow-up. J Pediatr 2002;141(2): 198–203.

14. Schilling F, Wagner AD. [Azithromycin: an anti-inflammatory effect in chronic recurrent multifocal osteomyelitis? A preliminary report]. Z Rheumatol 2000; 59(5):352–3.

15. Zimmermann P, Curtis N. The role of Cutibacterium acnes in auto-inflammatory bone disorders. Eur J Pediatr 2019;178(1):89–95.

16. Girschick HJ, Huppertz HI, Harmsen D, et al. Chronic recurrent multifocal osteomyelitis in children: diagnostic value of histopathology and microbial testing. Hum Pathol 1999;30(1):59–65.

17. Zeus M, Janssen S, Fischer U, et al. THU0514 Role of the oral microbiome in chronic non-baterial osteomyelitis in children. Ann Rheum Dis 2019;78:546–8.

18. Hofmann SR, Kubasch AS, Ioannidis C, et al. Altered expression of IL-10 family cytokines in monocytes from CRMO patients result in enhanced IL-1beta expression and release. Clin Immunol 2015;161(2):300–7.

19. Hofmann SR, Kubasch AS, Range U, et al. Serum biomarkers for the diagnosis and monitoring of chronic recurrent multifocal osteomyelitis (CRMO). Rheumatol Int 2016;36(6):769–79.

20. Hofmann SR, Morbach H, Schwarz T, et al. Attenuated TLR4/MAPK signaling in monocytes from patients with CRMO results in impaired IL-10 expression. Clin Immunol 2012;145(1):69–76.

21. Hofmann SR, Schwarz T, Moller JC, et al. Chronic non-bacterial osteomyelitis is associated with impaired Sp1 signaling, reduced IL10 promoter phosphorylation, and reduced myeloid IL-10 expression. Clin Immunol 2011;141(3):317–27.

22. Surace AEA, Hedrich CM. The Role of Epigenetics in Autoimmune/Inflammatory Disease. Front Immunol 2019;10:1525.

23. Brandt D, Sohr E, Pablik J, et al. CD14(+) monocytes contribute to inflammation in chronic nonbacterial osteomyelitis (CNO) through increased NLRP3 inflammasome expression. Clin Immunol 2018;196:77–84.

24. Scianaro R, Insalaco A, Bracci Laudiero L, et al. Deregulation of the IL-1beta axis in chronic recurrent multifocal osteomyelitis. Pediatr Rheumatol Online J 2014; 12:30.

25. Cox AJ, Darbro BW, Laxer RM, et al. Recessive coding and regulatory mutations in FBLIM1 underlie the pathogenesis of chronic recurrent multifocal osteomyelitis (CRMO). PLoS One 2017;12(3):e0169687.

26. Abe K, Cox A, Takamatsu N, et al. Gain-of-function mutations in a member of the Src family kinases cause autoinflammatory bone disease in mice and humans. Proc Natl Acad Sci U S A 2019;116(24):11872–7.

27. Hildebrand JM, Kauppi M, Majewski IJ, et al. A missense mutation in the MLKL brace region promotes lethal neonatal inflammation and hematopoietic dysfunction. Nat Commun 2020;11(1):3150.
28. King SM, Laxer RM, Manson D, et al. Chronic recurrent multifocal osteomyelitis: a noninfectious inflammatory process. Pediatr Infect Dis J 1987;6(10):907–11.
29. Bjorksten B, Gustavson KH, Eriksson B, et al. Chronic recurrent multifocal osteomyelitis and pustulosis palmoplantaris. J Pediatr 1978;93(2):227–31.
30. Oliver M, Lee TC, Halpern-Felsher B, et al. Disease burden and social impact of pediatric chronic nonbacterial osteomyelitis from the patient and family perspective. Pediatr Rheumatol Online J 2018;16(1):78.
31. von Kalle T, Heim N, Hospach T, et al. Typical patterns of bone involvement in whole-body MRI of patients with chronic recurrent multifocal osteomyelitis (CRMO). Rofo 2013;185(7):655–61.
32. Andronikou S, Mendes da Costa T, Hussien M, et al. Radiological diagnosis of chronic recurrent multifocal osteomyelitis using whole-body MRI-based lesion distribution patterns. Clin Radiol 2019;74(9):737.e3-15.
33. Bhat CS, Anderson C, Harbinson A, et al. Chronic non bacterial osteitis- a multicentre study. Pediatr Rheumatol Online J 2018;16(1):74.
34. Miettunen PM, Wei X, Kaura D, et al. Dramatic pain relief and resolution of bone inflammation following pamidronate in 9 pediatric patients with persistent chronic recurrent multifocal osteomyelitis (CRMO). Pediatr Rheumatol Online J 2009;7:2.
35. Hirano D, Chiba K, Yamada S, et al. Oral alendronate in pediatric chronic recurrent multifocal osteomyelitis. Pediatr Int 2017;59(4):506–8.
36. Perkins A, Stevens AM, Ferguson PJ, et al. Urinary N-telopeptide as a Biomarker of Disease Activity in Patients with Chronic Nonbacterial Osteomyelitis Who Have Not Received Bisphosphonates. J Rheumatol 2020;47(12):1842–4.
37. Fritz J, Tzaribatchev N, Claussen CD, et al. Chronic recurrent multifocal osteomyelitis: comparison of whole-body MR imaging with radiography and correlation with clinical and laboratory data. Radiology 2009;252(3):842–51.
38. Duffy CM, Lam PY, Ditchfield M, et al. Chronic recurrent multifocal osteomyelitis: review of orthopaedic complications at maturity. J Pediatr Orthop 2002;22(4):501–5.
39. Sato TS, Watal P, Ferguson PJ. Imaging mimics of chronic recurrent multifocal osteomyelitis: avoiding pitfalls in a diagnosis of exclusion. Pediatr Radiol 2020;50(1):124–36.
40. Khanna G, Sato TS, Ferguson P. Imaging of chronic recurrent multifocal osteomyelitis. Radiographics 2009;29(4):1159–77.
41. Jurik AG. Chronic recurrent multifocal osteomyelitis. Semin Musculoskelet Radiol 2004;8(3):243–53.
42. Kahn MF. Chronic recurrent multifocal osteomyelitis. Association with vertebra plana. J Bone Joint Surg Am 1990;72(2):305–6.
43. Anderson SE, Heini P, Sauvain MJ, et al. Imaging of chronic recurrent multifocal osteomyelitis of childhood first presenting with isolated primary spinal involvement. Skeletal Radiol 2003;32(6):328–36.
44. Acikgoz G, Averill LW. Chronic recurrent multifocal osteomyelitis: typical patterns of bone involvement in whole-body bone scintigraphy. Nucl Med Commun 2014;35(8):797–807.
45. Morbach H, Schneider P, Schwarz T, et al. Comparison of magnetic resonance imaging and 99mTechnetium-labelled methylene diphosphonate bone scintigraphy in the initial assessment of chronic non-bacterial osteomyelitis of childhood and adolescents. Clin Exp Rheumatol 2012;30(4):578–82.

46. Himuro H, Kurata S, Nagata S, et al. Imaging features in patients with SAPHO/CRMO: a pictorial review. Jpn J Radiol 2020;38(7):622–9.

47. Hedrich CM, Hofmann SR, Pablik J, et al. Autoinflammatory bone disorders with special focus on chronic recurrent multifocal osteomyelitis (CRMO). Pediatr Rheumatol Online J 2013;11(1):47.

48. Zhao Y, Dedeoglu F, Ferguson PJ, et al. Physicians' Perspectives on the Diagnosis and Treatment of Chronic Nonbacterial Osteomyelitis. Int J Rheumatol 2017;2017:7694942.

49. Beck C, Morbach H, Beer M, et al. Chronic nonbacterial osteomyelitis in childhood: prospective follow-up during the first year of anti-inflammatory treatment. Arthritis Res Ther 2010;12(2):R74.

50. Zhao Y, Wu EY, Oliver MS, et al. Consensus Treatment Plans for Chronic Nonbacterial Osteomyelitis Refractory to Nonsteroidal Antiinflammatory Drugs and/or With Active Spinal Lesions. Arthritis Care Res (Hoboken) 2018;70(8):1228–37.

51. Voit AM, Arnoldi AP, Douis H, et al. Whole-body Magnetic Resonance Imaging in Chronic Recurrent Multifocal Osteomyelitis: Clinical Longterm Assessment May Underestimate Activity. J Rheumatol 2015;42(8):1455–62.

52. Hofmann C, Wurm M, Schwarz T, et al. A standardized clinical and radiological follow-up of patients with chronic non-bacterial osteomyelitis treated with pamidronate. Clin Exp Rheumatol 2014;32(4):604–9.

53. Schnabel A, Range U, Hahn G, et al. Treatment Response and Longterm Outcomes in Children with Chronic Nonbacterial Osteomyelitis. J Rheumatol 2017;44(7):1058–65.

54. Leclair N, Thormer G, Sorge I, et al. Whole-Body Diffusion-Weighted Imaging in Chronic Recurrent Multifocal Osteomyelitis in Children. PLoS One 2016;11(1):e0147523.

55. Zhao YCN, Jaramillo D, Burnham JM. Aggressive therapy reduces disease activity without skeletal damage progression in chronic nonbacterial osteomyelitis. J Rheumatol 2015;42:1245–51.

56. Kellenberger CJ, Epelman M, Miller SF, et al. Fast STIR whole-body MR imaging in children. Radiographics 2004;24(5):1317–30.

57. Zhao Y, Iyer RS, Reichley L, et al. A Pilot Study of Infrared Thermal Imaging to Detect Active Bone Lesions in Children With Chronic Nonbacterial Osteomyelitis. Arthritis Care Res (Hoboken) 2019;71(11):1430–5.

58. d'Angelo P, de Horatio LT, Toma P, et al. Chronic nonbacterial osteomyelitis - clinical and magnetic resonance imaging features. Pediatr Radiol 2021;51(2):282–8.

59. Arnoldi AP, Schlett CL, Douis H, et al. Whole-body MRI in patients with Non-bacterial Osteitis: Radiological findings and correlation with clinical data. Eur Radiol 2017;27(6):2391–9.

60. Zhao Y, Sato TS, Nielsen SM, et al. Development of a Scoring Tool for Chronic Nonbacterial Osteomyelitis Magnetic Resonance Imaging and Evaluation of its Interrater Reliability. J Rheumatol 2020;47(5):739–47.

61. Capponi M, Marafon DP, Rivosecchi F, et al. Correlation of a whole-body MRI derived radiological activity index with disease activity in chronic nonbacterial osteomyelitis. Pediatr Rheumatol 2020;18:83.

62. Rheumatology OMi. OMERACT Handbook. Secondary OMERACT Handbook 2018. Available at: https://omeracthandbook.org/handbook.

63. Jansson AF, Muller TH, Gliera L, et al. Clinical score for nonbacterial osteitis in children and adults. Arthritis Rheum 2009;60(4):1152–9.

64. Zhao YNR, Oliver M, Wang Z, et al. Comparison of Clinicopathologic and Imaging Features Between Chronic Nonbacterial Osteomyelitis and Its Mimickers: A Multinational 450 Case-Control Study [abstract]. Arthritis Rheumatol 2020;72.

65. Kostik MM, Kopchak OL, Chikova IA, et al. Comparison of different treatment approaches of pediatric chronic non-bacterial osteomyelitis. Rheumatol Int 2019; 39(1):89–96.

66. Borzutzky A, Stern S, Reiff A, et al. Pediatric chronic nonbacterial osteomyelitis. Pediatrics 2012;130(5):e1190–7.

67. Bellido T, Plotkin LI. Novel actions of bisphosphonates in bone: preservation of osteoblast and osteocyte viability. Bone 2011;49(1):50–5.

68. Bhat CS, Roderick M, Sen ES, et al. Efficacy of pamidronate in children with chronic non-bacterial osteitis using whole body MRI as a marker of disease activity. Pediatr Rheumatol Online J 2019;17(1):35.

69. Andreasen CM, Jurik AG, Glerup MB, et al. Response to Early-onset Pamidronate Treatment in Chronic Nonbacterial Osteomyelitis: A Retrospective Single-center Study. J Rheumatol 2019;46(11):1515–23.

70. Andreasen CM, Jurik AG, Deleuran BW, et al. Pamidronate in chronic non-bacterial osteomyelitis: a randomized, double-blinded, placebo-controlled pilot trial. Scand J Rheumatol 2020;49(4):312–22.

71. Pardeo M, Pires Marafon D, Messia V, et al. Anakinra in a Cohort of Children with Chronic Nonbacterial Osteomyelitis. J Rheumatol 2017;44(8):1231–8.

72. Goenka A, Roderick M, Finn A, et al. The jigsaw puzzle of chronic non-bacterial osteomyelitis: are anti-IL17 therapies the next piece? Rheumatology (Oxford) 2020;59(3):459–61.

73. Gaal A, Basiaga ML, Zhao Y, et al. Pediatric chronic nonbacterial osteomyelitis of the mandible: Seattle Children's hospital 22-patient experience. Pediatr Rheumatol Online J 2020;18(1):4.

74. Kostik MM, Kopchak OL, Maletin AS, et al. The peculiarities and treatment outcomes of the spinal form of chronic non-bacterial osteomyelitis in children: a retrospective cohort study. Rheumatol Int 2020;40(1):97–105.

Unique Aspects of Pediatric Sjögren Disease

Rachel L. Randell, MD[a],*, Scott M. Lieberman, MD, PhD[b]

KEYWORDS

- Sjögren syndrome • Pediatric Sjögren syndrome • Parotitis • Sjögren disease

KEY POINTS

- Sjögren disease is increasingly recognized in pediatric patients, who present with more glandular swelling (parotitis) and less dryness (sicca symptoms) than do adults.
- Diagnosis is challenging because young patients may present with different features and diagnostic testing results than adults.
- Most pediatric patients do not meet adult criteria, and pediatric-specific criteria are urgently needed.
- Symptomatic therapies as used in adults should be used to treat dryness symptoms.
- Systemic immunomodulators may be uniquely beneficial to pediatric patients, but studies are needed to evaluate the effect on symptoms and course of progressive glandular dysfunction.

INTRODUCTION

Sjögren disease (SD) is a chronic, systemic autoimmune disease marked by immune-mediated exocrine gland destruction that affects approximately 4 million individuals in the United States. Although pediatric SD (pedSD), or diagnosis of SD before the age of 18 years, previously was considered rare, cases increasingly are reported. Primary SD refers to SD in the absence of comorbid autoimmune disease,[1,2] although co-occurrence is common.[3] SD characteristically manifests with the sicca syndrome of xerostomia (dry mouth) and xerophthalmia (dry eye), but other exocrine glands and organ systems can be affected. Chronic glandular dysfunction and other symptoms reduce quality of life and cause significant morbidity.[2,4] SD also increases risk of malignancy, specifically non-Hodgkin lymphoma,[5] and a subset of patients have increased mortality.[6] Long-term daily use of symptomatic therapies can alleviate

[a] Department of Pediatrics, Duke University School of Medicine, 2301 Erwin Road Box #3212, Durham, NC 27705, USA; [b] Division of Rheumatology, Allergy, and Immunology, Stead Family Department of Pediatrics, Carver College of Medicine, University of Iowa, 500 Newton Road, 2191 ML, Iowa City, IA 52242, USA
* Corresponding author.
E-mail address: rachel.randell@duke.edu

Rheum Dis Clin N Am 47 (2021) 707–723
https://doi.org/10.1016/j.rdc.2021.07.008
0889-857X/21/© 2021 Elsevier Inc. All rights reserved.

dryness symptoms, and systemic immunosuppression may be warranted to treat some patients.[7] Although a vast majority of studies focus on SD in adults, an increasing number of pediatric cases are reported. Distinct features of pediatric disease are noted, although the pathophysiology likely is similar to that of adult disease, with pediatric cases representing early-onset disease. This review summarizes key clinical concepts of SD, primarily drawn from adult data. Where available, data from pediatric studies are noted.

EPIDEMIOLOGY

SD is the second most common rheumatologic disease in adults in the United States.[2] Exact prevalence and incidence of pedSD are unknown. In a large, multinational cohort of primary SD, only 1.3% of cases were diagnosed before the age of 19 years.[8] Between the mid 1960s[9,10] and 2019,[11] a few hundred cases of pedSD had been reported in the literature. In 2020, 3 large studies[8,12,13] reported greater than 500 cases. The dramatic increase in number of reported cases over the past year could reflect the increasing prevalence of autoimmunity,[14] increasing recognition and diagnosis of pedSD, or a combination of several factors.

As with other autoimmune diseases, there is a strong female predominance, with approximately 90% of adult cases female.[2] Among pediatric studies, the proportion of female patients is 80% to 87%.[8,11–13,15] Most adult studies draw from European and/or Asian populations, but SD has been reported across racial and ethnic groups.[16] The distribution across racial and ethnic groups of pedSD is unknown; however, in a multinational cohort study of 158 patients diagnosed with SD before 19 years of age, a majority (68%) were white, followed by Asian (17%) and Hispanic (12%).[8] Diagnosis typically occurs between 30 years and 50 years of age in adults.[1] In large pedSD studies, diagnosis typically occurred between 12 years and 14 years of age.[8,12,13,15]

HISTORY, CONTROVERSY, AND TERMINOLOGY

Sicca syndrome has been recognized dating back to the 1920s.[1] Dr Henrik Sjögren first described the association between sicca syndrome and systemic features in his thesis, "On knowledge of keratoconjunctivitis sicca" in 1933. Major advances in diagnosis of SD were made in the late 1960s and 1970s, with the discovery of inflammatory infiltrates on salivary gland biopsy, circulating antibodies (Sjögren syndrome A [SSA] and Sjögren syndrome B [SSB], also referred to as Ro and La, respectively), and the technique of salivary scintigraphy. In 1981, Chudwin and colleagues[17] first compared clinical findings in adults and children with SD and concluded that pedSD largely was similar to adult disease. Over the following years, however, several pediatric cases reported a high prevalence of parotitis,[18] with cases of parotitis often preceding sicca syndrome by several years[19] and unusual clinical features, including central nervous system (CNS) manifestations.[20] In 1999, Bartunkova and colleagues[21] proposed pediatric diagnostic criteria unique from adult criteria, but the criteria were never validated or widely accepted for use in research or clinical care. Until recently, a paucity of pediatric-specific data contributed to controversy surrounding the diagnosis of pedSD. Although some studies conclude that pedSD closely resembles adult disease,[18] other retrospective and survey-based studies highlight differences, such as high prevalence of parotitis and systemic features at onset of pedSD.[22,23] Additionally, several studies conclude that children do not fulfill adult SD criteria[12,23,24] and advocate for pediatric-specific criteria.[12,23] The recently published large pediatric studies support the notion that pediatric disease presents differently than adult disease.[8,12] Key findings of these studies are summarized later.

Several terms describe diagnosis of SD before 18 years of age, including pediatric Sjögren syndrome, Sjögren disease, juvenile Sjögren Syndrome, childhood or childhood-onset Sjögren syndrome, Sjögren syndrome in childhood, and others, but no consensus terminology exists. Patient advocacy groups and leaders in the field have proposed removing "syndrome" from the name of the condition to reduce stigma,[25] and the Sjögren's Syndrome Foundation recently changed its name to the Sjögren's Foundation.[26] This article uses pedSD to describe individuals diagnosed with SD before the age of 18 years.

PATHOPHYSIOLOGY

The pathophysiology of SD is complex and incompletely understood but likely results from a combination of host and environmental factors triggering robust immune activation in epithelial and glandular tissues that bridges both innate and adaptive immunity.[1] Genetic susceptibility has been linked to common immune-related genes implicating interferon signaling, innate immunity, lymphocyte activation, and the X chromosome.[2] Lymphocytes have long been recognized as key mediators of inflammation in SD, beginning with observation of lymphocytic sialadenitis on oral tissue biopsy dating back to the 1960s.[1] Subsequent identification of specific autoantibodies and germinal centers in affected tissues highlight the pathogenic role of B cells in disease manifestations, including the risk of lymphoma.[1]

CLINICAL FEATURES

Clinical features typically are categorized as glandular, if involving exocrine tissues, or as extraglandular manifestations. Prevalence of manifestations in adults with SD in comparison to prevalence in recent large pediatric studies is reported in **Tables 1** and **2**.

Glandular Manifestations

Xerostomia (dry mouth)
Immune-mediated infiltration and dysfunction of the salivary glands result in decreased saliva production. Patients may complain of dry mouth, which tends to worsen throughout the day, increased water intake, and inability to swallow food without drinking. Additional symptoms include halitosis, dysgeusia, cheilosis, dysphonia, mucositis, odynophagia, and weight loss. Patients may present with numerous caries and/or caries in unusual locations. On examination, oral mucosa may have a dry appearance and/or decreased salivary pooling.[2,27] Oral symptoms occur in 34% to 80% of pedSD cases.[8,11–13,15]

Xerophthalmia (dry eye)
Immune-mediated infiltration and dysfunction of lacrimal glands result in decreased tear production and keratoconjunctivitis sicca, or damage to corneal and bulbar epithelium. This dysfunction can lead to vision-threatening complications (eg, corneal ulceration, scarring).[4] Patients may report a sandy, gritty, or burning sensation in the eye, itching, redness, and photosensitivity. Examination may reveal conjunctival vessel dilation and/or pericorneal irritation.[2,27] The prevalence of ocular symptoms in pedSD cases ranges from 35% to 70%.[8,11–13,15]

Parotitis and submandibular salivary gland swelling
Recurrent or persistent swelling of the major salivary glands is a heralding symptom of pedSD.[11,12,28] The parotid glands, the largest of the major salivary glands, are most

Table 1
Clinical features of Sjögren disease in adults and children

Clinical feature	Adult From Brito-Zeron and Colleagues, 2016,[1] and Vivino and Colleagues, 2019[2]	Pediatric				
		Means and Colleagues, 2017[11]	Hammenfors and Colleagues, 2020[13]	Basiaga and Colleagues, 2020[12]	Ramos-Casals and Colleagues, 2020[8] c	Marino and Colleagues, 2020[15]
Age at diagnosis, mean (y)	30–50	12.4	12.1	12 (median)	14.2	10.2 (median)
Age at symptom onset, mean (y)		8.4	10.2		13.2	
Female (%)	90	83	87	83	86	80
Primary SD (%)	50	50	86	85	100	85
Oral symptom (%)	~100	34	80	52	80	35
Ocular symptom (%)		35	63	48	70	37
Parotitis (%)	33	53	64 a	47	47	56
CNS (%)d	3	9	5	9 b	1	17
Renal (%)	5	10	5	8	5	13
Musculoskeletal, all (%)		21	58		27	37
Arthritis (%)	10–30			24		
Arthralgia (%)	50–75			54		
Cutaneous (%)	6	6	29	9	12	18
Constitutional or fever (%)	6–13 (not including fatigue)	9	41	11	22	22
Lymphadenopathy (%)	8–32	8	59	18	25	
Pulmonary (%)	16	2	2	8	5	
Hematologic/cytopenia (%)	30–60	28	28	17	28	13
Lymphoma (no. cases)				5	1	2

a Any salivary gland enlargement.
b Includes headache, seizure, NMO, CNS vasculitis, and other neurologic.
c Features reported at time of diagnosis.
d Not including brain fog or mild cognitive dysfunction.

Note: clinical features are defined as positive reported findings divided by total number of cases. For Hammenfors and colleagues and for Ramos-Casals and colleagues, clinical features are defined as positive domain on EULAR Sjögren's Syndrome Disease Activity Index (constitutional, cutaneous, lymphadenopathy, articular, pulmonary, renal, CNS, and hematologic). NMO, neuromyelitis optica.

Table 2
Laboratory and diagnostic testing in adult and pediatric Sjögren disease

Laboratory and diagnostic test	Adult	Pediatric				
	From Brito-Zeron and Colleagues, 2016,[1] and 2020,[16] and Vivino and Colleagues, 2019[2]	Means and Colleagues, 2017[11]	Hammenfors and Colleagues, 2020[13]	Basiaga and Colleagues, 2020[12]	Ramos-Casals and Colleagues, 2020[8a]	Marino and colleagues, 2020[15]
Antinuclear antibody (%)	80–90		93	88	90	89
Anti-Ro/SSA (%)	70	75	75	74	83	82
Anti-La/SSB (%)	50	65	40	45	62	62
Rheumatoid factor (%)	50		45	60	68	70
Cryoglobulins (%)	10			3	5	
Hypergammaglobulinemia (%)	20–50			54		84
Salivary flow test (%)	74		33	30	79	
Schirmer test (%)	77		42	42	51	60[a]
Ocular stain (%)	74		54	19	36	
Salivary gland biopsy (%)	82		82	53	97	92
Ultrasound (%)	50–90		61	82	94	96[b]

Note: laboratory features are defined as percent of positive/abnormal test out of number of patients tested.
[a] Any abnormal ophthalmologic test.
[b] Any abnormal imaging.

commonly involved, although swelling of the submandibular glands also is reported.[11] Parotitis may be unilateral or bilateral. Swelling may be accompanied by tenderness and pain, which may worsen with jaw movement. Examination may reveal enlarged, tender parotid glands with swelling that obscures the angle of the mandible.[27] Parotid gland enlargement is associated with increased mortality in adults with primary SD,[29] but a similar risk has not been defined for children. Parotitis is present in approximately 33% of adults with SD but occurs in approximately 50 to 60% of pediatric cases.[8,11–13,15]

Other glandular involvement

Vaginal dryness and/or recurrent vaginitis may result from decreased vaginal lubrication due to immune infiltration of periepithelial cervicovaginal mucosa[30] and potentially Bartholin glands. Patients who are sexually active may experience dyspareunia and sexual dysfunction.[30] Pancreatic dysfunction and pancreatitis may occur. Dry skin may result from dysfunction of cutaneous exocrine glands.[27] Glandular dysfunction and immune infiltration of the upper airways can lead to xerotrachea and chronic dry cough.[2] Although these symptoms occur in pediatric patients, the prevalence is unknown.

Extraglandular Manifestations

Musculoskeletal

Musculoskeletal manifestations range from nonspecific arthralgias and myalgias to inflammatory arthritis and myositis.[27] Arthralgias are common, reported in approximately 50% of pedSD cases, whereas inflammatory arthritis affects approximately 25%.[8,11–13] Inflammatory arthritis can affect small and large joints and typically is nonerosive.[2]

Renal

Renal manifestations include primarily glomerulonephritis, from immune complex deposition, and interstitial nephritis, from direct infiltration of lymphocytes, which can lead to distal renal tubular acidosis.[11,27,31] Renal tubular acidosis may lead to hypokalemia and even hypokalemic periodic paralysis.[32] Renal involvement is reported in approximately 5% to 10% of pedSD cases.[8,11–13]

Pulmonary

Pulmonary manifestations of SD primarily include interstitial lung disease (ILD) but also can include pulmonary arterial hypertension and airway hyperreactivity due to lymphocytic infiltration of bronchi and bronchioles.[2,27] ILD subtypes reported include nonspecific interstitial pneumonia, usual interstitial pneumonia, lymphocytic interstitial pneumonia, and others.[2] Patients may be asymptomatic or may present with chronic cough, dyspnea, and abnormal findings on imaging and/or pulmonary function testing. In adults with SD, ILD can be life threatening[6] and contributes to disease-specific mortality.[2] Pulmonary involvement is reported in less than 10% of pedSD cases.[8,11–13]

Neurologic

Neurologic involvement, including both CNS and peripheral nervous system (PNS), can be dramatic. CNS manifestations occurred in 1% to 9% of cases included in large pedSD studies[8,11–13] and include encephalitis,[33,34] meningitis,[35] encephalopathy, optic neuritis, and demyelinating lesions.[2] Specifically, several cases of comorbid SD and neuromyelitis spectrum disorder are reported in adults and in children.[36] PNS manifestations include cranial neuropathies, demyelinating polyneuropathy, and mononeuritis multiplex.[2] Patients may present with a variety of symptoms including headache, altered mental status, seizure,[2] chorea,[37] numbness, weakness, paralysis, dysarthria, dysmetria, and others.[35] Dysautonomia, cognitive dysfunction,[2] mental disturbance,[35] hallucinations, and psychosis also have been reported.[38]

Cutaneous
Cutaneous manifestations are diverse and varied and include cutaneous vasculitis and purpura, annular erythema, erythema nodosum, cutaneous amyloidosis, and other lesions.[2] Raynaud phenomenon also may occur. In adults with SD, purpura and vasculitis are associated with increased mortality.[2,29] Prevalence is difficult to determine in pedSD because definitions vary, but cutaneous involvement is present in up to 30% of reported cases.[8,11–13]

Gastrointestinal
Beyond the oral and pancreatic manifestations, other gastrointestinal manifestations include gastritis,[39] primary biliary cirrhosis, hepatitis,[2,15,40] chronic diarrhea, and constipation.[2] Nonalcoholic steatohepatitis has been reported in pedSD.[39]

Hematologic
Hematologic manifestations typically are mild and include anemia of chronic disease,[2] leukopenia, and thrombocytopenia. Severe anemia, including hemolytic anemia, neutropenia, and thrombocytopenia, can occur.[2,41] Prevalence among pedSD cases ranges 17% to 28%.[8,12,13]

Systemic inflammatory/constitutional symptoms
Fevers range in frequency and severity and may be associated with other symptoms, including malaise and fatigue. Fevers and constitutional symptoms occurred in 20% to 40% of pedSD cases.[8,13,15]

Fatigue
Fatigue is common and often persistent in SD,[2] but the etiology is unclear. Depression and pain may contribute.[2] Data are limited but suggest that fatigue is less common in pedSD, reported in 5% to 13%.[8,15]

Congenital heart block
Congenital heart block and an array of immune phenomena, known as neonatal lupus, can affect infants born to mothers with SD and other connective tissue diseases. Anti-SSA/Ro and anti-SSB/La antibodies can cross the placenta and block signal conduction at the atrioventricular node of infants, even if mothers are asymptomatic and lack a diagnosis of SD or other connective tissue disease.[42]

LABORATORY AND DIAGNOSTIC TESTING

A majority of children with SD have a positive antinuclear antibody, although approximately 10% are negative.[8,11–13,15] Anti-SSA/Ro and anti-SSB/La are less sensitive, with anti-SSA/Ro present in up to 70% of adult cases[1] and 74% to 83% of pediatric cases,[8,11–13,15] and anti-SSB/La present in approximately 50%[1] of adult and 40% to 65% of pediatric cases.[8,11–13,15] Rheumatoid factor is present in approximately 50% of adults[1] and 45% to 70% of pediatric cases, with higher positivity among children with parotitis.[8,12,13,15] Cryoglobulinemia is less common but may indicate a poor prognosis.[2,6] Although reported in up to 10% of adult cases,[1,2] cryoglobulins were positive in less than 5% of the small fraction of those tested in 2 large pedSD studies.[8,12]

Although nonspecific, approximately 20% of patients have elevated erythrocyte sedimentation rate.[2] Hypergammaglobulinemia is present in approximately 50% of adult and pediatric patients.[2,12]

Hypocomplementemia is present in up to 20% of adult patients. Low complement 4 (C4) is more common in severe disease[6] and is a risk factor for lymphoma among adult patients.[43] In 1 study of pedSD, low C4 was present in 12% of patients and did not vary based on disease severity, however the number tested was small.[8]

Diagnostic testing for SD includes (1) objective markers of dryness, (2) histologic evidence of inflammation, (3) anatomic evaluation, and (4) functional studies.

Objective Markers of Dryness

Sialometry, or salivary flow testing, is a simple, in-office test that measures the volume of saliva accumulated over 5 minutes to 15 minutes. A flow rate of less than or equal to 0.1 mL/min is abnormal in adults. No age-adjusted normal values exist for children. The Schirmer test is an in-office test of tear volume, in which a specialized strip of filter paper is placed between the lower eyelid and the eye for 5 minutes. A wet length of paper less than or equal to 5 mm indicates decreased tear production in adults. No age-adjusted normal values exist for children. Ocular surface stain assesses for keratoconjunctivitis sicca. An ocular stain score (OSS) greater than or equal to 5 or van Bijsterveld score greater than or equal to 4 in at least 1 eye indicates ocular surface inflammation. OSS and other objective measures lack normative, age-adjusted values for pediatric patients.

Histologic Evidence of Inflammation

Salivary gland biopsy often is considered the gold standard for diagnosis of SD. Hematoxylin-eosin (H&E) stain revealing dense periductal mononuclear cell aggregates, or focal lymphocytic sialadenitis, is characteristic of SD (**Fig. 1**). Adult criteria define a focus score greater than or equal to 1 focus/4 mm^2 consistent with SD.[44] Labial salivary gland biopsies in children with SD often demonstrate focal lymphocytic

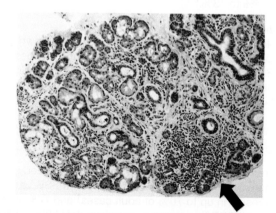

Fig. 1. Focal sialadenitis on labial minor salivary gland biopsy in a child with SD. This H&E-stained section of a minor salivary gland from an 8-year-old girl demonstrates normal glandular architecture with a focus of mononuclear cells (*arrow*) in the typical periductal distribution. A focus is defined as an aggregate of greater than or equal to 50 mononuclear cells. The focus score is defined as the number of foci per 4 mm^2 of tissue, with a score of greater than or equal to 1 focus/4 mm^2 meeting histopathologic criteria for SD in adults. (Courtesy of Scott Steward-Tharp, DDS, PhD, University of Iowa.)

sialadenitis but with a focus score less than the adult cutoff. Some investigators suggest that any focal sialadenits (ie, focus score >0 foci/4 mm^2) may be sufficient for diagnosis of pedSD.[12] Additionally, although labial minor salivary gland biopsy is considered equivalent to major salivary gland biopsy in adults,[45] parotid biopsy may be more sensitive in children.[46]

Anatomic Evaluation

Historically, sialography has been used to evaluate anatomy of the parotid ductal system using radiocontrast injected into Stensen duct or Wharton duct. Findings of sialectasis, ductal narrowing, and parenchymal abnormalities (eg, inhomogeneous parenchymal blushing) suggest SD.[47] Over the past few decades, however, sialography has been used less frequently, likely due to the invasiveness and radiation involved, and is no longer included in SD criteria. Salivary gland changes consistent with SD, including enlargement and architectural abnormalities (eg, cystic changes and calcifications), are visualized on magnetic resonance imaging (MRI) and computed tomography (CT). Findings may be incidental or part of diagnostic evaluation and occur in both adult and pediatric patients.[48] Neither MRI nor CT findings currently are included in SD criteria. Salivary gland ultrasound (SGUS) increasingly is utilized for diagnostic evaluation of SD. Abnormal salivary gland architecture in SD is seen as areas of hypoechogenicity within the submandibular and parotid glands. Several scoring systems exist,[49–51] although they generally grade the parenchymal inhomogeneity of each parotid and submandibular gland on a scale of 0 to 3, with 0 being normal and 3 being gross inhomogeneity. SGUS is highly sensitive and specific for primary SD,[52] can detect early onset-disease,[53] and is favorable due to the lack of radiation, noninvasive nature and relative ease of performance in the outpatient setting. SGUS has been proposed as an addition to or replacement for other diagnostic tests in the most recent SD criteria.[54] Although most studies on SGUS involve primary SD, SGUS also has been used successfully in diagnosis of nonprimary SD[51] and pedSD.[13,15]

Functional Tests

Salivary scintigraphy, a radiolabeled functional test, can show delayed or absent isotope uptake and secretion in SD.[55] Although this test is reported in a small number of pedSD cases, a majority (81%–94%) were abnormal.[8,13] The degree of dysfunction by scintigraphy may indicate a worse prognosis in adults.[55]

EVOLUTION OF DISEASE FEATURES OVER TIME

SD is not a static disease, and disease features vary with age at presentation. Compared with adults, children present more often with glandular swelling and less often with dryness symptoms. In the study by Basiaga and colleagues,[12] parotid swelling was present in 100% of cases diagnosed with pedSD at the youngest ages (1–4 y), and the prevalence decreased with increasing age at diagnosis. Similar findings were reported for parotitis[15] and any glandular swelling.[8] In contrast, patients less than 15 years old at diagnosis were less likely to report dry eyes compared with patients 15 years to 18 years old.[8] These findings support the notion that glandular inflammation represents an earlier stage of disease; glandular dysfunction and dryness symptoms require time to develop and thus are less common in childhood disease. Other inflammatory symptoms may occur more frequently in childhood disease, as well. In the study by Ramos-Casals and colleagues,[8] younger patients had higher mean disease activity scores, higher frequency of active disease, and higher frequency of lymphadenopathy. These findings have significant implications for treatment, as young patients with active inflammatory disease could present an opportunity for successful treatment with systemic immunotherapy.

DIFFERENTIAL DIAGNOSIS

The spectrum of clinical manifestations of SD leads to a broad differential diagnosis. Xerostomia and xerophthalmia may be side effects of commonly used medications, such as antidepressants and anticholinergics, including over-the-counter antihistamines. The most common cause of parotitis in childhood is infection, and mumps must be considered, especially in a patient without routine childhood vaccinations. Anatomic causes, such as stones, may cause parotid pain and swelling. Juvenile recurrent parotitis (JRP) is a benign condition of nonobstructive sialectasia, resulting in recurrent, usually unilateral parotitis, without other signs or symptoms of pedSD.[56] Sialendoscopy can be both diagnostic and therapeutic for JRP.[56] Other organ manifestations, such as pulmonary, renal, and cutaneous disease, with systemic inflammation should prompt evaluation for connective tissue disease, such as systemic lupus erythematosus as well as malignancy and chronic infection. Neurologic manifestations should be evaluated broadly for infectious, traumatic, toxic, malignant, primary neurologic, and primary autoimmune etiologies and may require referral to a specialized center.

DIAGNOSIS AND CLASSIFICATION

In 2002, the American-European Consensus Group developed classification criteria for primary SD requiring 4 of 6 standardized features, including oral and ocular dryness symptoms, ocular signs (Schirmer test or OSS), evidence of salivary gland involvement (salivary flow test, sialography, and scintigraphy), positive salivary gland biopsy, and/or positive serologies (ie, anti-SSA/Ro and/or anti-SSB/La). In 2016, the American College of Rheumatology (ACR) and European League Against Rheumatism (EULAR) developed updated classification criteria (**Table 3**). Key differences from prior criteria are the addition of extra-glandular manifestations to the inclusion criteria and a weighted scoring system.[44]

Adult criteria fail to capture a large proportion, if not the majority, of pedSD cases diagnosed by a pediatric rheumatologist.[12,13,57] Potential explanations for failure include different clinical features in young patients, different diagnostic testing results,[12] and lower utilization of diagnostic tests. Basiaga and colleagues[12] found that only two-thirds of the pedSD cohort underwent enough diagnostic testing to achieve a classifiable score, and, of those cases, only 36% met 2016 ACR/EULAR criteria. Proposed pediatric modifications to the 2016 ACR/EULAR criteria include addition of parotitis as inclusion criteria,[57] any focal sialadenitis on biopsy (eg, focus score >0 foci/4 mm^2),[12,57] and/or characteristic ultrasound findings[12,13] as diagnostic test. Advancing understanding of the natural history of disease, identifying prognostic and risk factors, and rigorously studying the effects of intervention on disease outcomes urgently require pediatric-specific normative values for diagnostic tests and classification criteria.[8,12]

Additional guidance for clinical diagnosis of pedSD is urgently needed, because classification criteria serve primarily for entry into clinical trials and may fail to capture early and/or atypical disease. Diagnosis often is delayed up to 2 years to 4 years from time of symptom onset.[11,15] The large proportion of pediatric patients diagnosed by a pediatric rheumatologist as having pedSD but failing to meet adult criteria[12,13,57] highlights the pressing need for improved diagnostic guidance. In 1999, Bartunkova and

Table 3
The 2016 American College of Rheumatology and European League Against Rheumatism classification criteria for primary Sjögren disease

The classification of primary Sjögren syndrome applies to any individual who meets the inclusion criteria, does not have any of the conditions listed as exclusion criteria, and has a score of ≥4 when the weights from the 5 criteria items below are summed.

Inclusion	Exclusion
Any patient with at least 1 symptom of ocular or oral dryness, defined as a positive response to at least 1 of the following questions:	Prior diagnosis of
1. Have you had daily, persistent, troublesome dry eyes for more than 3 mo?	1. History of head and neck radiation treatment
2. Do you have a recurrent sensation of sand or gravel in the eyes?	2. Active hepatitis C infection (with confirmation by PCR)
3. Do you use tear substitutes more than 3 times a day?	3. AIDS
4. Have you had a daily feeling of dry mouth for more than 3 mo?	4. Sarcoidosis
5. Do you frequently drink liquids to aid in swallowing dry food?	5. Amyloidosis
or in whom there is suspicion of Sjögren syndrome from the EULAR Sjögren Syndrome Disease Activity Index questionnaire	6. Graft-versus-host disease
	7. IgG4-related disease

Item	Weight
Labial salivary gland with focal lymphocytic sialadenitis and focus score of ≥1 foci/4 mm^2	3
Anti–SSA/Ro-positive	3
OSS ≥5 (or van Bijsterveld score ≥4) in at least 1 eye	1
Schirmer test ≤5 mm/5 min in at least 1 eye	1
Unstimulated whole saliva flow rate ≤0.1 mL/min	1

Abbreviations: AIDS, acquired immunodeficiency syndrome; PCR, polymerase chain reaction.

Adapted from Shiboski CH, Shiboski SC, Seror R, et al. 2016 American College of Rheumatology/European League Against Rheumatism classification criteria for primary Sjogren's syndrome: A consensus and data-driven methodology involving three international patient cohorts. Ann Rheum Dis. 2017;76(1):9-16.

colleagues[21] proposed pediatric-specific diagnostic criteria, which included not only the characteristic sicca symptoms plus serologic and diagnostic testing abnormalities but also several nonspecific symptoms (eg, fever and abdominal pain) and testing abnormalities (eg, leukopenia). The Bartunkova criteria never were validated or widely used. More recently, the Japanese Pediatric Sjögren's Syndrome Study Group developed criteria relying exclusively on laboratory and diagnostic testing to classify patients as definite, probable, possible, needing follow-up, or non-SD.[58] These criteria have been used in a limited number of Japanese patients but have not been evaluated in larger pedSD studies and are not used widely in practice. Guidance for clinical evaluation and diagnosis from an International Childhood Sjögren Workgroup currently is under way and should be available soon. Diagnostic pearls for pedSD are included in **Table 4**.

Table 4
Care points for diagnosis of Sjögren disease in a pediatric patient

Presenting Symptom	History	Diagnostic Evaluation
Sicca/dryness	• Obtain careful history to elicit symptoms. • Review medications to screen for drug side effects (anticholinergics, antidepressants).	• All patients need evaluation by dentist and ophthalmologist to establish objective findings of dryness[a] and assist with symptomatic treatment.
Parotitis	• Exclude infection (mumps; viral infection, including EBV, CMV, and HIV, especially if persistent rather than recurrent). • Exclude stones and anatomic abnormalities. • Consider JRP.	• Collaborate with otolaryngologist and/or oral pathologist. • Consider referral to center that can perform sialendoscopy (which can be diagnostic and therapeutic). • If persistent enlargement, consider biopsy of gland to evaluate for malignancy.
Lymphadenopathy	• Exclude malignancy, infection, IgG4 disease.	
Neurologic symptom	• Maintain broad differential diagnosis, including infection, malignancy, and other autoimmune brain disease.	• Consider referral to specialized center.
All	• Evaluate for secondary or comorbid autoimmune disease (systemic lupus erythematosus and others).	• Consider ultrasonography even in absence of glandular swelling. • Negative serologies or diagnostic test results should not preclude diagnosis in setting of high clinical suspicion. • May consider positive biopsy any focal sialadenitis (focus score >0 foci/4 mm^2).

Abbreviations: CMV, cytomegalovirus; EBV, epstein barr virus; HIV, human immunodeficiency virus.
   [a] Note that objective tests (Schirmer test, salivary flow test, and so forth) are not standardized to pediatric patients and adult normative values may not apply.

TREATMENT

For symptoms of dryness, topical therapies are well tolerated and can improve symptoms[59]; however, no therapies have been shown to reverse glandular dysfunction or cure sicca symptoms.[2] Although systemic therapy, including hydroxychloroquine (HCQ), is widely used, the limited number of randomized trials in adults largely have shown mixed results or failed to reach primary efficacy endpoints.[59] Rituximab may have a role,[59] however, and belimumab[60] and iscalimab[61] have promising early results for systemic disease manifestations.

In 2020, a EULAR task force published recommendations for topical and systemic therapies in adults.[7] The overarching recommendations include (1) management at centers of expertise using a multidisciplinary approach, (2) use of topical therapies for symptomatic relief of dryness, and (3) consideration of systemic therapy for active systemic disease. A stepwise therapeutic approach is provided based on organ involvement. Systemic therapies range from HCQ for articular involvement, to glucocorticoids and cyclophosphamide for refractory and severe disease, such as neurologic involvement.[7]

No pediatric-specific treatment recommendations exist. Reports of treatments used for pedSD are limited. In the study by Hammenfors and colleagues,[13] a vast majority of patients received symptomatic (80%) or systemic (95%) therapy during follow-up. The most commonly prescribed systemic therapy was HCQ (92%), followed by systemic steroids (up to 77%), methotrexate (39%), and azathioprine (21%).[13] Other treatments, including rituximab, cyclophosphamide, and mycophenolate mofetil, have been reported in pedSD.[35] Compared with adults, young patients may present a unique opportunity to modify the natural history of disease, prevent chronic glandular dysfunction, and improve other outcomes; however, measures demonstrating response to treatment and prevention of progressive glandular dysfunction are needed.

OUTCOMES

SD causes significant morbidity and reduces quality of life.[62] Primary SD also is associated with an increased risk of lymphoma, primarily low-grade B-cell non-Hodgkin lymphoma.[5] Although SD traditionally was not thought to impact mortality, a subset of adults with primary SD develop severe systemic disease with a mortality rate of 20%.[6] Adult studies have identified risk factors for malignancy and other unfavorable outcomes. Persistent parotid enlargement and lymphadenopathy are among the risk factors for lymphoma.[5] Cryoglobulinemia, low C4, and cytopenias, among other features, predict lymphoma and are seen more commonly in the severe systemic disease phenotype.[5,6] Early-onset adult disease (age at diagnosis <35 y) is associated with these risk factors along with worsening disease activity over time.[63] It is unknown but certainly worrisome that the high prevalences of parotid swelling and lymphadenopathy in pedSD may indicate an increased risk of poor outcomes. Fewer than a dozen cases of lymphoma have been reported in pedSD,[12,64,65] and other long-term outcomes have not been characterized. Given the long disease duration in pedSD, high representation of adult risk factors for severe disease, and unique opportunities for intervention, prospective and longitudinal studies are of paramount importance in pedSD.

SUMMARY

Although previously considered rare in children, pedSD increasingly is reported. Distinct clinical features, including higher prevalence of parotitis and lower prevalence of sicca symptoms compared with adults, and failure to meet adult criteria highlight the need for pediatric-specific studies and criteria. Risk factors for poor outcomes in adults have been established, and many of these features are more common in young patients; however, whether they portend worse outcomes for these children is not known. Rigorous prospective and longitudinal studies will define pedSD better. Ultimately, diagnosis of SD in young patients may provide a unique opportunity to modify disease course through therapeutic intervention.

DISCLOSURE

RLR receives support from the National Institute of General Medical Sciences and the Eunice Kennedy Shriver National Institute of Child Health and Human Development (NICHD) of the National Institutes of Health (NIH) under Award Number

T32GM086330. RLR's spouse has current or prior employment and/or stock ownership in Merck & Co and in Biogen.

SML receives support from the National Eye Institute (NEI) of the NIH under Award Number R01EY027731.

REFERENCES

1. Brito-Zeron P, Baldini C, Bootsma H, et al. Sjogren syndrome. Nat Rev Dis Primers 2016;2:16047.
2. Vivino FB, Bunya VY, Massaro-Giordano G, et al. Sjogren's syndrome: an update on disease pathogenesis, clinical manifestations and treatment. Clin Immunol 2019;203:81–121.
3. Alani H, Henty JR, Thompson NL, et al. Systematic review and meta-analysis of the epidemiology of polyautoimmunity in Sjogren's syndrome (secondary Sjogren's syndrome) focusing on autoimmune rheumatic diseases. Scand J Rheumatol 2018;47(2):141–54.
4. Akpek EK, Mathews P, Hahn S, et al. Ocular and systemic morbidity in a longitudinal cohort of Sjogren's syndrome. Ophthalmology 2015;122(1):56–61.
5. Nocturne G, Mariette X. Sjogren Syndrome-associated lymphomas: an update on pathogenesis and management. Br J Haematol 2015;168(3):317–27.
6. Flores-Chavez A, Kostov B, Solans R, et al. Severe, life-threatening phenotype of primary Sjogren's syndrome: clinical characterisation and outcomes in 1580 patients (GEAS-SS Registry). Clin Exp Rheumatol 2018;36 Suppl 112(3):121–9.
7. Ramos-Casals M, Brito-Zeron P, Bombardieri S, et al. EULAR recommendations for the management of Sjogren's syndrome with topical and systemic therapies. Ann Rheum Dis 2020;79(1):3–18.
8. Ramos-Casals M, Acar-Denizli N, Vissink A, et al. Childhood-onset of primary Sjögren's syndrome: phenotypic characterization at diagnosis of 158 children. Rheumatology (Oxford). 2021 Jan 25:keab032. doi:10.1093/rheumatology/keab032. Epub ahead of print.
9. O'Neill EM. Sjogren's syndrome with onset at ten years of age. Proc Rox Soc Med 1965;58(9):689–90.
10. Duncan H, Epker BN, Sheldon GM. Sjögren's syndrome in childhood: report of a case. Henry Ford Hosp Med J 1969;17(1):35–42.
11. Means C, Aldape MA, King E. Pediatric primary Sjogren syndrome presenting with bilateral ranulas: a case report and systematic review of the literature. Int J Pediatr Otorhinolaryngol 2017;101:11–9.
12. Basiaga ML, Stern SM, Mehta JJ, et al. Childhood Arthritis and Rheumatology Research Alliance and the International Childhood Sjögren Syndrome Workgroup. Childhood Sjögren syndrome: features of an international cohort and application of the 2016 ACR/EULAR classification criteria. Rheumatology (Oxford). 2021 Jul 1;60(7):3144-3155. doi:10.1093/rheumatology/keaa757.
13. Hammenfors DS, Valim V, Bica B, et al. Juvenile Sjogren's syndrome: clinical characteristics with focus on salivary gland ultrasonography. Arthritis Care Res (Hoboken) 2020;72(1):78–87.
14. Dinse GE, Parks CG, Weinberg CR, et al. Increasing prevalence of antinuclear antibodies in the United States. Arthritis Rheumatol 2020;72(6):1026–35.
15. Marino A, Romano M, Giani T, et al. Childhood Sjogren's syndrome: An Italian case series and a literature review-based cohort. Semin Arthritis Rheum. 2020 Nov 21:S0049-0172(20)30279-1. doi:10.1016/j.semarthrit.2020.11.004. Epub ahead of print.

16. Brito-Zeron P, Acar-Denizli N, Ng WF, et al. Epidemiological profile and north-south gradient driving baseline systemic involvement of primary Sjogren's syndrome. Rheumatology (Oxford) 2020;59(9):2350–9.
17. Chudwin DS, Daniels TE, Wara DW, et al. Spectrum of Sjögren syndrome in children. J Pediatr 1981;98(2):213–7.
18. Ostuni PA, Ianniello A, Sfriso P, et al. Juvenile onset of primary Sjögren's syndrome: report of 10 cases. Clin Exp Rheumatol 1996;14(6):689–93.
19. Mizuno Y, Hara T, Hatae K, et al. Recurrent parotid gland enlargement as an initial manifestation of Sjogren syndrome in children. Eur J Pediatr 1989;148(5):414–6.
20. Berman JL, Kashii S, Trachtman MS, et al. Optic Neuropathy and Central Nervous System Disease Secondary to Sjögren's Syndrome in a Child. Ophthalmology 1990;97(12):1606–9.
21. Bartunkova J, Sediva A, Vencovsky J, et al. Primary Sjögren's syndrome in children and adolescents: proposal for diagnostic criteria. Clin Exp Rheumatol 1999;17(3):381–6.
22. Virdee S, Greenan-Barrett J, Ciurtin C. A systematic review of primary Sjögren's syndrome in male and paediatric populations. Clin Rheumatol 2017;36(10): 2225–36.
23. Houghton K, Malleson P, Cabral D, et al. Primary Sjögren's syndrome in children and adolescents: are proposed diagnostic criteria applicable? J Rheumatol 2005;32(11):2225–32.
24. Cimaz R, Casadei A, Rose C, et al. Primary Sjogren syndrome in the paediatric age: a multicentre survey. Eur J Pediatr 2003;162(10):661–5.
25. Baer AN, Hammitt KM. Sjögren's Disease, Not Syndrome. Arthritis Rheumatol 2021 Jul;73(7):1347–8. https://doi.org/10.1002/art.41676. Epub 2021 Jun 1.
26. The Sjogren's Foundation. 2021. Available at: https://www.sjogrens.org/about-us. Accessed January 6, 2021.
27. Lieberman SM, Stern SM, Basiaga ML. Approach to children with Sjogren's syndrome. In: Vivino FB, ed. [ital]Sjogren's Syndrome: A Clinical Handbook [/ital]. Elsevier; 2020:75-91.
28. Baszis K, Toib D, Cooper M, et al. Recurrent parotitis as a presentation of primary pediatric Sjogren syndrome. Pediatrics 2012;129(1):e179–82.
29. Singh AG, Singh S, Matteson EL. Rate, risk factors and causes of mortality in patients with Sjogren's syndrome: a systematic review and meta-analysis of cohort studies. Rheumatology (Oxford) 2016;55(3):450–60.
30. van Nimwegen JF, van der Tuuk K, Liefers SC, et al. Vaginal dryness in primary Sjogren's syndrome: a histopathological case-control study. Rheumatology (Oxford) 2020;59(10):2806–15.
31. Bogdanovic R, Basta-Jovanovic G, Putnik J, et al. Renal involvement in primary Sjogren syndrome of childhood: case report and literature review. Mod Rheumatol 2013;23(1):182–9.
32. Garza-Alpirez A, Arana-Guajardo AC, Esquivel-Valerio JA, et al. Hypokalemic paralysis due to primary Sjogren syndrome: case report and review of the literature. Case Rep Rheumatol 2017;2017:7509238.
33. Matsui Y, Takenouchi T, Narabayashi A, et al. Childhood Sjogren syndrome presenting as acute brainstem encephalitis. Brain Dev 2016;38(1):158–62.
34. Iwai K, Amo K, Kuki I, et al. An unusual manifestation of Sjogren syndrome encephalitis. Brain Dev 2019;41(2):217–20.
35. Zhao J, Chen Q, Zhu Y, et al. Nephrological disorders and neurological involvement in pediatric primary Sjogren syndrome:a case report and review of literature. Pediatr Rheumatol Online J 2020;18(1):39.

36. Kornitzer JM, Kimura Y, Janow GL. Primary Sjogren syndrome in a child with a neuromyelitis optica spectrum disorder. J Rheumatol 2016;43(6):1260–1.
37. Delorme C, Cohen F, Hubsch C, et al. Chorea as the initial manifestation of Sjogren syndrome. Pediatr Neurol 2015;52(6):647–8.
38. Hammett EK, Fernandez-Carbonell C, Crayne C, et al. Adolescent Sjogren's syndrome presenting as psychosis: a case series. Pediatr Rheumatol Online J 2020; 18(1):15.
39. Kashiwagi Y, Hatsushika T, Tsutsumi N, et al. Gastrointestinal and liver lesions in primary childhood Sjogren syndrome. Clin Rheumatol 2017;36(6):1433–5.
40. Popov Y, Salomon-Escoto K. Gastrointestinal and hepatic disease in sjogren syndrome. Rheum Dis Clin North Am 2018;44(1):143–51.
41. Nakahara E, Yagasaki H, Shimozawa K, et al. Severe thrombocytopenia as initial signs of primary sjogren syndrome in a 9-Year-old female. Pediatr Blood Cancer 2016;63(7):1312–3.
42. Brito-Zeron P, Pasoto SG, Robles-Marhuenda A, et al. Autoimmune congenital heart block and primary Sjogren's syndrome: characterisation and outcomes of 49 cases. Clin Exp Rheumatol 2020;38 Suppl 126(4):95–102.
43. Fragkioudaki S, Mavragani CP, Moutsopoulos HM. Predicting the risk for lymphoma development in Sjogren syndrome: an easy tool for clinical use. Medicine (Baltimore) 2016;95(25):e3766.
44. Shiboski CH, Shiboski SC, Seror R, et al. 2016 American College of Rheumatology/European League Against Rheumatism classification criteria for primary Sjogren's syndrome: a consensus and data-driven methodology involving three international patient cohorts. Ann Rheum Dis 2017;76(1):9–16.
45. Wise CM, Agudelo CA, Semble EL, et al. Comparison of parotid and minor salivary gland biopsy specimens in the diagnosis of Sjogren's syndrome. Arthritis Rheum 1988;31(5):662–6.
46. McGuirt WF Jr, Whang C, Moreland W. The role of parotid biopsy in the diagnosis of pediatric Sjogren syndrome. Arch Otolaryngol Head Neck Surg 2002;128(11): 1279–81.
47. Stiller M, Golder W, Doring E, et al. Primary and secondary Sjogren's syndrome in children–a comparative study. Clin Oral Investig 2000;4(3):176–82.
48. Kumar KJ, Kudakesseril AS, Sheeladevi CS, et al. Primary Sjogrens syndrome in a child. Iran J Pediatr 2015;25(2):e254.
49. Hocevar A, Ambrozic A, Rozman B, et al. Ultrasonographic changes of major salivary glands in primary Sjogren's syndrome. Diagnostic value of a novel scoring system. Rheumatology (Oxford) 2005;44(6):768–72.
50. Milic VD, Petrovic RR, Boricic IV, et al. Diagnostic value of salivary gland ultrasonographic scoring system in primary Sjogren's syndrome: a comparison with scintigraphy and biopsy. J Rheumatol 2009;36(7):1495–500.
51. Martel A, Coiffier G, Bleuzen A, et al. What is the best salivary gland ultrasonography scoring methods for the diagnosis of primary or secondary Sjogren's syndromes? Joint Bone Spine 2019;86(2):211–7.
52. Ramsubeik K, Motilal S, Sanchez-Ramos L, et al. Diagnostic accuracy of salivary gland ultrasound in Sjogren's syndrome: A systematic review and meta-analysis. Ther Adv Musculoskelet Dis 2020;12. 1759720X20973560.
53. Baldini C, Luciano N, Tarantini G, et al. Salivary gland ultrasonography: a highly specific tool for the early diagnosis of primary Sjogren's syndrome. Arthritis Res Ther 2015;17:146.
54. van Nimwegen JF, Mossel E, Delli K, et al. Incorporation of Salivary Gland Ultrasonography Into the American College of Rheumatology/European League

Against Rheumatism Criteria for Primary Sjögren's Syndrome. Arthritis Care Res (Hoboken) 2020 Apr;72(4):583–90. https://doi.org/10.1002/acr.24017.

55. Ramos-Casals M, Brito-Zeron P, Perez DELM, et al. Clinical and prognostic significance of parotid scintigraphy in 405 patients with primary Sjogren's syndrome. J Rheumatol 2010;37(3):585–90.

56. Tucci FM, Roma R, Bianchi A, et al. Juvenile recurrent parotitis: diagnostic and therapeutic effectiveness of sialography. Retrospective study on 110 children. Int J Pediatr Otorhinolaryngol 2019;124:179–84.

57. Yokogawa NLS, Sherry DD, Vivino FB. Features of childhood Sjögren's syndrome in comparison to adult Sjögren's syndrome: considerations in establishing child-specific diagnostic criteria. Clin Exp Rheumatol 2016;34:343–51.

58. Tomiita M, Kobayashi I, Itoh Y, et al. Clinical practice guidance for Sjögren's syndrome in pediatric patients (2018) - summarized and updated. Mod Rheumatol 2020;1–11.

59. Brito-Zeron P, Retamozo S, Kostov B, et al. Efficacy and safety of topical and systemic medications: a systematic literature review informing the EULAR recommendations for the management of Sjogren's syndrome. RMD Open 2019;5(2):e001064.

60. Mariette X, Seror R, Quartuccio L, et al. Efficacy and safety of belimumab in primary Sjogren's syndrome: results of the BELISS open-label phase II study. Ann Rheum Dis 2015;74(3):526–31.

61. Fisher BA, Szanto A, Ng W-F, et al. Assessment of the anti-CD40 antibody iscalimab in patients with primary Sjögren's syndrome: a multicentre, randomised, double-blind, placebo-controlled, proof-of-concept study. Lancet Rheumatol 2020;2(3):e142–52.

62. Cornec D, Devauchelle-Pensec V, Mariette X, et al. Severe health-related quality of life impairment in active primary Sjogren's syndrome and patient-reported outcomes: data from a large therapeutic trial. Arthritis Care Res (Hoboken) 2017;69(4):528–35.

63. Anquetil C, Hachulla E, Machuron F, et al. Is early-onset primary Sjogren's syndrome a worse prognosis form of the disease? Rheumatology (Oxford) 2019;58(7):1163–7.

64. Tesher MS, Esteban Y, Henderson TO, et al. Mucosal-associated Lymphoid Tissue (MALT) lymphoma in association with pediatric primary Sjogren syndrome: 2 cases and review. J Pediatr Hematol Oncol 2019;41(5):413–6.

65. Fukumoto Y, Hosoi H, Kawakita A, et al. [Sjögren's syndrome with MALT (mucosa-associated lymphoid tissue) lymphoma in a 13-year-old girl: a case report]. Nihon Rinsho Meneki Gakkai Kaishi 2000;23(1):49–56.

Juvenile Fibromyalgia

Jennifer E. Weiss, MD[a,*], Susmita Kashikar-Zuck, PhD[b,c]

KEYWORDS

- Juvenile fibromyalgia • Chronic musculoskeletal pain • Cognitive-behavioral therapy
- Physical exercise • Combined treatments • Multidisciplinary treatment

KEY POINTS

- Juvenile fibromyalgia is a chronic musculoskeletal pain condition commonly seen in pediatric rheumatology practice.
- Juvenile fibromyalgia is more prevalent in adolescent females.
- Juvenile fibromyalgia is characterized by widespread pain and associated symptoms including fatigue, sleep disturbance, anxiety, dysautonomia, headaches, and abdominal pain.
- Multidisciplinary treatment is recommended for juvenile fibromyalgia with studies showing beneficial effects from cognitive-behavioral therapy, physical exercise, and combined treatments.

INTRODUCTION

Juvenile fibromyalgia syndrome (JFM) is a chronic musculoskeletal (MSK) pain syndrome commonly seen in pediatric rheumatology practice. JFM is a noninflammatory condition and typically presents as a primary chronic pain disorder, but can also be present as a secondary pain syndrome in patients who have an underlying inflammatory or autoimmune condition such as juvenile idiopathic arthritis or systemic lupus erythematosus. In patients with secondary JFM, pain symptoms exceed clinical expectations based on the severity of disease activity and may persist even when peripheral (eg, joint) inflammation is well-controlled. Based on current knowledge, JFM is characterized as a centralized or nociplastic (ie, altered nociception in the absence of tissue damage or lesion) pain condition. In this article, we focus on primary JFM, how it is diagnosed, the potential pathophysiologic and contributory factors, its impact on patients' lives, and evidence-based treatment approaches.

Patients suffering from JFM experience widespread MSK pain (ie, pain in the bones, joints, and tissues of the body) that persists longer than 3 months.[1] The etiology of JFM is unknown, but frequently there is a family history of chronic pain, suggesting

[a] Pediatric Rheumatology, Hackensack Meridian School of Medicine, Hackensack University Medical Center, 30 Prospect Avenue, Hackensack, NJ 07601, USA; [b] Department of Pediatrics, University of Cincinnati College of Medicine; [c] Cincinnati Children's Hospital Medical Center, Cincinnati, OH, USA
* Corresponding author.
E-mail address: Jennifer.Weiss@hmhn.org

Rheum Dis Clin N Am 47 (2021) 725–736
https://doi.org/10.1016/j.rdc.2021.07.002
0889-857X/21/© 2021 Elsevier Inc. All rights reserved.

rheumatic.theclinics.com

a genetic component. The onset of JFM symptoms may be preceded by injury, illness, or a stressful event, implicating possible environmental triggers. Although widespread pain is the cardinal feature of JFM, it is usually accompanied by a number of additional symptoms such as fatigue, sleep disturbance, dysautonomia, anxiety and depression, headaches, abdominal pain, and irritable bowel syndrome (IBS).[2] Pain is characterized by central sensitization and wind-up (ie, increasing pain sensitivity to repeated stimulation) and allodynia (pain with light touch).[3] The pain may be sponta- neous (eg, throbbing, burning, or tingling) or evoked in response to noxious (hyperal- gesia) or non-noxious stimuli that can arise from everyday daily activities.[4] The constellation of unexplained symptoms in JFM makes it one of the more complex chronic pain conditions to treat. JFM may cause marked impairment, including poor school attendance and performance, as well as a decrease in physical activities and social engagement.[5,6] Heightened emotional distress, particularly increased anx- iety, is common in youth with JFM.[7] The negative impact of JFM on patients' daily lives is significantly greater than that of other chronic childhood rheumatic diseases such as juvenile idiopathic arthritis and systemic lupus erythematosus[8] and may affect quality of life well into adulthood.[9,10]

The diagnosis of JFM can be challenging because physical examination and labo- ratory findings do not reveal clear abnormalities, making it difficult to explain the diag- nosis to patients and families. Patients may, therefore, see multiple specialists resulting in unnecessary tests and costs in the hopes that a definitive medical diag- nosis can be found. Inconsistencies in diagnostic terminology also contribute to pa- tients and families' confusion. Health care professionals use various umbrella terms including chronic widespread pain and amplified MSK pain syndrome, under which is JFM. Sherry[11] defines amplified MSK pain syndrome, a descriptive term, as pain disproportionate to the stimulus without other medical explanation, such as inflamma- tion or injury (similar to the more recent terminology of nociplastic pain). Amplified MSK pain syndrome can be diffuse (as in JFM) or localized (as in complex regional pain syndrome). Chronic widespread pain is a similarly broad term that encompasses pain in multiple areas of the body but it does not assume the presence of other symp- toms (eg, dysautonomia and fatigue). Perhaps the best way to conceptualize JFM is as a subset of widespread or amplified MSK pain disorders, typified by a particular constellation of symptoms that accompany pain, including fatigue and sleep and cognitive difficulties, as well as other somatic and mood symptoms. Currently, the diagnosis of JFM is based either on the Yunus and Masi classification criteria for JFM[1] or the 2010 American College of Rheumatology (ACR) fibromyalgia syndrome criteria[12] described in detail elsewhere in this article.

PREVALENCE AND CLINICAL FEATURES OF JUVENILE FIBROMYALGIA

There are no population-based prevalence studies of JFM within the United States, but adult fibromyalgia (FM) is reported to have a prevalence rate of about 2.5%.[13] Chil- dren and adolescents with JFM form between 7% and 15% of new visits to pediatric rheumatology clinics.[14,15] Studies in other countries have reported that JFM or chronic widespread pain affects up to 6% of children and adolescents,[16,17] with females affected more than males (4:1). Age at first diagnosis is typically between 13 and 15 years of age, although JFM has been reported in children of younger ages as well. In a study of more than 200 patients with JFM enrolled between 2010 and 2014 in the Childhood Arthritis and Rheumatology Research Alliance (CARRA) Legacy Registry, a patient registry of 56 pediatric rheumatology clinics in North America (https://carragroup.org), the majority of the patients were Caucasian or White (85%), non-Hispanic (83%), and female (84%) with an average age of 15.4 ± 2.2 years.[18] Patients tended to be symptomatic for more than 1 year before their first visit to a pediatric rheumatologist. The most common presenting symptoms in the CARRA Legacy Registry (**Table 1**) are representative of the JFM population at large. In the CARRA cohort, 18% of patients endorsed a family history of FM. Higher household income was associated with less time between symptom onset and evaluation by a pediatric rheumatologist. Symptoms such as sleep difficulties, headaches and IBS were similar between males and females, except for numbness and tingling, which was more common in females. Males with JFM reported significantly greater functional impairment and had worse health-related quality of life compared with females.

ETIOLOGY AND PATHOGENESIS

Most of what is known about FM comes from the adult FM and chronic pain literature, which has consistently shown augmented pain sensitivity and disruption in endogenous pain modulation, resulting in hypersensitivity to painful and nonpainful stimuli.[19–21] The strongest evidence of altered pain processing in FM comes from neuroimaging studies that have shown alterations in brain structure, metabolic activity, and resting state functional connectivity in regions of the brain associated with pain processing, as well as augmented responses to painful as well as nonpainful stimuli.[22] Emerging research suggests that similar alterations are present in adolescents with JFM.[23] Familial aggregation of chronic pain syndromes (FM, low back pain, IBS, and temporomandibular jaw dysfunction) suggests that genetics may play a role in the pathophysiology of FM and JFM. Furthermore, a significant concordance between a FM diagnosis in children and their mothers and other family members has been

Table 1
Symptoms associated with JFM in the CARRA legacy registry (N = 201)

	n (%)
Widespread MSK pain	164 (91%)
Pain modulation with anxiety or stress	121 (80%)
Pain modulation with physical activity	117 (75%)
Frequent headaches	111 (68%)
Pain modulation with weather change	86 (61%)
Nonrestorative sleep	94 (52%)
Frequent awakenings	75 (42%)
Increased sleep latency	74 (41%)
Numbness and tingling of extremities	48 (32%)
Anxiety and/or depression	40 (28%)
Hypermobility on examination	35 (28%)
Subjective soft tissue swelling of extremities	32 (22%)
Irritable bowel symptoms	24 (16%)
Hypersomnia	25 (14%)

Adapted from Weiss JE, Schikler KN, Boneparth AD, Connelly M, Investigators CR. Demographic, clinical, and treatment characteristics of the juvenile primary fibromyalgia syndrome cohort enrolled in the Childhood Arthritis and Rheumatology Research Alliance Legacy Registry. *Pediatr Rheumatol Online J.* 2019;17(1):51.*This article is distributed under the terms of the Creative Commons Attribution 4.0 International License* (http://creativecommons.org/licenses/by/4.0/).

found.[24,25] Candidate genes such as *COMT* (catechol O-methyltransferase), *ADRB2* (β2 adrenergic receptor), *HTR2A* (5-hydroxytryptamine receptor 2A, also known as serotonin receptor 2A), and *Dopamine D4 receptor exon III repeat polymorphism* have been associated with FM. However, Ablin and colleagues propose that genetic associations no longer be thought of in terms such as "identifying the gene or genes responsible for FM," but rather as incorporating genetic data relevant to the processing of pain into the spectrum of centralized pain.[26,27] Patients with JFM commonly suffer comorbid psychiatric symptoms along with chronic pain and the overlap may be related to common triggers (such as stress or trauma), and their common neurobiological basis, including neural pathways and neurotransmitters that are involved in both pain and emotional distress circuitry.[28]

Although JFM is considered a noninflammatory condition by rheumatologists, there seems to be evidence of neuroinflammation, which is thought to drive chronic widespread pain via central sensitization. The release of proinflammatory cytokines and chemokines[4] promotes chronic widespread pain at multiple body sites. Some researchers have proposed that bacterial and viral infections and injury may predispose to the development of chronic pain syndromes.[29,30] A possible role for small fiber polyneuropathy in the etiology of chronic pain syndromes such as JFM has been suggested.[31,32] The last decade has brought a great deal of progress in understanding the pathophysiology of FM and, although research in JFM is still sparse, recent studies are beginning to corroborate similarities between FM and JFM with regards to underlying abnormalities in pain processing.

PROGNOSIS FOR JUVENILE FIBROMYALGIA

There are variable reports on the prognosis of JFM, likely owing to differences in methodology, including the JFM case definition and the populations studied. Community-based studies report a positive prognosis with approximately 70% of children no longer meeting JFM criteria after 2 years.[33,34] However, more recent clinic-based studies of those seeking treatment at tertiary pediatric rheumatology or pain clinics found a high likelihood of continued symptoms into young adulthood, with about 50% meeting FM criteria in adulthood and the majority of others having continued (but less severe) symptoms.[35] A subset of patients with JFM (approximately 15%) showed long-term functional impairment associated with worsening depressive symptoms over time. Conversely, pain severity remained stable or decreased slightly. Approximately one-third of the CARRA Legacy Registry JFM cohort reported pain symptoms that persisted and measures of function and well-being either worsened or remained relatively unchanged over time.[18] Thus, converging evidence shows that patients with JFM seen in pediatric rheumatology clinics tend to experience a chronic course, with a small proportion experiencing worsening disability. Worsening function over time may be driven by poorly controlled mood symptoms rather than worsening pain, underscoring the importance of early recognition and multidisciplinary management of JFM.

EVALUATION OF JUVENILE FIBROMYALGIA IN A RHEUMATOLOGY CLINIC

Children and adolescents with complaints of joint pain are routinely referred to pediatric rheumatology for the evaluation of potential rheumatic or autoimmune disease. From a rheumatology perspective, the differential diagnosis of joint pain is broad and ranges from benign pain to serious disease owing to infection, inflammation, or malignancy. A comprehensive history is extremely important to making the diagnosis. A past medical history of psoriasis, enthesitis or inflammatory bowel disease may be clues to the diagnosis of inflammatory arthritis. In addition, it is helpful to have prior laboratory testing and imaging results at the time of the visit, not only to help make a diagnosis, but also to minimize duplicate testing. When assessing pain, it is important to ask about onset, aggravating or alleviating factors, pain quality (ie, throbbing, stabbing), pain location (including body areas involved), pain severity (a 0–10 visual analog or numeric rating scale can be used), and the time of day, frequency, and duration of the pain. An assessment of pain interference or impact of pain on daily activities (school, physical, and social activities) should also be included.

The review of systems provides additional critical information such as the presence of fever, fatigue, weight loss, rashes, gastrointestinal symptoms, headache, sleep disturbance, and mood changes. Patients with joint complaints may endorse diffuse or more localized pain, stiffness, swelling, or limp. The reported pain intensity in patients with JFM tends to be moderate to severe, but expressions of pain can vary from minimal outward discomfort to high levels of pain behavior and impairment. It is imperative for the therapeutic alliance that the clinician accept the patient's report of pain at face value. Pain is a subjective experience by definition and encompasses both sensory and affective components. Most important, it is important to validate that the patient is experiencing real pain and that they are believed.

In addition to a complete physical examination, including a joint examination, a tender point evaluation can be done by palpating 18 specific tender points with application of up to 4 kg of pressure.[36] Although the tender point examination is no longer a required component for the diagnosis of JFM, it can be helpful to evaluate pain sensitivity and the extent of widespread pain. The joint examination may reveal laxity or hypermobility (excessive range of movement in 1 or more joints), a common finding in patients with and without JFM. Joint hypermobility is prevalent in children in the general population and, although most children with joint hypermobility are asymptomatic, it is routinely present in patients with chronic MSK pain and JFM. Pediatric patients with hypermobility as part of Ehlers–Danlos syndrome frequently report pain.[37] In the CARRA Legacy Registry, almost one-third of patients with JFM had joint hypermobility. The diagnosis of benign joint hypermobility syndrome, is made using the revised Brighton criteria, which include arthralgia, joint dislocation or subluxation, abnormal skin changes (ie, striae), Marfanoid habitus, eye signs (ie, drooping eyelids), soft tissue changes (ie, tenosynovitis) and varicose veins, uterine prolapse, or hernia.[38] Although the association between joint hypermobility and chronic MSK pain is known, more study is needed to identify a possible relationship between genetic connective tissue disorders (such as Ehlers–Danlos syndrome and Marfan syndromes) and chronic MSK pain.[39]

A comprehensive assessment for JFM should always include an assessment of mood symptoms, because of the strong overlap of chronic pain and emotional distress, which can augment pain sensitivity and the ability to cope with pain. If the patient has anxiety or depression, is the patient under the care of a psychiatrist or therapist? Psychological symptoms are common in JFM and range in severity. Anxiety disorders are most prevalent, but depressive symptoms, which can include suicidal ideation, are reported in about 20% of patients with JFM.[40] Hence, at least a brief assessment or screening of emotional functioning is essential to optimize treatment planning. Other essential parts of the history include a social and family history. Is the patient attending school, sporting, and social activities? The clinician may want to know if the patient is a competitive athlete or described as type A personality or a straight A student to identify potential sources of stress. Are there any recent trauma, major life changes, or stressors? What is the parent–patient interaction like? Are there indications of family conflict or overprotectiveness? If a parent also has a chronic pain condition, how has it affected their lives? The presence of stressors and adaptive versus maladaptive coping may be factors that exacerbate symptoms or pain-related disability.

The diagnosis of JFM should be considered in all patients with chronic pain who also report marked functional impairment, sleep disturbance and fatigue, psychological impairments, headache, and abdominal pain or other somatic symptoms that are not clearly associated with an underlying disease condition.[2] When explaining the diagnosis to patients, it is recommended that providers acknowledge the biologic components of JFM, but aim to decrease its overmedicalization[41] and refrain from ordering unnecessary additional testing and procedures. A holistic approach to assessment, which includes ruling out underlying disease, a careful assessment of symptoms including pain and the known associated features of JFM, as well as the impact of symptoms on their daily lives and functioning will provide a comprehensive picture to guide treatment recommendations.

DIAGNOSTIC CRITERIA FOR JUVENILE FIBROMYALGIA

Over the past few decades, classification criteria for adult FM have been revised and validated; however, there has been limited research on JFM. The Yunus and Masi JFM classification criteria described in 1985[1] are still in use today. These criteria include the hallmark triad of pain, associated symptoms and tender points. Specifically, the criteria include symptoms of widespread MSK pain for greater than 3 months in 3 or more sites plus 3 of 10 associated symptoms: fatigue, nonrestorative sleep, chronic anxiety, chronic headaches, subjective soft tissue swelling, numbness, IBS, and worsening pain owing to physical activity, weather, or stress. A minimum of 5 of 18 painful tender points (heightened pain sensitivity upon palpation) are required.

The ACR criteria for FM published in 2010 and 2011 included the Widespread Pain Index (the number of painful body locations over the past week) and a Symptom Severity scale of cardinal symptoms (fatigue, waking unrefreshed, and cognitive symptoms) and other associated symptoms over the past week (such as dizziness, depression, nausea, blurred vision, and fatigue).[12] The tender point examination had no additive value and, as such, was removed from the diagnostic criteria. In 2016, the Widespread Pain Index and Symptom Severity scale were modified to allow for self-report and the recommendation regarding diagnostic exclusions was changed.[42]

A recent study assessing the utility of the 2010 ACR FM criteria for adolescents with JFM was published in 2016, providing preliminary evidence that the ACR criteria can be applied to pediatric populations with minor modifications.[43] The ACR 2010 criteria had 89.4% sensitivity and 87.5% specificity, with no additional improvement in accuracy when the results of the tender point examination were included. The pediatric version of the ACR 2010 criteria consists of the identical Widespread Pain Index and a slightly shorter Symptom Severity checklist, which together form the Pain and Symptom Assessment Tool.[44] The Pain and Symptom Assessment Tool offers a simple, quick, and standardized approach to classifying JFM in a manner consistent with adult FM criteria. Recent studies have begun to use the Pain and Symptom Assessment Tool for research purposes[45,46] and a subcommittee of CARRA researchers are planning further validation studies that will lay the groundwork for greater adoption of these criteria for clinical diagnostic purposes.

TREATMENT OF JUVENILE FIBROMYALGIA

Once the diagnosis of JFM is made and properly explained as a pain condition that arises from disturbances in pain processing and without judgment or implication of a purely psychological origin, there is often a decrease in patient (and parent) anxiety, allowing for a discussion of initiating multidisciplinary treatment. As with many idiopathic chronic MSK pain conditions, the primary goal of JFM treatment is to improve pain and symptom management through therapies that focus on improving function so they can resume their usual social, school, and family activities. In fact, research has shown that a return to everyday activities and overall improvement in functioning precedes decreases in pain intensity in multidisciplinary pain management and treatment.[47] Stressing pharmacotherapies as a sole recommendation should be avoided, because this tactic may imply a curative fix. Instead, active engagement in multidisciplinary care should be encouraged. Most pediatric rheumatologists approach the treatment of JFM with education about pain syndromes, providing guidelines for improving sleep hygiene, and increasing physical activity with a graded aerobic exercise program or low-impact exercise such as aquatic therapy.[41] Recommendations for sleep hygiene include eliminating caffeine, having a bedtime routine with consistent bedtimes and wake times, sleeping in a cool comfortable dark room without electronics, and advising the patient try a quiet activity such as reading a book or other non–screen-related activity to wind down if they are unable to fall asleep within 30 minutes.

The optimal standard of care for JFM includes both intensive physical therapy and psychological therapies (such as cognitive-behavioral therapy [CBT] or mindfulness-based approaches[48,49]). patients with JFM with arthralgia may think that painful extremity(ies) are injury or exercise related and therefore avoid movement. In addition, deconditioned patients may interpret pain with activity as an indication of a JFM flare. It is imperative that the physician or health care provider reassure the patient and family that no harm or damage will occur from engaging in physical activity, but that they should pace themselves as they initiate new activities or exercises. Patients may improve with education, reassurance, and restoring normal daily activities.[50] Typical physical exercise programs include starting a graduated aerobic exercise program with the goal of working up to 30 minutes of vigorous exercise at least 2 to 3 times a week, if not more. It is important to monitor progress measured by pain severity, especially pain interference and impact on functioning. If the patient responds poorly to outpatient physical therapy, a more rigorous day or inpatient program may be needed. Sherry and colleagues[51] found that patients with JFM treated with 5 to 6 hours per day of physical therapy in an intensive day treatment program showed great benefit. Other complimentary or adjunctive therapies such as acupuncture, massage or use of transcutaneous electric nerve stimulation may also be helpful.[51]

The strongest evidence for treatment efficacy in JFM comes from clinical trials of CBT, which have shown that CBT is effective in decreasing pain and significantly improving function in children and adolescents with JFM.[49,52] CBT was also effective in decreasing depressive symptoms. Typical outpatient CBT programs involve 8 to 10 weekly sessions with a trained therapist who teaches patients a menu of adaptive pain coping skills, including muscle relaxation techniques, guided imagery, activity pacing, cognitive reframing, problem solving, and other skills. Parents are often included in sessions to learn how to help their child manage pain more independently using behavior management skills. Although CBT is quite effective at improving coping and decreasing disability, it has somewhat smaller effects on pain reduction. Thus, newer studies are testing the benefits of combining CBT with specialized exercise training programs to improve fitness, strength, and biomechanics (via neuromuscular training) to promote exercise participation, which is necessary to achieve sustained pain reduction.[45,53] Although the research studying CBT and other nonpharmacologic approaches for JFM show significant benefits for treating JFM, these services may not be readily accessible for all patients owing to the need for trained pediatric CBT providers, proximity to medical centers with multidisciplinary programs, and insurance coverage for behavioral services.

Medications prescribed to patients by pediatric rheumatologists primarily provide minimal pain relief but more successfully treat associated mood or sleep difficulties. These include, selective serotonin reuptake inhibitors, selective norepinephrine reuptake inhibitors, anticonvulsants (such as gabapentin or pregabalin), and low-dose tricyclic antidepressants. Many medications prescribed for FM are not approved for use in children.[54] Although a small number of clinical trials have shown that medications such as duloxetine, fluoxetine, and pregabalin may be beneficial for some patients,[55–58] there remains relatively little evidence supporting the use of medications in JFM, and many young patients have difficulties with tolerability. Physicians must also be cautious when prescribing selective serotonin reuptake inhibitors to adolescents because of the October 2004 US Food and Drug Administration black box warning advising of the increased risk of suicidal behavior among pediatric users of selective serotonin reuptake inhibitors.[59] Low-dose amitriptyline, cyclobenzaprine, or pregabalin may be used to treat sleep disturbance.[60] Nonresponding patients may be referred to a pediatric pain clinic, psychiatrist, or integrative medicine specialist to help better manage symptoms and prescription medications. Opioid medications and nonsteroidal anti-inflammatory drugs are not recommended for JFM and the use of cannabinoid substances remains unproven at the current time.

FUTURE RESEARCH

Evidence supporting the proper identification and treatment of JFM has been increasing in the past decade, but there is still a large gap in what we know about the pathophysiology of this poorly understood condition. Studies in adult FM illuminate potential genetic, neurobiological, and environmental factors that play a role in the etiology and maintenance of FM but require further investigation into their relevance to JFM in children and adolescents. In recognition of the significant burden, cost, and suffering of poorly managed chronic pain (including opioid misuse and addiction), the National Institutes of Health have put forward several funding opportunities under the HEAL initiative (heal.nih.gov) to promote epidemiologic, clinical, and translational research for chronic pain conditions, including FM and JFM. Increased focus on pain research will undoubtedly lead to the better identification of treatment targets and more effective therapeutic approaches for patients with these conditions across the lifespan. Studies that specifically focus on chronic pain conditions early in life, such as JFM, are vital to gain a deeper understanding of how abnormalities in pain processing unfold and whether developmental factors such as neuroplasticity of the developing nervous system create the possibility of attenuating pain sensitization via early intervention. If that is, the case, targeting modifiable behavioral, lifestyle, or other triggering factors early in life could potentially alter the course of the disease and thereby eliminate the long-term impact of JFM.

SUMMARY

JFM in children and adolescents is a common referral in pediatric rheumatology settings. Providing patients with a clear diagnosis of JFM and an explanation of altered pain processing offers reassurance to patients and families that pain has a biologic basis and that the patient's symptoms are part of a recognized pain syndrome. Physicians should acknowledge the impact of chronic pain and associated symptoms such as fatigue and sleep difficulty on patient's lives and take time to understand contributing factors including stress, mood, inactivity, and lifestyle factors. The optimal treatment for JFM is multidisciplinary, focusing on education about JFM, along with physical therapy, CBT, recommendations for sleep hygiene, healthy lifestyle habits, and medications for symptom management as appropriate.

CLINICS CARE POINTS

- JFM diagnosis can be made using the ACR 2010 diagnostic criteria and performing a thorough history and physical examination.
- Physicians should educate patients and families about the biologic basis of JFM as a pain processing disorder that is distinct from rheumatic disease.
- Psychological and lifestyle factors may contribute to heightened pain and disability in JFM.
- Multidisciplinary treatment including CBT or similar behavioral interventions, and physical exercise, are vital to the successful treatment of JFM, along with medications for symptom management as indicated.
- Physicians should reassure the patient and family that it is safe to engage in gradually increasing physical activity and resume their usual school and daily activities while engaging in multidisciplinary pain management.

DISCLOSURE

S. Kashikar-Zuck receives funding for her research in JFM from the National Institute of Arthritis and Musculoskeletal and Skin Diseases (NIAMS) of the National Institutes of Health, USA. Drs J.E. Weiss and S. Kashikar-Zuck receive support from the Arthritis Foundation for their work on the Steering Committee of the Childhood Arthritis and Rheumatology Research Alliance (CARRA) of North America.

REFERENCES

1. Yunus MB, Masi AT. Juvenile primary fibromyalgia syndrome. A clinical study of thirty-three patients and matched normal controls. Arthritis Rheum 1985;28(2): 138–45.
2. Kashikar-Zuck S, Ting TV. Juvenile fibromyalgia: current status of research and future developments. Nat Rev Rheumatol 2014;10(2):89–96.
3. Sluka KA, Clauw DJ. Neurobiology of fibromyalgia and chronic widespread pain. Neuroscience 2016;338:114–29.
4. Ji RR, Nackley A, Huh Y, et al. Neuroinflammation and central sensitization in chronic and widespread pain. Anesthesiology 2018;129(2):343–66.
5. Kashikar-Zuck S, Johnston M, Ting TV, et al. Relationship between school absenteeism and depressive symptoms among adolescents with juvenile fibromyalgia. J Pediatr Psychol 2010;35(9):996–1004.
6. Kashikar-Zuck S, Lynch AM, Slater S, et al. Family factors, emotional functioning, and functional impairment in juvenile fibromyalgia syndrome. Arthritis Rheum 2008;59(10):1392–8.
7. Kashikar-Zuck S, Parkins IS, Graham TB, et al. Anxiety, mood, and behavioral disorders among pediatric patients with juvenile fibromyalgia syndrome. Clin J Pain 2008;24(7):620–6.
8. Varni JW, Seid M, Kurtin PS. PedsQL 4.0: reliability and validity of the Pediatric Quality of Life Inventory version 4.0 generic core scales in healthy and patient populations. Med Care 2001;39(8):800–12.

9. Kashikar-Zuck S, Cunningham N, Sil S, et al. Long-term outcomes of adolescents with juvenile-onset fibromyalgia in early adulthood. Pediatrics 2014;133(3): e592–600.

10. Kashikar-Zuck S, Parkins IS, Ting TV, et al. Controlled follow-up study of physical and psychosocial functioning of adolescents with juvenile primary fibromyalgia syndrome. Rheumatology (Oxford) 2010;49(11):2204–9.

11. Sherry DD. Amplified musculoskeletal pain: treatment approach and outcomes. J Pediatr Gastroenterol Nutr 2008;47(5):693–4.

12. Wolfe F, Clauw DJ, Fitzcharles MA, et al. The American College of Rheumatology preliminary diagnostic criteria for fibromyalgia and measurement of symptom severity. Arthritis Care Res (Hoboken) 2010;62(5):600–10.

13. Wolfe F, Brahler E, Hinz A, et al. Fibromyalgia prevalence, somatic symptom reporting, and the dimensionality of polysymptomatic distress: results from a survey of the general population. Arthritis Care Res (Hoboken) 2013;65(5):777–85.

14. Gare BA. Epidemiology of rheumatic disease in children. Curr Opin Rheumatol 1996;8(5):449–54.

15. Siegel DM, Janeway D, Baum J. Fibromyalgia syndrome in children and adolescents: clinical features at presentation and status at follow-up. Pediatrics 1998; 101(3 Pt 1):377–82.

16. Buskila D, Press J, Gedalia A, et al. Assessment of nonarticular tenderness and prevalence of fibromyalgia in children. J Rheumatol 1993;20(2):368–70.

17. King S, Chambers CT, Huguet A, et al. The epidemiology of chronic pain in children and adolescents revisited: a systematic review. Pain 2011;152(12):2729–38.

18. Weiss JE, Schikler KN, Boneparth AD, et al. Demographic, clinical, and treatment characteristics of the juvenile primary fibromyalgia syndrome cohort enrolled in the Childhood Arthritis and Rheumatology Research Alliance Legacy Registry. Pediatr Rheumatol Online J 2019;17(1):51.

19. Gracely RH, Petzke F, Wolf JM, et al. Functional magnetic resonance imaging evidence of augmented pain processing in fibromyalgia. Arthritis Rheum 2002; 46(5):1333–43.

20. Neblett R, Cohen H, Choi Y, et al. The Central Sensitization Inventory (CSI): establishing clinically significant values for identifying central sensitivity syndromes in an outpatient chronic pain sample. J Pain 2013;14(5):438–45.

21. Staud R. Abnormal endogenous pain modulation is a shared characteristic of many chronic pain conditions. Expert Rev Neurother 2012;12(5):577–85.

22. Lopez-Sola M, Woo CW, Pujol J, et al. Towards a neurophysiological signature for fibromyalgia. Pain 2017;158(1):34–47.

23. Suñol M, PM, Tong H, et al. Brain Structural Correlates of Juvenile Fibromyalgia. Poster presented at: IASP 2021 Virtual World Congress on Pain. June 9-11 and 16-18, 2021. Available at: https://iaspvirtualcongress.evareg.com/poster/brain-structural-correlates-of-juvenile-fibromyalgia. Accessed July 29, 2021.

24. Arnold LM, Hudson JI, Hess EV, et al. Family study of fibromyalgia. Arthritis Rheum 2004;50(3):944–52.

25. Roizenblatt S, Tufik S, Goldenberg J, et al. Juvenile fibromyalgia: clinical and polysomnographic aspects. J Rheumatol 1997;24(3):579–85.

26. Ablin JN, Buskila D. Update on the genetics of the fibromyalgia syndrome. Best Pract Res Clin Rheumatol 2015;29(1):20–8.

27. Buskila D, Sarzi-Puttini P, Ablin JN. The genetics of fibromyalgia syndrome. Pharmacogenomics 2007;8(1):67–74.

28. Diatchenko L, Fillingim RB, Smith SB, et al. The phenotypic and genetic signatures of common musculoskeletal pain conditions. Nat Rev Rheumatol 2013; 9(6):340–50.
29. Buskila D, Atzeni F, Sarzi-Puttini P. Etiology of fibromyalgia: the possible role of infection and vaccination. Autoimmun Rev 2008;8(1):41–3.
30. McLean SA, Diatchenko L, Lee YM, et al. Catechol O-methyltransferase haplotype predicts immediate musculoskeletal neck pain and psychological symptoms after motor vehicle collision. J Pain 2011;12(1):101–7.
31. Boneparth A, Chen S, Horton DB, et al. Epidermal neurite density in skin biopsies from patients with juvenile fibromyalgia. J Rheumatol 2020;48(4):575–8.
32. Oaklander AL, Klein MM. Evidence of small-fiber polyneuropathy in unexplained, juvenile-onset, widespread pain syndromes. Pediatrics 2013;131(4):e1091–100.
33. Buskila D, Neumann L, Hershman E, et al. Fibromyalgia syndrome in children–an outcome study. J Rheumatol 1995;22(3):525–8.
34. Mikkelsson M. One year outcome of preadolescents with fibromyalgia. J Rheumatol 1999;26(3):674–82.
35. Kashikar-Zuck S, Cunningham N, Peugh J, et al. Long-term outcomes of adolescents with juvenile-onset fibromyalgia into adulthood and impact of depressive symptoms on functioning over time. Pain 2019;160(2):433–41.
36. Wolfe F, Smythe HA, Yunus MB, et al. The American College of Rheumatology 1990 Criteria for the classification of fibromyalgia. Report of the Multicenter Criteria Committee. Arthritis Rheum 1990;33(2):160–72.
37. Feldman ECH, Hivick DP, Slepian PM, et al. Pain symptomatology and management in pediatric Ehlers-Danlos syndrome: a review. Children (Basel) 2020; 7(9):146.
38. Grahame R, Bird HA, Child A. The revised (Brighton 1998) criteria for the diagnosis of benign joint hypermobility syndrome (BJHS). J Rheumatol 2000;27(7): 1777–9.
39. Grahame R. Joint hypermobility and genetic collagen disorders: are they related? Arch Dis Child 1999;80(2):188–91.
40. Gmuca S, Sonagra M, Xiao R, et al. Suicidal risk and resilience in juvenile fibromyalgia syndrome: a cross-sectional cohort study. Pediatr Rheumatol Online J 2021;19(1):3.
41. Gmuca S, Sherry DD. Fibromyalgia: treating pain in the juvenile patient. Paediatr Drugs 2017;19(4):325–38.
42. Wolfe F, Clauw DJ, Fitzcharles MA, et al. 2016 Revisions to the 2010/2011 fibromyalgia diagnostic criteria. Semin Arthritis Rheum 2016;46(3):319–29.
43. Ting TV, Barnett K, Lynch-Jordan A, et al. 2010 American College of Rheumatology adult fibromyalgia criteria for use in an adolescent female population with juvenile fibromyalgia. J Pediatr 2016;169:181–7.e1.
44. Daffin M, Gibler RC, Kashikar-Zuck S. Measures of juvenile fibromyalgia. Arthritis Care Res (Hoboken) 2020;72(Suppl 10):171–82.
45. Kashikar-Zuck S, Black WR, Pfeiffer M, et al. Pilot randomized trial of integrated cognitive-behavioral therapy and neuromuscular training for juvenile fibromyalgia: the FIT Teens Program. J Pain 2018;19(9):1049–62.
46. Kashikar-Zuck S, Briggs MS, Bout-Tabaku S, et al. Randomized clinical trial of Fibromyalgia Integrative Training (FIT teens) for adolescents with juvenile fibromyalgia - study design and protocol. Contemp Clin Trials 2021;103:106321.
47. Lynch-Jordan AM, Sil S, Peugh J, et al. Differential changes in functional disability and pain intensity over the course of psychological treatment for children with chronic pain. Pain 2014;155(10):1955–61.

48. Ali A, Weiss TR, Dutton A, et al. Mindfulness-based stress reduction for adolescents with functional somatic syndromes: a pilot cohort study. J Pediatr 2017; 183:184–90.

49. Kashikar-Zuck S, Ting TV, Arnold LM, et al. Cognitive behavioral therapy for the treatment of juvenile fibromyalgia: a multisite, single-blind, randomized, controlled clinical trial. Arthritis Rheum 2012;64(1):297–305.

50. Sherry DD, Wallace CA, Kelley C, et al. Short- and long-term outcomes of children with complex regional pain syndrome type I treated with exercise therapy. Clin J pain 1999;15(3):218–23.

51. Weiss JE, Stinson JN. Pediatric pain syndromes and noninflammatory musculoskeletal pain. Pediatr Clin North Am 2018;65(4):801–26.

52. Degotardi PJ, Klass ES, Rosenberg BS, et al. Development and evaluation of a cognitive-behavioral intervention for juvenile fibromyalgia. J Pediatr Psychol 2006;31(7):714–23.

53. Tran ST, Guite JW, Pantaleao A, et al. Preliminary outcomes of a cross-site cognitive-behavioral and neuromuscular integrative training intervention for juvenile fibromyalgia. Arthritis Care Res (Hoboken) 2017;69(3):413–20.

54. Grégoire M-C, Finley GA. Why were we abandoned? Orphan drugs in paediatric pain. Paediatrics Child Health 2007;12(2):95–6.

55. Arnold LM, Bateman L, Palmer RH, et al. Preliminary experience using milnacipran in patients with juvenile fibromyalgia: lessons from a clinical trial program. Pediatr Rheumatol Online J 2015;13:27.

56. Mariutto EN, Stanford SB, Kashikar-Zuck S, et al. An exploratory, open trial of fluoxetine treatment of juvenile fibromyalgia. J Clin Psychopharmacol 2012; 32(2):293–5.

57. Upadhyaya HP, Arnold LM, Alaka K, et al. Efficacy and safety of duloxetine versus placebo in adolescents with juvenile fibromyalgia: results from a randomized controlled trial. Pediatr Rheumatol Online J 2019;17(1):27.

58. Arnold LM, Schikler KN, Bateman L, et al. Safety and efficacy of pregabalin in adolescents with fibromyalgia: a randomized, double-blind, placebo-controlled trial and a 6-month open-label extension study. Pediatr Rheumatol Online J 2016; 14(1):46.

59. Kondro W. FDA urges "black box" warning on pediatric antidepressants. CMAJ 2004;171(8):837–8.

60. Anthony KK, Schanberg LE. Pediatric pain syndromes and management of pain in children and adolescents with rheumatic disease. Pediatr Clin North Am 2005; 52(2):611–39, vii.

Juvenile Localized Scleroderma
Updates and Differences from Adult-Onset Disease

Natalia Vasquez-Canizares, MD, MS[a], Suzanne C. Li, MD, PhD[b],*

KEYWORDS

- Pediatric scleroderma • Morphea • Linear scleroderma • en coup de sabre
- Extracutaneous involvement • Pathophysiology • Treatment • Outcome

KEY POINTS

- Juvenile localized scleroderma (jLS) is associated with a high risk for functional impairment from musculoskeletal, neurologic, and other extracutaneous involvement (ECI).
- ECI is twice as prevalent and often more severe in juvenile-onset than adult-onset linear scleroderma.
- LS pathogenesis involves vascular alterations, fibrosis, and immune dysregulation. Key processes include T-helper cell 1 and interferon gamma–induced responses and the fibroblast secretome.
- Methotrexate is the standard-of-care treatment of patients with jLS at risk for moderate to severe disease and morbidity.
- Because skin and extracutaneous activities are frequently discordant, and ECI often presents years later, long-term monitoring by rheumatology is essential for optimal outcome.

INTRODUCTION

Localized scleroderma (LS), also known as morphea, is an idiopathic inflammatory and sclerosing disorder affecting the skin and subcutaneous structures.[1,2] Although skin fibrosis pathology can be identical to systemic sclerosis (SSc), LS usually has unilateral skin involvement and a different extracutaneous involvement (ECI) pattern.[1,3] ECI complicates the disease in a high proportion of patients and is the main cause

[a] Department of Pediatrics, Division of Pediatric Rheumatology, Children's Hospital at Montefiore, Albert Einstein College of Medicine, 3415 Bainbridge Avenue, Bronx, NY 10467, USA;
[b] Department of Pediatrics, Division of Pediatric Rheumatology, Joseph M. Sanzari Children's Hospital, Hackensack University Medical Center, Hackensack Meridian School of Medicine, 30 Prospect Avenue, WFAN PC337, Hackensack, NJ 07601, USA
* Corresponding author.
E-mail address: Suzanne.li@hmhn.org

Rheum Dis Clin N Am 47 (2021) 737–755
https://doi.org/10.1016/j.rdc.2021.07.014
0889-857X/21/© 2021 Elsevier Inc. All rights reserved.

rheumatic.theclinics.com

of severe morbidity.[1] This review provides an overview of the pathophysiology and clinical aspects of juvenile LS (jLS) with an emphasis on recent advances and its differences from adult-onset LS (aLS).

EPIDEMIOLOGY

LS is rare, with an estimated incidence of 0.34 to 2.7 cases/100,000/y.[3,4] Twenty to thirty percent of patients have onset in childhood, most commonly in the first decade (**Table 1**). Women are more often affected than men, with disease more prevalent in Caucasians (73%–82%).[5,6]

PATHOGENESIS

Disease pathogenesis involves genetic, environmental, immunologic, and vascular factors with several identified mechanisms shared with SSc.[3,7,8] In a genetically susceptible individual, epigenetic mechanisms and environmental triggers result in microvascular injury, keratinocyte activation, and subsequent inflammation (**Fig. 1**). Dysregulation of fibrotic and antifibrotic pathways leads to persistent fibroblast activation and epithelial-mesenchymal transition, resulting in excessive extracellular matrix synthesis and collagen deposition.[7,9] Advances in transcriptomics and proteomics have identified key processes, including the T-helper cell 1 (Th1) and interferon (IFN)γ gene–induced responses, and the LS fibroblast secretome.

Immunophenotype of Localized Scleroderma

A characteristic inflammatory phenotype in the peripheral blood and skin of LS has been identified.[3,10] Specifically, a Th1 response with increased IFN-γ–expressing T cells, and elevation of Th1-related cytokines, chemokines, and their receptors, has been seen with active disease.[3] Th2, regulator T cells (Tregs), B, and natural killer cells are decreased with a reduced number of functional Tregs likely explaining a "permissive state."[10] After the Th1-associated inflammatory state, a Th2-induced fibrotic signature occurs, resembling that seen in long-term SSc disease profiles.[3]

Transcriptome of Localized Scleroderma

Differential expression of IFNγ-related genes has been identified in the skin of a subset of active patients with jLS by transcriptomic analysis.[3] CCL18 has been found to be a specific predictor of disease activity, performing better than CXCL9 or CXCL10, with CCL18 gene expression increased at the inflammatory lesion border compared with the sclerotic center, unaffected skin, or healthy control biopsies.[11]

Fibroblasts and the Secretome

The secretome is a subset of proteomes that are actively secreted into the extracellular space.[12] A specific fibroblast cell phenotype and secretome was characterized in the lesional skin of children with linear scleroderma compared with nonlesional skin.[13] Fibroblasts with altered collagen processing were hyperproliferative and had hypermigratory properties. Fibroblasts were also less responsive to transforming growth factor beta 1 (TGF-β1) and more had differentiated into myofibroblasts. Key modulators of the TGF-β superfamily members (SOSTDC1 and FRAS1) were also found dysregulated. Importantly, modification of the secretome was able to change the fibroblast phenotype, suggesting secretome modulation as a potential therapeutic target.

Table 1
Subtype frequency in pediatric and adult-onset localized scleroderma

Onset of LS (No. Patients)	Age of Onset, Mean or Median, Years	Female: Male	Circumscribed Morphea No. (%)	Linear Scleroderma No. (%)	Generalized Morphea No. (%)	Pansclerotic and Deep Morphea No. (%)	Mixed Morphea No. (%)
Pediatric (1997)	7–8.7	1448: 545 2.7:1	431 (21.6)	1127 (56.4)	146 (7.3)	22 (1.1)	271 (13.6)
Adult (893)	44.1–47	680: 192 3.4:1	548 (61.4)	87 (9.7)	194 (21.7)	37 (4.1)	23 (2.6)
P-value of pediatric to adult	<0.001	0.003	<0.001	<0.001	<0.001	<0.001	<0.001

Studies were selected if they reported on their entire cohort, only one study per site included. Deep and pansclerotic morphea were grouped together because some classifications list pansclerotic under deep morphea. In those studies, circumscribed deep morphea may also be listed under deep rather than circumscribed morphea. P-values calculated by Z-score and t-test; significant P-values <0.05.

Abbreviation: No, number.

Data from Kreuter et al,[20] 2012; Leitenberger et al,[6] 2009; Marzano et al,[21] 2003; Mertens et al,[22] 2015; Peterson et al,[4] 1997;Christen-Zaech et al,[23] 2008; Lythgoe et al,[24] 2018; Pequet et al,[25] 2014; Wu et al,[5] 2019; Zulian et al,[26] 2006.

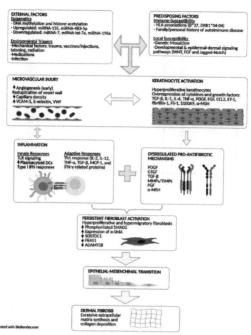

Fig. 1. Possible LS pathogenesis model. External stimuli and intrinsic susceptibility factors lead to activation and dysregulation of vascular, inflammatory, and fibrogenic pathways, resulting in excessive tissue collagen deposition and fibrosis. α-MSH, melanocyte stimulating hormone; α-SMA, smooth muscle actin; ADAMTS8, a disintegrin and metalloproteinase with thrombospondin motifs 8; CCL2, chemokine ligand 2; CTGF, connective tissue growth factor; DCs, dendritic cells; ET-1, endothelin-1; FGF, fibroblast growth factor; Fli-1; friend leukemia integrated transcription factor; FRAS1, fraser extracellular matrix complex subunit 1; HLA, human leukocyte antigen; IL, interleukin; IFN; interferon; MCP, monocyte chemoattractant protein-1; miRNA, microRNA; MMPs, matrix metalloproteinases; PDGF, platelet-derived growth factor; S100A, S100 calcium-binding protein A1; SMAD2, mothers against decapentaplegic homolog 2; SOSTDC1, sclerostin domain-containing protein 1; TGF-β, transforming growth factor-β; TIMPs; tissue inhibitors of metalloproteinases; TLR, toll-like receptor; TNF-α, tumor necrosis factor-α; VCAM-1, vascular cell adhesion molecule 1; VWF; von Willebrand factor; WNT, wingless and int.

Vascular Factors

Microvascular alterations including vasculopathic and vasculitic changes in the skin and other affected tissues of patients with LS have been documented.[8,14] Increased angiogenesis has been identified in the early inflammatory stage, whereas inactive lesions show disturbed vascular architecture, with enlarged vessels showing reduplication of the vessel wall that suggests endothelial cell injury, and reduced capillary density.[15]

Markers of endothelial activation

Both sera and endothelial cells from patients with SSc and LS show overexpression of endothelial cell adhesion molecules.[16,17] Levels of vascular cell adhesion molecule 1 (VCAM-1) and E-selectin were significantly higher in patients with LS than healthy controls and correlated with the number of sclerotic lesions and areas involved.[17] Serum levels of von Willebrand factor (VWF) antigen were similarly found to correlate with disease severity in patients with LS and SSc.[18] In LS and SSc, increased tissue expression of VWF in extravascular areas colocalized with inflammatory cell infiltrates and collagens I and III, suggesting VWF may participate in fibrosis.[18]

PATIENT EVALUATION OVERVIEW: MANIFESTATIONS
Classification

Several classification systems have been proposed that group patients based on lesion location, appearance, and size. The Pediatric Rheumatology European Society criteria (**Fig. 2**) performed better than the Mayo Clinic or German criteria in classifying 944 adults and children.[19] **Table 1** presents data from 10 pediatric rheumatology and/ or dermatology cohorts,[4–6,20–26] including the largest international jLS cohort (750 patients)[2] and 5 pediatric and adult-onset cohorts.[4,6,20–22] Most patients with jLS (56%) had linear scleroderma, with trunk or limb more often affected than the head (**Table 2**). Another 14% had mixed morphea, which usually included linear scleroderma. aLS had different subtype frequencies, with circumscribed morphea (61%) and generalized morphea (22%) the most common and linear scleroderma and mixed morphea rare (P <.001, see **Table 1**). Female predominance was also higher in aLS (P = .003).

Cutaneous Features

LS lesions change over time, reflecting changes in disease state. Early lesions may show subtle erythema (**Fig. 3**A) that can later become pronounced (**Fig. 3**B–D). Other lesions develop a lilac, violaceous, or bruiselike appearance (**Fig. 3**E, F). Early skin thickening reflects edema more than fibrosis. Lesions can then develop a thickened, white or yellow waxy appearance, reflecting robust fibrosis with ongoing inflammation (see **Fig. 3**B–F). Active lesions can also have tactile warmth.[27] Still later, only aberrant fibrosis (sclerosis) persists, often associated with damage features of dyspigmentation and atrophy (epidermal, dermal, and/or subcutaneous) (**Fig. 3**G–J).

Extracutaneous Features

ECI has been associated with functional impairment and lower quality of life (**Fig. 4**).[5,28] Unlike SSc, vascular manifestations or visceral organ involvement are uncommon, and typically mild or asymptomatic, even in patients with LS with Raynaud phenomenon.[1,2,21]

ECI has been reported in 22% to 75% of patients with jLS, with musculoskeletal the most common.[2,29] Higher frequencies (46%–74%) found in prospective studies may reflect more complete ECI capture (see **Fig. 4**).[2,29] For most patients, onset of ECI follows skin disease, with neurologic manifestations occurring a mean of 4.3 years later.[30] Decades later onset[14,31] and onset before skin disease[21,30,32] also occur. ECI usually presents near the skin lesion site especially for sclerosis-related problems (ie, joint contractures). But involvement remote from the skin lesion occurs for about 25% to 30% of neurologic and ocular ECI[2] and for 25% of most of the inflammatory arthritis.[2,33]

Musculoskeletal manifestations are associated with linear scleroderma of the trunk or limb, either isolated or as part of mixed morphea.[2,21,25,29] A major complication is bony undergrowth (hemiatrophy, see **Fig. 4**), identified in 25% of patients in a recent study.[29] Before widespread use of methotrexate, bone growth disturbances were more common and worse, often necessitating surgical intervention including amputation.[1]

Neurologic, ocular, and oral involvement are more common in craniofacial linear scleroderma.[2,6,21,25] Headaches, including migraines and hemiplegic migraines, and

Subtype Examples	Pediatric Rheumatology European Society (PReS) Padua Preliminary Criteria,2006
Superficial (Trunk) Deep (Trunk)	Circumscribed Morphea -**Superficial**: Ovoid/round lesions limited to epidermis and dermis, often with altered pigmentation and violaceous, erythematous halo ('lilac ring') Can be single or multiple, affect trunk > limbs, face. Includes plaque, guttate and keloid morphea forms. -**Deep**: Ovoid/round lesions with deep induration of the skin involving subcutaneous tissue extending to fascia, can involve underlying muscle Lesions can be single or multiple and affect trunk > limbs, face. The primary involvement can be of the subcutaneous tissue with sparing of the skin. Includes morphea profunda and subcutaneous morphea forms.
Linear (limb) Head/face (ECDS and PRS)	Linear Scleroderma -**Trunk or limbs**: Linear induration involving dermis, subcutaneous tissue, and sometimes muscle and underlying bone, and affecting the limbs and/or the trunk -**Head**: two forms o En Coup de Sabre (ECDS): Linear induration that affects the face and the scalp. Can affect muscle and bone, and cause scarring alopecia o Parry-Romberg Syndrome (PRS) or progressive hemifacial atrophy: unilateral loss of underlying tissues, often overlying skin appears normal. Skin is mobile, not bound down
Large lesions on arms and back, some with cliff-drop atrophy	Generalized Morphea 4 or more indurated plaques of at least 3 cm in size that become confluent and involve at least 2 anatomic sites Anatomic sites: head/neck, right or left upper extremity, right or left lower extremity, anterior or posterior trunk. Unilateral generalized morphea usually begins in childhood
	Pansclerotic Morphea Most severe form with circumferential involvement of limb(s) affecting the skin and underlying tissues. Often widespread involvement of other parts of the body, usually sparing fingers and toes. Normal nailbed capillaries on exam, no Raynaud's phenomenon, and usually no significant internal organ involvement. Can lead to severe ulcerations with subsequent life-threatening infections or development of squamous cell carcinoma
Linear (upper arm) and circumscribed (trunk) morphea in the same patient	Mixed Morphea Combination of 2 or more of the previous subtypes. Most commonly, linear scleroderma and circumscribed morphea, or linear scleroderma and generalized morphea.
Exclusion of Other Forms	Eosinophilic fasciitis, atrophoderma of Pasini and Pierini, and bullous morphea

Fig. 2. Padua preliminary classification criteria for LS. PReS classification criteria from Laxer RM and Zulian F, Curr Opin Rheumatol. 2006;18:606 with patient examples. (*B*) Circumscribed deep morphea republished with permission from Browning JC. *Dermatol Clin.* 2013;31:229. (*D*) PRS. Republished under the CC BY 4.0 license agreement copyright c2019 Khatri, Torok, Mirizio, Liu and Astakhova, Front. Immunol 2019;10:1487. (*E*) Generalized morphea republished with permission from Torok KS. Pediatr Clin North Am. 2012;59(2):381-405. (*H*) republished with permission from Hong JH, et al. *J Cutan Pathol.* 2015;42:929.

Table 2
Linear scleroderma in pediatric and adult-onset localized scleroderma

LS Onset (No. Patients)	Age Onset, Mean Years[a]	Female: Male[b]	Trunk or Limb No. (%)	Head No. (%)	Mixed Morphea[d] No. (%)	>1 Linear Lesion[e] No. (%)	>2 sites[f] No. (%)	ECI[g] No. (%)	Joint Contracture or LROM No. (%)
Pediatric (552)	7.95	2.9:1	355[c] (68)	182[c] (35)	52 (26)	139 (57)	196 (42)	136 (46.7)	135[h] (31)
Adult (224)	32.4	4.7:1	139 (62)	93 (41.5)	11 (31)	48 (41.7)	63 (30.3)	24 (18.8)	34 (15.2)
P-value	<0.001	0.080	NS	0.084	NS	0.005	0.005	<0.001	<0.001

Studies were selected if they reported on their entire linear scleroderma cohort, only one study per site included; pediatric references.[21,23,38-45] ECI may be an underestimate, as Falanga and colleagues[37], Arkachaisri and colleagues[39], Vancheeswaran and colleagues[43], and Rubin and colleagues[38] did not specify nonjoint ECI. P-values calculated by Z-score and t-test. Superscripts indicate data not available from listed studies.

Abbreviations: ECI, extracutaneous involvement; LROM, limited range of motion; LS, localized scleroderma; No, number.

[a] Marzano et al,[21] 2003.
[b] Marzano et al,[21] 2003; Kunzler et al,[40] 2019.
[c] Vancheeswaran et al,[43] 1996.
[d] Arkachaisri et al,[39] 2008; Kunzler et al,[40] 2019; Weibel et al,[41] 2008; Piram et al,[42] 2013; Mazori et al,[44] 2016.
[e] Marzano et al,[21] 2003; Arkachaisri et al,[39] 2008; Mazori et al,[44] 2016; Weibel et al,[41] 2008; Piram et al,[42] 2013; Vancheeswaran et al,[43] 1996; Christen-Zaech et al,[23] 2008.
[f] Marzano et al,[21] 2003; Vancheeswaran et al,[43] 1996.
[g] Kunzler et al,[40] 2019; Weibel et al,[41] 2008.
[h] Weibel et al,[41] 2008; Piram et al,[42] 2013.

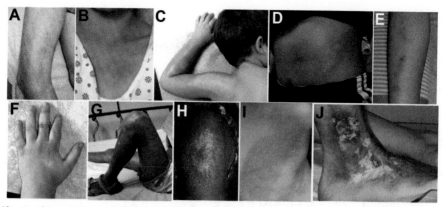

Fig. 3. Skin activity and damage features. (*A*) Mild erythema in linear scleroderma of leg. Photo courtesy of G. Higgins. (*B*) Moderate erythema in circumscribed lesion on lower neck to chest, with yellow waxy lesion with hyperpigmentation. (*C*) Mild erythema and waxy white lesion in linear scleroderma lesion extending to back. (*D*) Moderate erythema, hyperpigmentation, and waxy center in truncal circumscribed lesion in a patient with darker skin. (*E*) Deep violaceous nodular lesions in a linear array; distal lesion has waxy center. (*F*) Lilac ring around a waxy center on hand. (*G*) Skin thickening, dyspigmentation, atrophy, and contractures in pansclerotic morphea. (*H*) Skin atrophy, dyspigmentation, and telangiectasia in pansclerotic morphea. (*I*) Hyperpigmentation and dermal atrophy with visible veins. (*J*) Sclerosis, atrophy, dyspigmentation, and telangiectasia from linear scleroderma.

seizures (often complex partial and refractory to antiepileptics) are the most common neurologic problems.[30,34] Younger age at onset ($\leq$5.4 years) is associated with a higher risk for bony undergrowth that begets global alterations including dental and jaw hypoplasia, muscle impairment (palate, extraocular, mastication), and enophthalmos.[35,36]

Extracutaneous involvement in pediatric versus adult-onset linear scleroderma

Table 2 presents linear scleroderma data from 10 studies,[21,23,37–44] including 5 pediatric and adult-onset cohorts.[21,37–40] Pediatric onset disease had a greater cutaneous burden, both for number of lesions and sites affected (*P* = .005 for both). In addition, ECI were 2.5-fold more prevalent in pediatric than adult-onset disease (*P* <.001).

Pediatric and adult-onset craniofacial linear scleroderma (en coup de sabre [ECDS], Parry-Romberg syndrome [PRS], and both combined [ECDS/PRS]) also differ (**Table 3**).[21,23,31,34,44–53] ECDS/PRS was more prevalent and ECDS less prevalent in jLS than aLS (*P* = .005, .019, respectively). Gender differences were even larger for craniofacial linear scleroderma than other subtypes, with a 3-fold lower female predominance for pediatric-onset disease (see **Tables 1** and **3**). Neurologic symptoms, including headache and seizures, were more prevalent in jLS than aLS (*P* <.001, see **Table 3**). Pediatric-onset disease was associated with a wide range of severe neurologic problems such as hemiparesis (5), pyramidal signs (4), Rasmussen encephalitis, stroke, and dysmetria, whereas problems reported for aLS were depression, syncope, and tinnitus (see **Table 3**). The higher prevalence of neurologic symptoms and neuroimaging abnormalities found in jLS, which is also associated with ECDS/PRS, supports the association identified by Kreuter and colleagues.[45] In their study of 96 craniofacial patients, Kreuter and colleagues found a higher frequency of neurologic symptoms and imaging abnormalities in patients with ECDS/PRS overlap than ECDS.[45]

Organ system	Tissue	Specific problem	Int'l: No. (%)	N. Am: No. (%)
Musculoskeletal (MSK)			**91 (12.1)**	**45 (52)**
	Joint		91 (12.1)	32 (37)
		Arthritis	91 (12.1)	8 (9.3)
		Arthralgia	ND	15 (17.4)
		Joint limitation or contracture	ND	26 (30.2)
	Muscle		ND	34 (39.5)
		Muscle atrophy, decreased mass	ND	25 (29.1)
		Myalgia	ND	8 (9.3)
		Myositis	ND	3 (3.5)
	Bone	Size difference: hemiatrophy of face, trunk, and/or limb	ND	22 (25.6)
	Other msk	*Angular deformities, Tenosynovitis, fasciitis, enthesitis, fibrous arthropathy* *Arthritis can mimic juvenile idiopathic arthritis presenting as:* *- arthralgia, morning stiffness and effusions, or* *- enthesitis, dactylitis, and back pain*		
Neurologic			**33 (4.4)**	**5 (5.8)**
		Headache, migraines	7 (0.9)	1 (1.2)
		Seizures	10 (1.3)	0
		Peripheral neuropathy	3 (0.4)	2 (2.3)
		Imaging abnormality	5 (0.7)	2 (2.3)
		CNS vasculitis, EEG alterations, vascular malformations, behavioral changes	8 (1.1)	0
	Other neurologic	*Cognitive impairment, Focal neurological deficits, mood problems, movement disorders, Rasmussen's encephalitis*		
Ocular			**16 (2.1)**	**1 (1.2)**
		Xerophthalmia	2 (0.3)	1 (1.2)
		Anterior uveitis	4 (0.5)	0
		Episcleritis, acquired glaucoma, keratitis, mydriasis, papilledema, strabismus	10 (1.2)	0
	Other ocular	*Anisocoria, enophthalmos, lid atrophy, optic neuritis, orbital myositis, ptosis, panuveitis, photophobia, retinal vasculitis*		
Odontostomatologic		Dental crowding, Tongue hemiatrophy	ND	1 (1.2)
	Other oral	*Dental hypoplasia, jaw hypoplasia, malalignment teeth and jaw, masseter muscle spasms, palate deficiencies*		
Vascular			**18 (2.4)**	**6 (7)**
		Cold fingers	ND	3 (3.5)
		Deep vein thrombosis	1 (0.1)	0
		Raynaud Phenomenon	16 (2.1)	0
		Vasculitic rash	1 (0.1)	3 (3.5)
Gastrointestinal		Dyspepsia, dysphagia, esophagitis, GERD	12 (1.6)	4 (4.7)
Pulmonary			**5 (0.7)**	**3 (3.5)**
		Abnormal PFT	3 (0.4)	3 (3.5)
		Dyspnea on exertion	5 (0.7)	1 (1.2)
Cardiac		Arrythmia, pericarditis, pulmonary hypertension	2 (0.3)	1 (1.2)
Renal		Nephritis	2 (0.3)	1 (1.2)

DISEASE MONITORING
Outcome Measures

Several LS cutaneous measures have been developed. Among the whole-body activity measures, the modified Localized Scleroderma Skin Index (mLoSSI) and Localized Scleroderma Cutaneous Activity Measure (LSCAM) were found valid and reliable, with mLoSSI the most widely used.[54–56] LSCAM differs from mLoSSI in including more skin variables and weighing them all equally.[54] In a prospective 1-year study, LSCAM was found to better correlate with physician assessment of disease activity at more time-points than the mLoSSI,[57] so further LSCAM study is warranted.

The CARRA LS group developed the Total Morbidity Score (TMS) to provide a global level of cutaneous damage and extracutaneous morbidity.[55] This measure may aid tracking of changes in ECI in response to treatment.

Imaging

Several imaging modalities have been used to evaluate and monitor skin and ECI, especially musculoskeletal and neurologic (**Table 4**).[58] Although more work is needed to compare these tools, many of which still need protocol standardization and validation,[56] multimodal evaluations may provide a more complete disease assessment.

Fig. 4. The pattern of ECI for two jLS cohorts, an international one of 750 patients (Zulian et al[26], 2005) and a N. American one of 86 patients (Li et al[29], 2021) are shown. Additional ECI from Kister et al[30], 2008; Magro et al[14], 2019; Bucher et al[35], 2016. (*A*) Polyarthritis in linear scleroderma. (*B*) Joint contractures, and leg length and girth differences from linear scleroderma. (*C*) Hemifacial atrophy in a patient with PRS, with progressive atrophy of soft tissues, eyeball, zygomatic arch, and maxillary bone on left side since disease onset around age 6 years. Republished under the CC license agreement copyright © 2014 Mesut Kaya et al. Case Reports in Otolaryngology 2014; https://doi.org/10.1155/2014/703017. (*D*) Myokymia and hemifacial dystonia in ECDS. Republished under the CC 3.0 license agreement, copyright Ó2012 Carlos A. Cañas et al. Case Rep Med. 2012:691314. (*E*) T1- weighted gadolinium enhanced MRI of patient with mixed morphea including ECDS, who developed intractable seizures, cognitive deficits, and personality changes more than 20 years after skin disease onset. There are enhancing white matter lesions and global volume loss; arrow points to an area of enhancement. (*F*) Brain biopsy of patient in E, showing lymphocytic vasculopathy. Figures E-F republished under the CC 4.0 license agreement, copyright Ó2019 Magro CM et al. Orphanet J Rare Dis. 2019; 14:110. (*G*) Young adult with onset PRS at age 7 years, who has had multiple left eye problems including enopthalmos, pseudoptosis, uveitis, iris atrophy, partial aniridia, phacodonesis and ciliary body hypotrophy. Republished under the CC BY 4.0 license agreement copyright ©2015, Fea AM et al, BMC Opthalmology 2015;15:119. (*H*) Atrophy of the left retrobulbar fat tissue and phthisis of the eyeball in patient with PRS, associated with vision loss. Arrow points to atrophy of temporalis muscle. Republished under the CC license agreement copyright © 2014 Mesut Kaya et al. Case Reports in Otolaryngology 2014;2014:703017. doi: 10.1155/2014/703017. (*I*) Enopthalmos of the left eye. Republished with permission from Bucher F, et al. Survey of Ophthalmology 2016;16:693. (*J*) ECDS affecting face, upper lip and gingiva, with asymmetrical malformation of gingiva identified after shedding of maxillary incisors. (*K*) Dental X-ray of patient with ECDS showing ectopic tooth eruption; tooth has a short, malformed root. J and K republished with permission from Hørberg M et al. Eur Arch Paediatr Dent 2015;16:227. Int'l, international; MRI, Magnetic resonance imaging. N. Am, North American; PRS, Parry Romberg syndrome.

Table 3
Craniofacial linear scleroderma in pediatric and adult-onset localized scleroderma

LS Onset (No. Patients)	Age Onset[a], Years (IQR)	Females: Males[b]	ECDS No. (%)	PRS No. (%)	ECDS/PRS, No. (%)	Eye[c] No. (%)	Neuro sx[d] No. (%)	Abnormal Imaging[e] No. (%)	Headache[d] No. (%)	Seizures[d] No. (%)	Other Neuro sx[d] No. (%)
Pediatric (285)	6.1 (4,10)	139: 76 1.8:1	171 (60.6)	54 (19.1)	57 (20.2)	24 (19.5)	120 (45.1)	80 (42.6)	70 (26.3)	40 (15.0)	26 (9.8)
Adult (116)	29.5 (24.8, 41.8)	58:10 5.8:1	85 (73.3)	19 (16.4)	11 (9.5)	2 (8.0)	17 (23.3)	11 (28.9)	11 (15.1)	4 (5.5)	6 (8.2)
	<0.001	<0.001	0.019	NS	0.005	NS	<0.001	<0.001	0.046	0.032	NS

Studies were selected if they reported sufficient detail on their site craniofacial cohort, only one study per site included; pediatric references,[21,23,31,36,45-53] adult references.[21,31,44-48] P-values calculated by Z-score and t-test. Other problems (number reported if >1) for jLS: neuropathy (12), hemiparesis (5), pyramidal signs (4), abnormal EEG without overt seizures (3), dysphagia or gastroparesis (2), Rasmussen encephalitis, stroke, developmental delay, mental retardation, dysmetria, slurred speech, cognitive and behavioral issues; and for adults: neuropathy (2), dizziness (2), syncope, tinnitus, depression. Superscripts indicate data not available from listed studies.

Abbreviations: ECDS, en coup de sabre; HA, headache; IQR, interquartile range; neuro, neurologic; No., number; PRS, Parry-Romberg syndrome; sx, symptoms.

[a] Marzano et al,[21] 2003; Mazori et al,[44] 2016; Kreuter et al,[45] 2018.
[b] Marzano et al,[21] 2003; Kreuter et al,[45] 2018.
[c] Appenzeller et al,[31] 2004; Mazori et al,[44] 2016; Kreuter et al,[45] 2018; Blaszczyk et al,[48] 1999.
[d] Partial reporting for Doolittle et al,[46] 2015; Mazori et al,[44] 2016.
[e] Marzano et al,[21] 2003; Kreuter et al,[45] 2018; Blaszczyk et al,[48] 1999; Garcia-de la Torre et al,[53] 1995; partial for Mazori et al,[44] 2016; Kornreich et al,[52] 1977; Chiu et al,[51] 2012; Mazori et al,[44] 2016.

Table 4
Imaging modalities for localized scleroderma

Modality	Able to Detect Activity?	Uses
Infrared thermography	Yes	Evaluation of skin temperature in lesion in comparison to unaffected site. Active lesions found warmer
Ultrasound: gray scale and color Doppler	Yes	Evaluation of echogenicity, vascularity, and tissue thickness of skin and underlying superficial tissues in comparison to unaffected, preferably contralateral site
Radiographs	No	Evaluate joint and bone involvement
Computerized tomography (CT)	No	Evaluate neurologic, musculoskeletal, and some other extracutaneous involvement
Cone beam CT	No	Evaluate dental and facial bony involvement
Magnetic resonance imaging	Yes	Evaluate musculoskeletal, brain, and other deep structures. Can identify musculoskeletal tissue activity, and vasculitis
LDF/LDI	Yes	Higher dermal flow rates found in active lesions

Abbreviations: CT, computerized tomography; LDF, laser Doppler flowmetry; LDI, laser Doppler imaging.

TREATMENT

Goals of treatment are to reduce inflammation, prevent damage, and preserve function. Because current therapies primarily target the inflammatory phase of LS, recognizing active disease is critical. Both PReS and CARRA, and a recent Cochrane review, support methotrexate as first-line treatment of patients at risk for moderate to severe disease.[56,59,60] **Fig. 5** shows risk factors for worse disease, which includes patients with deeper tissue subtypes and ECI. For these patients, topical treatments with their limited depth of penetration are insufficient for controlling activity and reducing morbidity risk.[59] PReS and CARRA generated standardized regimens based on best available evidence, with PReS favoring inclusion of concurrent glucocorticoid treatment, whereas CARRA members were divided on its need.[56,60]

The algorithm in **Fig. 5** shows many of the factors delineated by CARRA[60] and the treatments recommended by CARRA and PReS.[56,60] This approach is favored by the investigators and is intended to serve as a guide but not prescriptive instructions. Treatment often needs to be individualized considering factors such as risk for growth impairment and other long-term problems.

Poorer outcomes, including a greater likelihood for incomplete remission and treatment failure, have been associated with treatment initiation delays for both jLS and

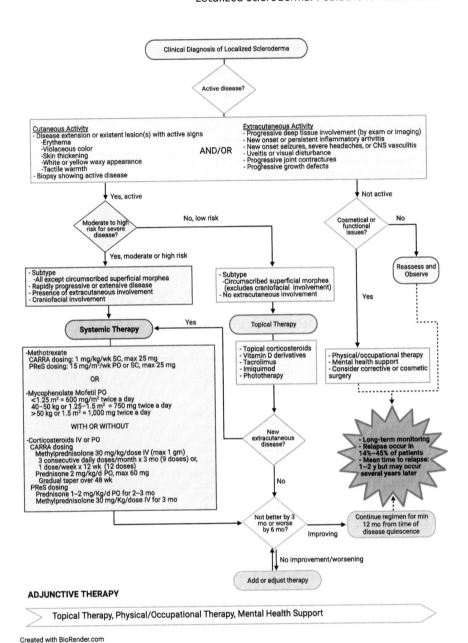

Fig. 5. LS treatment recommendations. This algorithm outlines factors to consider when deciding upon treatment, and CARRA and PReS recommended treatments. Careful and long-term monitoring for both cutaneous and extracutaneous activity is important. The algorithm is based upon the authors' experiences and not intended to serve as prescriptive instructions. Data from Li et al[60], 2012 and Zulian et al[56], 2019. CARRA, childhood arthritis and rheumatology research alliance; IV, intravenous; max, maximum; min, minimum; PO, by mouth; PReS, pediatric rheumatology European society; SC, subcutaneous.

Table 5
Consensus-based recommendations for the management of juvenile localized scleroderma from single hub and access point for pediatric rheumatology in Europe (SHARE)

Overarching Principle	L	S	% Agreement
1. All children with suspected LS should be referred to a specialized pediatric rheumatology center	4	D	100
2. LoSSI, which is part of LoSCAT, is a good clinical instrument to assess activity and severity in jLS lesions and is highly recommended in clinical practice LoSSI = Localized Scleroderma Skin Severity Index LoSCAT = Localized Scleroderma Cutaneous Assessment Tool	3	C	90
3. LoSDI, which is part of LoSCAT, is a good clinical instrument to assess damage in jLS and is highly recommended in clinical practice LoSDI = Localized Scleroderma Skin Damage Index	3	C	90
4. Infrared thermography can be used to assess activity of the lesions in jLS, but skin atrophy can give false-positive results	4	D	90
5. A specialized US imaging, using standardized assessment and color Doppler, may be a useful tool for assessing disease activity, extent of jLS, and response to treatment	4	D	100
6. All patients with jLS at diagnosis and during follow-up should be carefully evaluated with a complete joint examination, including the temporomandibular joint	2A	C	100
7. MRI can be considered a useful tool to assess musculoskeletal involvement in jLS, especially when the lesion crosses the joint	3	C	100
8. It is highly recommended that all patients with JLS involving face and head, with or without signs of neurologic involvement, have an MRI of the head at the time of the diagnosis	3	C	90
9. All patients with jLS involving face and head should undergo an orthodontic and maxillofacial evaluation at diagnosis and during follow-up	2B	B	90
10. Ophthalmologic assessment, including screening for uveitis, is recommended at diagnosis for every patient with jLS, especially in those with skin lesions on the face and scalp	2A	C	100
11. Ophthalmologic follow-up, including screening for uveitis, should be considered for every patient with jLS, especially in those with skin lesions on the face and scalp	3	C	100

Abbreviations: jLS, juvenile localized scleroderma; L, level of evidence; S, strength of recommendation; US, ultrasound.

Data from Zulian F, Culpo R, Sperotto F, et al. Consensus-based recommendations for the management of juvenile localised scleroderma. *Ann Rheum Dis.* 2019;78(8):1019-1024.

aLS.[61,62] Even a 79-day delay reduced remission likelihood in jLS.[62] Because half or more patients with jLS have ECI, and many dermatologists still favor topicals as solo treatment of linear scleroderma and other subtypes,[1] the authors recommend all patients with jLS be evaluated early in their disease by a rheumatologist. Patients also need long-term cutaneous and extracutaneous monitoring, potentially into and thru adulthood. **Table 5** shows recently generated consensus and evidence-based management recommendations from PReS.[56]

Treatment Resistance: Refractory Disease

About one-third of patients fail initial methotrexate treatment. Potential risk factors for refractory disease are disease subtype and ECI. In one study, treatment failure was associated with both mixed morphea and ECI,[57] whereas another found a more pro-tracted and complicated course associated with mixed morphea.[21] As ECI is also associated with larger cutaneous extent, refractory disease may be due to the greater disease burden in patients with jLS with ECI.[29]

Mycophenolate mofetil (MMF) is often used to treat patients with LS who have meth-otrexate refractory disease, with case series reporting it to be effective and well toler-ated.[63,64] The CARRA LS group also developed consensus treatment plans for MMF with dosing shown in **Fig. 5**[60] Other medicines that are reported beneficial for metho-trexate nonresponders in small case reports include tocilizumab,[24,65] abatacept,[66,67] infliximab,[68] and JAK inhibitors.[69]

SUMMARY

Outcomes in LS have improved significantly with the widespread implementation of methotrexate treatment since the early 2000s.[1] Mortality is rare, mainly related to com-plications from widespread skin involvement in pansclerotic morphea.[1] Unfortunately, functional impairment, permanent disfigurement, chronic pain, and the psychological impact of LS are still frequent problems. More work is needed to better assess disease impact on health-related quality of life in LS.[28]

Due to the high frequency of ECI, frequent asynchrony between cutaneous and extracutaneous activity, and often initially asymptomatic presentation of skin and ECI, monitoring of patients with pediatric-onset disease by rheumatology is essential. Because pediatric-onset LS has a long disease duration (mean 13.5 years versus 5.8 years for aLS)[21] and high relapse rate (>45% after $\geq$ 5 years of follow-up),[62] long-term monitoring is needed including into adult life. As with other rheumatic diseases, early aggressive treatment is likely to yield better outcomes for both remission and morbidity likelihood.1 While tremendous improvements in jLS outcome have been made, about a quarter of patients still have functional impairment. Continued valida-tion and refinement of reliable clinical, biomarker, imaging, and histologic outcomes is necessary to accurately measure disease activity, identify patients at risk for non-responsiveness, and enable trials that can identify more effective therapies. Recent advances in our understanding of scleroderma pathophysiology offer great hope for the discovery of sensitive biomarkers to track activity and identification of novel ther-apeutic targets to further advance outcome.

CLINICS CARE POINTS

- Most patients with jLS have both skin and extracutaneous tissue involvement, with a higher frequency of extracutaneous involvement found in pediatric versus aLS.

- Morbidity is primarily related to extracutaneous involvement and can be severe.

- Musculoskeletal is the most common type of extracutaneous involvement, with abnormal growth, including hemiatrophy, a major concern for growing children.

- Patients with craniofacial skin involvement have a higher risk for neurologic, ocular, and oral problems.

- Systemic immunosuppressants, especially methotrexate, are considered standard of care for jLS treatment by pediatric rheumatologists. Methotrexate treatment has greatly reduced morbidity frequency in jLS, including the need for orthopedic surgeries.

- Most patients respond to methotrexate treatment in the first 3 to 6 months, but about one-third are nonresponders.

- Nonresponders need additional treatment, often initiation or more glucocorticoids, with mycophenolate mofetil recommended as the next disease-modifying antirheumatic drug to use.

- Long-term monitoring of patients with jLS is needed because average disease duration is greater than 10 years, relapses are common, and extracutaneous involvement often presents years after skin disease onset. Skin and extracutaneous tissue activity patterns often differ.

ACKNOWLEDGMENTS

The authors thank Alexander Kreuter and Steffen Goldbach for kindly providing us with additional data from their study (Acta Derm Venereol. 2018;98(6):603-5) to use in **Table 3**.

DISCLOSURE

The authors have nothing to disclose.

REFERENCES

1. Li SC, O'Neil KM, Higgins GC. Morbidity and Disability in Juvenile Localized Scleroderma: The Case for Early Recognition and Systemic Immunosuppressive Treatment. J Pediatr 2021;234:245–56.
2. Zulian F, Vallongo C, Woo P, et al. Localized scleroderma in childhood is not just a skin disease. Arthritis Rheum 2005;52(9):2873–81.
3. Torok KS, Li SC, Jacobe HM, et al. Immunopathogenesis of Pediatric Localized Scleroderma. Front Immunol 2019;10:908.
4. Peterson L, Nelson A, Su W, et al. The epidemiology of morphea (localized scleroderma) in Olmstead County 1960-1993. J Rheumatol 1997;24:73–80.
5. Wu E, Li S, Torok K, et al. Baseline description of the juvenile localized scleroderma subgroup from the Childhood Arthritis and Rheumatology Research Alliance Legacy Registry. ACR Open Rheumatol 2019;1:119–24.
6. Leitenberger J, Cayce R, Haley R, et al. Distinct Autoimmune Syndromes in Morphea. Arch Dermatol 2009;145:545–50.
7. Saracino AM, Denton CP, Orteu CH. The molecular pathogenesis of morphoea: from genetics to future treatment targets. Br J Dermatol 2017;177(1):34–46.
8. Rongioletti F, Ferreli C, Atzori L, et al. Scleroderma with an update about clinicopathological correlation. G Ital Dermatol Venereol 2018;153(2):208–15.
9. Wolska-Gawron K, Bartosińska J, Krasowska D. MicroRNA in localized scleroderma: a review of literature. Arch Dermatol Res 2020;312(5):317–24.
10. Mirizio E, Marathi A, Hershey N, et al. Identifying the Signature Immune Phenotypes Present in Pediatric Localized Scleroderma. J Invest Dermatol 2019;139(3):715–8.
11. Mertens J, de Jong E, van den Hoogen L, et al. The identification of CCL18 as biomarker of disease activity in localized scleroderma. J Autoimmun 2019;10:86–93.
12. Uhlén M, Karlsson MJ, Hober A, et al. The human secretome. Sci Signal 2019;12(609):eaaz0274.
13. Badshah II, Brown S, Weibel L, et al. Differential expression of secreted factors SOSTDC1 and ADAMTS8 cause profibrotic changes in linear morphoea fibroblasts. Br J Dermatol 2019;180(5):1135–49.

14. Magro C, Halteh P, Olson L, et al. Linear scleroderma "en coup de sabre" with extensive brain involvement—Clinicopathologic correlations and response to anti-Interleukin-6 therapy. Orphanet J Rare Dis 2019;14:110.

15. Kowalewski C, Kozlowska A, Górska M, et al. Alterations of Basemement Membrane Zone and Cutaneous Microvasculature in Morphea and Extragenital Lichen Sclerosus. Am J Dermatopathol 2005;27:489–96.

16. Mostmans Y, Cutolo M, Giddelo C, et al. The role of endothelial cells in the vasculopathy of systemic sclerosis: A systematic review. Autoimmun Rev 2017;16(8): 774–86.

17. Yamane K, Ihn H, Kubo M, et al. Increased serum levels of soluble vascular cell adhesion molecule 1 and E-selectin in patients with localized scleroderma. J Am Acad Dermatol 2000;42(1 Pt 1):64–9.

18. Vasquez-Canizares N, Agarwal B, Rubinstein T, et al. Exploring the Use of Von Willebrand Factor as a Disease Biomarker in a Cohort of Patients with Juvenile Scleroderma: A Pilot Study [abstract]. Arthritis Rheumatol 2020;72.

19. Prasad S, Zhu JL, Schollaert-Fitch K, et al. An Evaluation of the Performance of Current Morphea Subtype Classifications. JAMA Dermatol 2021;157(4):1–8.

20. Kreuter A, Wischnewski J, Terras S, et al. Coexistence of lichen sclerosus and morphea: a retrospective analysis of 472 patients with localized scleroderma from a German tertiary referral center. J Am Acad Dermatol 2012;67:1157–62.

21. Marzano AV, Menni S, Parodi A, et al. Localized scleroderma in adults and children. Clinical and laboratory investigations on 239 cases. Eur J Dermatol 2003; 13(2):171–6.

22. Mertens JS, Seyger MM, Kievit W, et al. Disease recurrence in localized scleroderma: a retrospective analysis of 344 patients with paediatric- or adult-onset disease. Br J Dermatol 2015;172(3):722–8.

23. Christen-Zaech S, Hakim MD, Afsar FS, et al. Pediatric morphea (localized scleroderma): review of 136 patients. J Am Acad Dermatol 2008;59(3):385–96.

24. Lythgoe H, Almeida B, Bennett J, et al. Multi-centre national audit of juvenile localised scleroderma: describing current UK practice in disease assessment and management. Pediatr Rheumatol Online J 2018;16(1):80.

25. Pequet MS, Holland KE, Zhao S, et al. Risk factors for morphoea disease severity: a retrospective review of 114 paediatric patients. Br J Dermatol 2014;170(4): 895–900.

26. Zulian F, Athreya B, Laxer R, et al. Juvenile localized scleroderma: clinical and epidemiological features in 750 children. An international study. Rheumatology 2006;45:614–20.

27. Li SC, Li X, Pope E, et al. New Features for Measuring Disease Activity in Pediatric Localized Scleroderma. J Rheumatol 2018;45(12):1680–8.

28. Ardalan K, Zigler CK, Torok KS. Predictors of Longitudinal Quality of Life in Juvenile Localized Scleroderma. Arthritis Care Res (Hoboken) 2017;69(7):1082–7.

29. Li S, Higgins G, Chen M, et al. Extracutaneous Involvement Is Common and Associated with Prolonged Disease Activity and Greater Impact in Juvenile Localized Scleroderma. Rheumatology (Oxford) 2021. https://doi.org/10.1093/rheumatology/keab238.

30. Kister I, Inglese M, Laxer R, et al. Neurologic manifestations of localized scleroderma. A case report and literature review. Neurology 2008;71:1538–45.

31. Appenzeller S, Montenegro M, San Juan Dertkigil S, et al. Neuroimaging findings in scleroderma en coup de sabre. Neurology 2004;62:1585–9.

32. Reiff D, Crayne C, Mannion M, et al. Characteristics of coexisting localized scleroderma and inflammatory arthritis. Eur J Rheumatol 2020;7:567–71.

33. Kashem S, Correll C, Vehe R, et al. Inflammatory arthritis in pediatric patients with morphea. J Am Acad Dermatol 2018;79:47–51.
34. Maloney E, Menashe SJ, Iyer RS, et al. The central nervous system manifestations of localized craniofacial scleroderma: a study of 10 cases and literature review. Pediatr Radiol 2018;48(11):1642–54.
35. Bucher F, Fricke J, Neugebauer A, et al. Ophthalmological manifestations of Parry-Romberg syndrome. Surv Ophthalmol 2016;61(6):693–701.
36. Pensler JM, Murphy GF, Mulliken JB. Clinical and ultrastructural studies of Romberg's hemifacial atrophy. Plast Reconstr Surg 1990;85(5):669–74 [discussion: 675–6].
37. Falanga V, Medsger T Jr, Reichlin M, et al. Linear scleroderma. Clinical spectrum, prognosis, and laboratory abnormalities. Ann Intern Med 1986;104:849–57.
38. Rubin L. Linear scleroderma; association with abnomalities. Arch Derm Syphilol 1948;58:1–18.
39. Arkachaisri T, Fertig N, Pino S, et al. Serum Autoantibodies and Their Clinical Associations in Patients with Childhood- and Adult-Onset Linear Scleroderma. A Single-Center Study. J Rheumatol 2008;35:2439–44.
40. Kunzler E, Florez-Pollack S, Teske N, et al. Linear morphea: Clinical characteristics, disease course, and treatment of the Morphea in Adults and Children cohort. J Am Acad Dermatol 2019;80(6):1664–70.e1.
41. Weibel L, Harper JI. Linear morphoea follows Blaschko's lines. Br J Dermatol 2008;159(1):175–81.
42. Piram M, McCuaig CC, Saint-Cyr C, et al. Short- and long-term outcome of linear morphoea in children. Br J Dermatol 2013;169(6):1265–71.
43. Vancheeswaran R, Black C, David J, et al. Childhood-onset scleroderma. Arthritis Rheum 1996;39:1041–9.
44. Mazori D, Wright N, Patel M, et al. Characteristics and treatment of adult-onset linear morphea: A retrospective cohort study of 61 patients at 3 tertiary care centers. J Am Acad Dermatol 2016;74:577–9.
45. Kreuter A, Mitrakos G, Hofmann SC, et al. Localized Scleroderma of the Head and Face Area: A Retrospective Cross-sectional Study of 96 Patients from 5 German Tertiary Referral Centres. Acta Derm Venereol 2018;98(6):603–5.
46. Doolittle D, Lehman V, Schwartz K, et al. CNS imaging findings associated with Parry-Romberg syndrome and en coup de sabre: correlation to dermatologic and neurologic abnormalities. Neuroradiology 2015;57:21–34.
47. Lis-Swiety A, Brzezinska-Wcislo L, Arasiewicz H. Neurological abnormalities in localized scleroderma of the face and head: a case series study for evaluation of imaging findings and clinical course. Int J Neurosci 2017;127(9):835–9.
48. Blaszczyk M, Jablonska S. Linear scleroderma en Coup de Sabre. Relationship with progressive facial hemiatrophy (PFH). Adv Exp Med Biol 1999;455:101–4.
49. De Somer L, Morren MA, Muller PC, et al. Overlap between linear scleroderma, progressive facial hemiatrophy and immune-inflammatory encephalitis in a paediatric cohort. Eur J Pediatr 2015;174(9):1247–54.
50. Seese RR, Glaser D, Furtado A, et al. Unilateral Neuroimaging Findings in Pediatric Craniofacial Scleroderma: Parry-Romberg Syndrome and En Coup de Sabre. J Child Neurol 2020;35(11):753–62.
51. Chiu YE, Vora S, Kwon EK, et al. A significant proportion of children with morphea en coup de sabre and Parry-Romberg syndrome have neuroimaging findings. Pediatr Dermatol 2012;29(6):738–48.
52. Kornreich H, King K, Bernstein B, et al. Scleroderma in childhood. Arthritis Rheum 1977;20:343–50.

53. Garcia-de la Torre I, Castello-Sendra J, Esgleyes-Ribot T, et al. Autoantibodies in Parry-Romberg syndrome: a serologic study of 14 patients. J Rheumatol 1995; 22(1):73–7.

54. Arkachaisri T, Vilaiyuk S, Li S, et al. The localized scleroderma skin severity index and physician global assessment of disease activity: a work in progress toward development of localized scleroderma outcome measures. J Rheumatol 2009; 36(12):2819–29.

55. Li S, Patel A, Pope E, et al. Capturing the Range of Disease Involvement in Localized Scleroderma: The Total Morbidity Score [abstract]. Arthritis Rheumatol 2020;72.

56. Zulian F, Culpo R, Sperotto F, et al. Consensus-based recommendations for the management of juvenile localised scleroderma. Ann Rheum Dis 2019;78(8):1019–24.

57. Li SC, Torok KS, Rabinovich CE, et al. Initial Results from a Pilot Comparative Effectiveness Study of 3 Methotrexate-based Consensus Treatment Plans for Juvenile Localized Scleroderma. J Rheumatol 2020;47(8):1242–52.

58. Lis-Swiety A, Janicka I, Skrzypek-Salamon A, et al. A systematic review of tools for determining activity of localized scleroderma in paediatric and adult patients. J Eur Acad Dermatol Venereol 2017;31(1):30–7.

59. Albuquerque JV, Andriolo BN, Vasconcellos MR, et al. Interventions for morphea. Cochrane Database Syst Rev 2019;7:CD005027.

60. Li SC, Torok KS, Pope E, et al. Development of consensus treatment plans for juvenile localized scleroderma: a roadmap toward comparative effectiveness studies in juvenile localized scleroderma. Arthritis Care Res (Hoboken) 2012;64(8):1175–85.

61. Mertens J, van den Reek J, Kievit W, et al. Drug Survival and Predictors of Drug Survival for Methotrexate Treatment in a Retrospective Cohort of Adult Patients with Localized Scleroderma. Acta Derm Venereol 2016;96:943–7.

62. Martini G, Fadanelli G, Agazzi A, et al. Disease course and long-term outcome of juvenile localized scleroderma: Experience from a single pediatric rheumatology Centre and literature review. Autoimmun Rev 2018;17:727–34.

63. Martini G, Saggioro L, Culpo R, et al. Mycophenolate mofetil for methotrexate-resistant juvenile localized scleroderma. Rheumatology (Oxford) 2021;60(3): 1387–91.

64. Arthur M, Fett NM, Latour E, et al. Evaluation of the Effectiveness and Tolerability of Mycophenolate Mofetil and Mycophenolic Acid for the Treatment of Morphea. JAMA Dermatol 2020;156:1–8.

65. Foeldvari I, Anton J, Friswell M, et al. Tocilizumab is a promising treatment option for therapy resistant juvenile localized scleroderma patients. J Scleroderma Relat Disord 2017;2(3):203–7.

66. Kalampokis I, Yi BY, Smidt AC. Abatacept in the treatment of localized scleroderma: A pediatric case series and systematic literature review. Semin Arthritis Rheum 2020;50(4):645–56.

67. Li SC, Torok KS, Ishaq SS, et al. Preliminary Evidence on Abatacept Safety and Efficacy in Refractory Juvenile Localized Scleroderma. Rheumatology (Oxford) 2020;60(8):3817–25.

68. Ferguson ID, Weiser P, Torok KS. A Case Report of Successful Treatment of Recalcitrant Childhood Localized Scleroderma with Infliximab and Leflunomide. Open Rheumatol J 2015;9:30–5.

69. Damsky W, Patel D, Garelli CJ, et al. Jak Inhibition Prevents Bleomycin-Induced Fibrosis in Mice and Is Effective in Patients with Morphea. J Invest Dermatol 2020; 140(7):1446–9.e4.

Updates in Systemic Sclerosis Treatment and Applicability to Pediatric Scleroderma

Kathryn S. Torok, MD[a,b]

KEYWORDS

- Systemic sclerosis • Pediatric rheumatology • Juvenile-onset systemic sclerosis
- Scleroderma • Treatment • Clinical practice

KEY POINTS

- Most treatment pathways in juvenile-onset systemic sclerosis (SSc) are extrapolated from adult-SSc studies given the rarity of childhood-onset disease.
- A comprehensive approach with pharmaceutical and supportive care of all organ systems is recommended.
- There are now 2 Food and Drug Administration–approved medications for SSc, both for the treatment of SSc-associated interstitial lung disease.
- Biological therapies and autologous stem cell transplantation are on the horizon, with potential for administration earlier in disease course to reprogram the immune system.

INTRODUCTION

Juvenile-onset systemic sclerosis (jSSc) is a rare autoimmune condition with inflammation-driven fibrosis, accounting for less than 10% of all SSc cases, with an estimated annual incidence of 0.27 to 1 per million children and a prevalence of 3 per 1,000,000 children.[1–3] The average age of jSSc onset is 8 to 10.8 years, and rarely occurs before 5 years.[4–7] Because of its insidious nature, delay in diagnosis is common: older than or equal to 2 years in 20% of patients.[4,5,7,8] Girls are more commonly affected at a ratio of 4:1.[4,5,7,9] There seems to be a Caucasian predominance of 78% to 92%,[4,6,7,9] followed by African decent ranging from 6% to 19% in a larger cohorts.[6,9,7]

Clinical presentation, manifestations, and initial organ assessment in jSSc based on adult SSc guidelines and their applicability to jSSc were recently described (summarized in **Table 1**).[10] Overall, organ manifestations in jSSc are similar to adult-onset,

a Division of Pediatric Rheumatology, UPMC & University of Pittsburgh Scleroderma Center;
b Pediatric Scleroderma Clinic, University of Pittsburgh |UPMC Children's Hospital of Pittsburgh, 4401 Penn Ave, Pittsburgh, PA 15224, USA
E-mail address: kathryn.torok@chp.edu

Rheum Dis Clin N Am 47 (2021) 757–780
https://doi.org/10.1016/j.rdc.2021.07.004
0889-857X/21/© 2021 Elsevier Inc. All rights reserved.

rheumatic.theclinics.com

Table 1
Baseline evaluation for a patient with juvenile-onset systemic sclerosis[a]

	General Assessment			
Examination	General: Blood pressure Weight, body mass index, growth curve assessment Cardiopulmonary examination: Rales, split S2, friction rub	Orofacial: Oral aperture, gum, and oral health status Vasculopathy: Nailfold capillary, digital tip ulcer, digital tip pitting assessment	Joint assessment: Range of motion, arthritis, tenosynovitis, assessment Finger to palm measurements Presence of tendon friction rubs	Musculoskeletal: Truncal, proximal and distal muscle strength, weakness, atrophy Skin: Modified Rodnan skin score
Laboratory Evaluation	General: CBC with differential Comprehensive Metabolic Panel (Albumin, Total protein) ESR CRP	Cardiac: Pro-BNP/BNP Renal: Urinalysis Spot urine protein: creatine	Gastrointestinal: Fat soluble vitamins (A, D, E, K) B12 folate	Musculoskeletal: CPK Aldolase AST, ALT LDH
Other Supportive Assessment	Behavioral therapy/psychiatry	Respiratory therapy (for ILD and muscle weakness)	Nutrition Speech pathology (oral pharyngeal mechanics)	Occupational therapy (upper extremities) Physical therapy (lower extremities)

Evaluations by Organ System and Tier

	Cardiac	Pulmonary	Gastrointestinal	Musculoskeletal
Tier 1	Electrocardiogram Echocardiogram	Chest radiograph High-resolution chest CT[b] Pulmonary function tests • Spirometry (FVC) • Lung volume by plethysmography (TLC, RV) • Diffusing capacity (DLCO) • Respiratory muscle pressure (MIP, MEP) 6-minute walk test (distance, preoxygen/postoxygen saturation) • Forehead SpO2 probe • Monitor spO2 during test	Esophagram/upper GI Fluoroscopic swallow study with speech pathology Gastric emptying study (4 h, solid meals)	Hand radiograph (acrosteolysis)
Tier 2	Exercise ECG/echo Holter monitor Cardiac MRI	Exercise PFTs Right heart catheter (pulmonary arterial hypertension)	Esophageal manometry pH probe impendence Endoscopy with biopsies	MRI hips/pelvis for myositis MRI wrist/hand for arthritis/tenosynovitis

Abbreviations: ALT, alanine aminotransferase; AST, aspartate transaminase; BNP, B-type natriuretic peptide; CBC, complete blood count; CPK, creatine phosphokinase; CRP, C-reactive protein; ECG, electrocardiogram, ESR, erythrocyte sedimentation rate; LDH, lactate dehydrogenase; MEP, maximal expiratory pressure; MIP, maximal inspiratory pressure; RV, residual volume.

[a] Recommendations derived from the literature and adult SSc management, with additional input based on the author's clinical experience directing a pediatric scleroderma clinic cohort for more than 15 y, with input from multidisciplinary team in Acknowledgments.

[b] Can detect patulous esophagus.

with comparable frequencies of interstitial lung disease (ILD), gastrointestinal (GI) involvement, and pulmonary arterial hypertension, supported by recent larger jSSc cohort data.[6,7] The 2 main variations from adult disease are higher frequency of musculoskeletal (MSK) involvement, secondary to the higher frequency of overlap subtype of SSc with predominant dermatomyositis features, and the lack of renal crises (<5% all cohort studies). Therefore, general guidelines regarding baseline organ systems evaluation for pediatric patients are similar,[10] except for reserving more invasive testing for children with more significant symptoms or findings on first-pass (Tier 1) evaluations (**Table 1**).

A major advancement over the past 5 years is recognition of "silent" ILD and the need for baseline high-resolution chest computational radiograph (HRCT),[11,12] previously reserved due to radiation concerns. A recent international jSSc cohort study found up to 60% underdetection of ILD by relying on pulmonary function tests (PFTs) alone.[13] Esophageal dysfunction is common in both pediatric and adult SSc, but often unrecognized, manifesting as nausea (due to stasis) and decreased appetite with subsequent weight loss and in children, as failure to thrive.[14] Esophageal dysmotility and gastroesophageal reflux can lead to silent aspiration and propagate or promote ILD, with this relationship recently demonstrated in jSSc cohorts.[13,14] Given concerns for growth impact and association with ILD, baseline screening of all jSSc with fluoroscopic swallow study with speech pathology and an esophagram/upper GI study should be considered. Further GI monitoring and evaluation depends on symptoms and initial findings (**Table 2**).

In addition to these recent clinical guidelines of organ evaluation in jSSc,[10] the first set of consensus-based recommendations for jSSc management were published by the Single Hub and Access point for pediatric Rheumatology in Europe (SHARE) in 2020.[11] Updated review of SSc treatment to March 2021, primarily in adults, with potential applicability in children and clinical care points is provided in this chapter.

MEDICAL TREATMENT OPTIONS AND ADJUNCT CARE
General Management

Treatment options for SSc have advanced dramatically in the past decade, including US Food and Drug Administration (FDA) approval of 2 agents for SSc-associated ILD and growing evidence of better survival and efficacy in autologous stem cell transplantation for moderate-to-severe disease. These advances, with careful monitoring and intensive modulation of treatment plans including nonpharmacologic adjunct care, have improved survival and health of patients with SSc. In general, the approach depends on disease stage and organ specificity. The best outcomes result from early diagnosis and recognition of internal organ involvement, allowing treatment to prevent permanent organ damage. The European League Against Rheumatism (EULAR) Scleroderma Trials and Research (EUSTAR) group has established evidence-based recommendations to be used in clinical practice.[15] The Canadian Scleroderma Society also developed guidelines to provide algorithms endorsed by SSc experts.[16] The following review of treatment by affected organ systems is in agreement with these general recommendations (see **Table 2** for organ system summary), with additional updates from the literature and commentary when appropriate about application to jSSc.

ORGAN SYSTEM MANAGEMENT
Cutaneous

Cutaneous manifestations frequently bring children to medical attention, and in general, the skin transitions through 3 phases in SSc: edematous, sclerosis (or induration),

Table 2
Organ-specific treatment of systemic sclerosis[a]

Manifestation	First Line	Second Line	Third Line	Supportive
Cutaneous	Methotrexate Mycophenolate mofetil Corticosteroids (low dose)	Cyclophosphamide Tocilizumab Immune globulin	Abatacept Rituximab	Liberal use emollients Antihistamines Avoid extreme temperature exposure • Lack functional sebaceous glands, overheat • Prolonged cold exposure, ischemia and ulceration Topical antibiotics Laser therapy for telangiectasias
Musculoskeletal	NSAIDs Corticosteroids (low dose) Hydroxychloroquine Methotrexate	Rituximab Abatacept Tocilizumab	TNF-alpha inhibitors	Occupational therapy • Wax bath before sessions Physical therapy • Active and passive range of motion
Renal Crisis	ACE inhibitors			
Raynaud Phenomenon	Calcium channel blockers	Phosphodiesterase inhibitors Topical nitrates	Angiotensin II receptor antagonists Fluoxetine Prostacyclins (for severe, refractory) Endothelial stabilizers: Low dose aspirin Pentoxifylline Statins Surgical techniques: Digital sympathectomy Botulism toxin injection Fat grafting	Core body and peripheral body warm • Hand warmer, gloves, socks, hat • Home ambient temperature Avoid vasoactive medications/supplements • nasal decongestants, amphetamines, herbs with ephedra, smoking, serotonin agonists, attention deficit hyperactivity disorder stimulants

(continued on next page)

Table 2
(continued)

Manifestation	First Line	Second Line	Third Line	Supportive
Digital Ulcers	PDE5 inhibitors Calcium channel blockers	Endothelin receptor antagonists	Prostacyclins	MediHoney, Mupirocin ointment • fingertip cracks/peeling, early ulcers Oral antibiotics (Cephalexin) • open ulcer Wound care consult Pain control
Pulmonary Hypertension	Phosphodiesterase inhibitors Endothelin receptor antagonists	Prostacyclins Riociguat		
Interstitial Lung Disease	Mycophenolate mofetil Tocilizumab Cyclophosphamide Corticosteroids	Nintedanib Rituximab	Autologous hematopoietic stem cell transplantation Lung transplantation	Aggressively treat GERD Keep vaccines up to date Pulmonary rehabilitation • Inspiratory muscle training
Gastrointestinal	GERD: Proton pump inhibitor H2 receptor antagonist Dysmotility: Erythromycin Cyproheptadine Metoclopramide	Small intestine: Rotating antibiotics Vitamin supplementation Octreotide Large intestine: Polyethylene glycol Sparing use loperamide	Gastric antral vascular ectasia: Laser photocoagulation Stricture: Mechanical dilatation Malnutrition: Nasogastric or jejunostomy tube	Saliva substitutes Tooth brushing devices Speech pathologist consult • Oropharyngeal exercises Small, frequent meals, avoid meals 3 h before bed Raise head of bed 6 inches Nutritionist consult GI motility expert consult

[a] Medications listed by evidence first to third tier. Supportive care includes author's recommendations.

and atrophy. Treatment is directed toward the edematous phase (puffy fingers/hands, swollen feet/ankles and early sclerodactyly) and the sclerosis phase (loss of skin pliability with palpable thickness, causing appearance of shiny, taught, bound-down skin). Skin thickness can be quantified by the modified Rodnan Skin Score (mRSS), and in adults it has been used as a surrogate measure of total disease severity.[17,18] The mRSS progression rate can be used to predict timing of internal organ involvement,[19] whereas an improving skin score signifies stable disease status and increased survival,[20] supporting its use as an outcome measure in clinical trials. Further study is being conducted in children to assess mRSS correlation with disease severity and prognosis.[10]

Currently, either methotrexate (MTX) or mycophenolate mofetil (MMF) are standard therapies for diffuse skin involvement, with or without internal organ involvement, especially if given within the first 3 years of disease onset (see **Table 2**). Typically, the decision depends on extracutaneous disease manifestations: arthritis or myositis may prompt MTX use, whereas concomitant ILD supports the selection of MMF. MTX has shown efficacy for treating skin disease in patients with diffuse and progressive skin disease in 2 randomized, placebo-controlled, double-blind trials with a trend toward mRSS improvement.[21,22] Based on these trials as well as observational data, EULAR endorsed the use of MTX for progressive skin involvement in the early stages of disease.[15,23] MMF has proved beneficial clinically (reflected by mRSS improvement), histologically, and transcriptionally, with significant decreases in inflammatory infiltrate and microarray inflammatory gene expression profiles when comparing pretreatment andto posttreatment skin biopsy specimens.[24,25] Most of these studies of MMF are small observational cohorts of 15 to 20 subjects,[26–29] but some have found significant mRSS changes, and data from secondary analyses of 2 major scleroderma lung fibrosis trials further support the benefit of MMF for skin disease.[29]

In addition, these studies found that cyclophosphamide (CYC) was effective in lowering the skin score in diffuse cutaneous SSc.[29,30] CYC should be reserved for those with rapidly progressing skin thickening or poor response to MTX and MMF. Other therapies for refractory skin progression and severe disease include intravenous immunoglobulin, rituximab, tocilizumab (interleukin-6 inhibitor), abatacept, and Janus kinase inhibitors, which have shown efficacy in case reports or small case series.[31–35]

Supportive skin care is recommended, including frequent application of unscented emollients, applied immediately after showering to allow deeper penetration into the thickened dermis, and antihistamines are helpful during early edematous and sclerotic disease when skin is pruritic. Topical antibiotics are often used for digital tip cracking and pitting to avoid infection.

Musculoskeletal

MSK involvement is more common in jSSc than in adults. One-third of patients experience joint effusions in addition to the typical dry synovitis of scleroderma.[4,5] Joint contractures of small, medium, and large joints are evident in most patients later during disease, resultant from the initial skin, subcutis, and underlying connective tissue sclerosis. A "bland" myositis or myopathy is present in at least one-third of patients with jSSc, demonstrated by muscle weakness but relatively unimpressive elevation of muscle enzymes and/or signal on MRI. The goal of MSK treatment is to combine pharmacologic with physical and occupational therapy as soon as possible to limit weakness, joint contractures, and disability while maximizing range of motion.

There is no dedicated recommendation for arthritis or myositis in SSc. Overall, these manifestations are treated as if they would be for adult or juvenile arthritis or myositis,[36] including nonsteroidal antiinflammatory drugs for arthralgia, disease-modifying antirheumatic drugs such as hydroxychloroquine and MTX, and biologics such as TNF-alpha inhibitors, rituximab, abatacept, and tocilizumab, for arthritis and myositis (see **Table 2**).[37–39]

Low-dose glucocorticoids (GC) are used as adjunct therapy earlier in disease course for arthritis and myositis in SSc. Adult SSc providers tend to limit dose to 10 mg prednisone daily due to concerns for instigating scleroderma renal crisis (SRC).[40] Although this should be taken into consideration, SRC is very rare in children, with 2 recent large jSSc cohorts having zero cases.[6,7] Liberalizing GC use in jSSc is therefore reasonable and commonplace,[11] although providers should closely monitor for blood pressure changes, renal function, and CBC changes. SRC is a medical emergency characterized by accelerated arterial hypertension, renal insufficiency, microangiopathic hemolytic anemia, and thrombocytopenia, and if untreated, can be fatal.[41] Immediate treatment with angiotensin-converting enzyme (ACE) inhibitors, captopril or enalapril, are effective treatments for SRC.[42–44]

VASCULOPATHY
Raynaud Phenomenon

Almost all patients with jSSc have Raynaud phenomenon (RP) (97%), and digital ulcers (DU) will develop in up to half of patients[4–6,9,45,46]; this is the most common and refractory concern among patients with jSSc. RP results from transient vasospasm and vasoconstriction of the arterioles, causing color change of pallor from transient ischemia with pain, numbness, and tingling, then cyanosis from deoxygenation, with an erythematous phase on rewarming. In SSc, RP is compounded by vasculopathy causing a stiffer vessel and unhealthy thickened endothelia. This vasculopathy is visually demonstrated by nailfold capillaroscopy, with nailfold capillary loops that are often dilated and tortuous, display areas of hemorrhage and telangiectasia, and later, show drop-out and arborization.[47] RP can lead to episodes of recurrent and prolonged ischemia, which cause digital pitting and ulcers at the pulp of the fingertips and gangrene in extreme cases (**Fig. 1**).

Treatment of RP include both supportive and pharmacologic (see **Table 2**). Primary treatment is to avoid precipitating circumstances, such as cold and stress, and keeping peripheral and core body temperature warm with appropriate clothing.[48] Avoidance of sympathetic stimulants may prevent episodes of RP, including attention deficit hyperactivity disorder stimulants (particularly important in pediatrics).[49]

Medical therapy involves a variety of medications that promote vasodilation and/or endothelial stabilization, often starting with one medication, but commonly adding

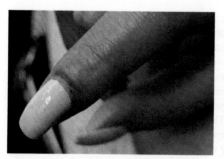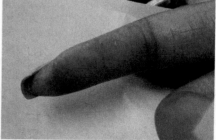

Fig. 1. Acute digital ischemia. Prolonged episode of uncontrolled Raynaud phenomenon can lead to tissue ischemia, denoted by sustained pallor at digital tip pad of finger with adjacent purple discoloration.

several together that take advantage of different mechanisms for cumulative effect, while counterbalancing the potential side effects, including lightheadedness from lowering the blood pressure. First-line therapy remains the dihydropyridine-type calcium channel blockers (CCBs) (see **Table 2**), which have been demonstrated to reduce the frequency and severity of ischemic attacks in patients with SSc.[50–52] Nifedipine is the most commonly studied, and sustained release is typically recommended for ease of administration and avoidance of reflex sinus tachycardia.[50–52] The increased convenience of a liquid preparation makes amlodipine an agent of choice in the younger pediatric population.[53]

Phosphodiesterase inhibitors, specifically phosphodiesterase-5 (PDE5) inhibitors, have been proposed to be effective agents for more moderate-to-severe RP, typically associated with DU, or in patients unable to tolerate or are refractory to CCB treatment. Reviewed in Phatak and colleagues,[54] a meta-analysis of randomized controlled trials on the efficacy of PDE5 inhibitors on RP included sildenafil, modified-release sildenafil, tadalafil, and vardenafil and demonstrated significant benefit for all agents, with reduction in frequency of RP attacks.[55]

Although clinically used for RP in the setting of connective tissue disease, there is no strong evidence for the use of other oral agents, such as ACE inhibitors, angiotensin II receptor antagonists, α-blockers, nitrates, and the selective serotonin receptor uptake inhibitor fluoxetine for RP.[48,56] An open-label controlled trial conferred losartan benefit in frequency and severity of RP attacks by the 12-week endpoint.[57] Fluoxetine is particularly useful for decreasing the frequency and severity of RP attacks in patients who already have low blood pressure and there is concern for hypotension with more traditional vasodilation medications.[15,58]

Topical nitrate therapy can be helpful for small, especially problematic areas of RP, for example, a recurrent single digit with RP pallor, although with heightened concern for systemic hypotension, especially when used with PDE-5 inhibitors.[59] It is best to apply these agents right away when having significant pallor and pain of an individual finger to avoid significant hypoperfusion.

Antiplatelet agents and statins have been used by clinicians in tandem to vasodilatory agents for RP in SSc with the concept of stabilizing a pathogenic endothelium and potentially augmenting microcirculatory flow.[60] Pentoxifylline, a blood viscosity reducing agent, may have this effect on the endothelium and has shown benefit with blood flow in patients with RP.[61] It is generally well tolerated and not associated with hypotension, and therefore a reasonable adjunct therapy, as would low-dose aspirin or statins, for moderate-to-severe RP.

Prostanoids and endothelin receptor antagonists are effective in RP associated with SSc but reserved for patients with DU and/or ischemia (Digital Ulcers section).[62] Intravenous prostanoids should be used only for severe cases in which pain is intractable or severe acute ischemia in which loss of digits is threatened.[63]

Digital Ulcers

DU associated with vasculopathy and RP are typically treated with vasodilators and endothelial stabilizers, as well as wound care management including topical and oral antibiotics when there is a concern for coinfection. CCBs themselves, as first-line therapy for RP, may prevent DU via increased microvasculature circulation. CCBs have been shown to reduce the number of RP-associated skin lesions including ulcers, fissures, and paronychia.[51]

The phosphodiesterase inhibitors (PDE-5), sildenafil and tadalafil, demonstrated a role in reducing DU number and promoting healing in a meta-analysis.[64] Subsequent trials of tadalafil supported these findings, and one even suggested efficacy in prevention of DU.[65] A more recent study of sildenafil demonstrated significant decrease in number of DU at weeks 8 and 12 but did not heal the ulcer quicker than placebo, with time to heal as the primary endpoint.[66]

The endothelin receptor antagonist, bosentan, is typically suggested for patients with recurrent ulcers despite the use of CCB and PDE-5 inhibitors. Bosentan has been demonstrated in 2 trials to *prevent* new DUs, especially in patients with more than 3 DU but was not shown to aid in healing of current ulcers.[64] Bosentan has been used in SSc primarily for the treatment of pulmonary arterial hypertension (PAH), with additional benefits for those with DU.

Acute Digital Ischemia

If acute digital ischemia occurs, this is an emergency requiring immediate hospitalization with special attention to wound care (debridement and/or antibiotics if necessary), pain control, anticoagulation, and maximizing vasodilator medication. If short-term CCB therapy is already maximized, typically titrated intravenous prostanoid in combination with other vasodilatory agents, such as PDE-5 inhibitors, are used.[62,67] Intravenous prostaglandins, iloprost in Europe and epoprostol in the United States, are infused continuously in the acute ischemia setting, similar to PAH protocols. These have been shown to rapidly reverse digital ischemia symptoms and provide several weeks of sustained benefit.[68–70] Those with recurrent but not acute severe DU and concern for ischemia can be scheduled for outpatient infusions of intravenous prostaglandins every 10 to 12 weeks. The adult EULAR and pediatric SHARE committees both recommend use of intravenous iloprost for treating severe RP in scleroderma after failure of oral therapy to reduce the frequency and severity of RP attacks.[11,15] There may be additional benefit from combination therapy of iloprost with bosentan, as seen in one prospective study.[71]

For moderate-to-severe RP and recurrent DU, surgical management may be necessary, especially when the patient has maximized or is intolerant of medical therapy. Digital sympathectomy (microsurgical technique[72]) or digital botulinum toxin injections (intradigital or palmar) have both been shown to be effective (including adolescents[73]).[74,75] Clinical trials with autologous fat grafting and its role in reducing RP and DU burden are underway with some demonstrating clear efficacy.[76] A hand surgeon with experience in patients with SSc and at a specialized hand center is recommended for any of these procedures.

Pulmonary Arterial Hypertension

Overall, guidelines and algorithms from the cardiology and respiratory specialty societies for idiopathic PAH are followed for SSc-associated PAH.[77] Treatment of PAH is directed toward 3 pathways: nitric oxide pathway via cyclic guanosine monophosphate enhancers (phosphodiesterase inhibitors and guanylate cyclase stimulants), endothelin pathway via endothelial receptor antagonists, and prostacyclin pathway via prostacyclin agonists, or combinations of these agents[77,78] (see **Table 2**). These include agents used for more severe Raynaud and DU discussed earlier, such as bosentan and iloprost. PAH is rare in pediatric SSc, with a frequency of 2% and 5% reported in recent North American[7] and international[6] prospective juvenile SSc cohorts, respectively.

Interstitial Lung Disease

ILD is present in approximately one-third of jSSc cohort patients,[6,7] with the presence of ground-glass opacities representing inflammatory alveolitis (**Fig. 2**, A and B) and coarse reticulations and traction bronchiectasis and honeycombing representing

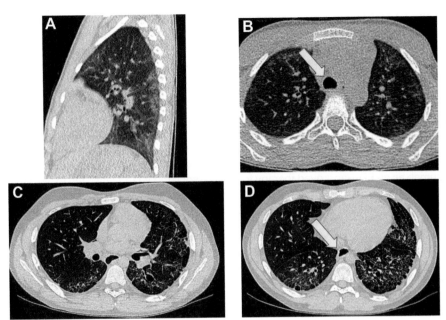

Fig. 2. Interstitial lung disease (ILD) phases in juvenile systemic sclerosis. (*A*) and (*B*) represent the acute inflammatory phase of ILD with associated ground glass opacities (GGO) and lack of reticulations in an 8-year-old patient. *Red arrows denote peripheral lung distribution of GGO.* (*C*) and (*D*) represent the fibrotic ILD changes with reticulations and honeycombing, predominant in posterior aspects of the lung, in a 17-year-old patient. The yellow arrows denote a patulous esophagus in both patients.

fibrotic lung disease on HRCT (see **Fig. 2**, C and D), as in adults.[79] ILD treatment primarily focuses on the inflammatory, alveolitis component with agents such as CYC, MMF, and tocilizumab, with more limited options for the fibrotic component, such as nintedanib. For the first time ever, 2 therapies for adult SSc–associated ILD recently received FDA approval: tocilizumab and nintedanib[80,81]; this is critical in the field because the main cause of SSc-related morbidity and death is ILD, both in adults and children.[46,82]

The initial treatment of choice in adult SSc for ILD was CYC, which stabilized lung decline evidenced by preserved the forced vital capacity (FVC) and total lung capacity, as well as improved dyspnea scoring and quality of life measures.[30,83,84] The greatest benefit was observed in those with more severe disease (FVC <50%, >50% lung involvement on HRCT and mRSS >23)[85] and was sustained up to 6 months after stopping CYC,[83] but without maintenance immunosuppression, ILD would progress afterward. Although 2 larger oral CYC clinical trials (Scleroderma Lung Study [SLS] I and II)[30,86] support these results, most SSc experts recommend intravenous CYC with intravenous hydration every 4 weeks for induction to avoid a high cumulative dose and reduce bladder toxicity.

The second study, SLS II, demonstrated noninferiority of MMF (1500 mg twice a day dosing), so most clinicians tend to use MMF as first-line treatment (see **Table 2**) based on comparable efficacy (preserving FVC in the same manner as CYC) and better adverse effect profile (less cytopenias and infections).[87,88] Several retrospective reviews and prospective case reports also support a modest improvement or stabilization in lung function and dyspnea with MMF.[89] Recommendations for length of MMF treatment are empiric, and most experts would treat at least 3 to 4 years after stabilization of lung function. Maintenance medication for SSc ILD after CYC induction used to be azathioprine[90] but now MMF has become the preferred agent of choice for maintenance, unless pregnancy is a consideration.

A new potential initial therapy may be tocilizumab, especially in those with earlier active disease (see **Fig. 2**, A and B), as demonstrated by FVC preservation in patients with SSc with ILD enrolled in the focuSSced tocilizumab trial.[80] SSc subjects with early, inflammatory disease were targeted for this placebo-controlled, double-blind study trial with an elevated ESR and CRP as part of the enrollment criteria. Although the primary endpoint of significant reduction of mRSS was not met, the secondary endpoint, change in FVC, was markedly preserved in those with ILD, advancing tocilizumab as an FDA-approved therapy for SSc-associated ILD. Overall, the tocilizumab group showed 0.1% mean FVC decline, whereas the placebo group had a 6.3% mean FVC decline over the 48-week study. When stratified by lung involvement, those with severe lung disease had a more notable difference in the treatment group versus placebo, with an *increase* of 2.1% versus a *decrease* of 6.7% FVC, respectively.[80]

When patients are refractory to the aforementioned treatments *or* they have evidence of fibrotic lung disease on HRCT (see **Fig. 2**, C and D), nintedanib should be considered. This tyrosine kinase inhibitor, which alters fibroblast and myofibroblast proliferation and thus limits extracellular matrix accumulation, has been shown to slow disease progression in idiopathic pulmonary fibrosis.[91] Recently, nintedanib has obtained approval for the treatment of adult SSc–associated ILD after the large randomized SENSCIS trial demonstrated a significant reduced rate of FVC decline.[92] Nausea, diarrhea, and weight loss are common with nintedanib (75% in SENSCIS trial) and limit its use in SSc. In general, most rheumatologists use nintedanib in addition to MMF or cyclophosphamide[92] and now tocilizumab. Another tyrosine kinase inhibitor, pirfenidone, has an acceptable safety profile in patients with SSc, but efficacy trials are ongoing.[93]

Second- or third-line therapy for SSc-related ILD (see **Table 2**) would be rituximab,[94] with rationale for its use evidenced that B lymphocytes have been found in the lung and skin of patients with SSc-ILD, implicating pathogenesis. There are no controlled trials, but multiple case series (including one pediatric[95]) and open-label studies suggest that rituximab may be beneficial by stabilizing lung disease.[96–99] Patients treated with rituximab and MMF seemed to have improved lung function (FVC, forced expiratory volume in the first second) and skin disease.[100,101] Abatacept could be considered as an alternative therapy in SSc-ILD but it is still under investigation, with only one small case report showing benefit and a phase II clinical trial of abatacept patients showing no benefit on FVC.[32] Although currently considered more third line, due to the nature of potential morbidity and mortality risk, autologous hematopoietic stem cell transplantation (ASCT) has shown pulmonary benefit in patients with severe diffuse cutaneous SSc.[102–104] ASCT is best performed in specialized centers with significant expertise in the procedure and with a multidisciplinary team, discussed in detail later. Lung transplantation at a multidisciplinary center is a last resort if all alternative therapies fail, given the higher mortality rate compared with ASCT, with mindful management of extrapulmonary manifestations such as esophageal and cardiac issues.[105–107] There are case reports of ASCT in jSSc but none having lung transplantation.

Autologous hematopoietic stem cell transplantation

There have now been 2 large multicenter trials examining the potential benefit and treatment-related risks of ASCT in patients with adult SSc. The Autologous Stem Cell Transplantation International Trial was performed in Europe[102] and the

Scleroderma: Cyclophosphamide or Transplantation (SCOT) trial in the United States.[104] Both trials enrolled subjects adult SSc with diffuse cutaneous SSc subtype and less than 5 years disease duration, comparing ASCT with intravenous CYC 12-month treatment. The ASCT regimen for both included high-dose CYC and antithymocyte globulin immunoablation followed by infusion of CD34+ autologous stem cells. SCOT also included total body irradiation in the ablation step. The significant benefit in the ASCT arm was demonstrated by year 3 in both trials with decreased pulmonary, renal, and cardiac morbidity, and superior survival in the ASCT arm was evident at the 5-year follow-up (86% vs 51%), overcoming initial transplantation-related events.[102,104]

Although the mortality rate in SSc-ILD seems to improve following ASCT, there remains significant initial transplant-related mortality (6%). Thus, ASCT should be reserved for refractory or rapidly progressive cases. There are currently 5 reported cases of ASCT in jSSc (4 females, 1 male), median age of 12 years (range 9–17 years), all with established lung disease.[108–110] General outcomes at approximately 3 years of follow-up include 3 patients in remission with catch up linear growth and weight along with increased general well-being, 1 in partial remission, and 1 relapse at 9 months after initial remission. These case reports along with recent efficacy and safety results from adult-onset SSc ASCT regimens[102,111,112] provide reasoning to use ASCT as a viable therapy for refractory jSSc.

Preventative measures cannot be underestimated for a patient with SSc-ILD and are recommended for all patients (see **Table 2**). These include adequate treatment of dysphagia and gastroesophageal reflux disease (GERD), which may prevent damage and inflammatory responses in the lung. Influenza and pneumococcal vaccinations (and now SARS-CoV-2 vaccination) can prevent pneumonia, which can have significant morbidity in a patient with compromised lung function. Pulmonary physical rehabilitation, for those with ILD and/or significant myopathy affecting respiratory muscles, is essential for strengthening respiratory muscles and is highly recommended with a therapist trained in pulmonary physiotherapy.[113,114]

Gastrointestinal Disease

The GI tract is affected in 42% to 74% patients with jSSc and may precede skin involvement.[4–7] Although frequently asymptomatic, GI manifestations have been associated with malnutrition, poor quality of life, and ILD.[4,5,7,14,82] Vasculopathy and inflammation leading to fibrosis can manifest in the entire GI tract, from mouth to anus. The most common GI problem encountered in jSSc and adult SSc is esophageal dysmotility, which causes poor weight gain and very low body mass index (BMI) (from nausea, dysphagia, and stasis), GERD with acid sequela, and silent aspiration of GI contents.[6,13,14] Routine assessment of nutritional status and referral to a nutritionist is helpful in growing children with SSc, especially those with low BMI. Medical treatment is directed at the area of GI tract involvement, and immunosuppressive therapy has not been shown to be beneficial (see **Table 2**). Surgical interventions should be avoided, as they are of high risk in patients with SSc, who are prone to perforation and postsurgical strictures.

Oral manifestations of SSc are best treated prophylactically. Xerostomia is common in SSc, and keeping the mouth hydrated is important to prevent cavities and to facilitate swallowing. Over-the-counter saliva substitutes, toothpastes and mouthwashes containing xylitol, or cellulose are recommended. Gingival and tooth care is important and may require devices to improve oral hygiene for patients with significant difficulty with mouth opening (**Fig. 3**). Referral to a speech pathologist can be considered for patients with small oral opening, dysphagia, or aspiration for orofacial exercise therapy and recommendations for safe foods.[115,116]

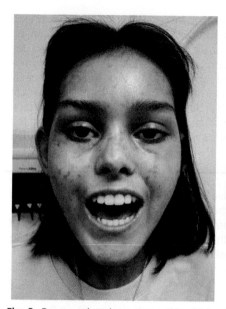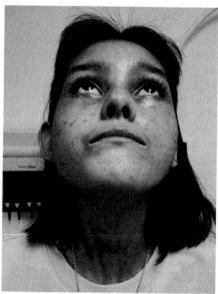

Fig. 3. Decreased oral aperture. Skin thickening and fibrosis of underlying tissue leads to decrease oral aperture, which compromises dental and gingival care and eating. A 2.5 cm maximal interlip distance is demonstrated in a 16-year-old patient with jSSc with a modified Rodnan skin score of 24.

GERD must be treated even in asymptomatic patients. GERD is managed in part by lifestyle and dietary changes, including nighttime routine to avoid chronic micro-aspiration while sleeping, which is associated with ILD in adults and children.[13,14] This is especially important in those who also have esophageal dysmotility and a patulous esophagus (see **Fig. 2**). Lifestyle changes include elevating the head of the bed[117]; avoiding meals 3 hours before bed; and small, frequent meals low in fat and low residue with plenty of water to facilitate passage of food. Medical therapy includes proton pump inhibitors,[118] taken 30 minutes before eating, up to twice a day, H2 blockers, given 30 minutes before bed to reduce residual acid of gastric contents, and promotility agents, such as erythromycin or cyproheptadine. GERD-induced esophagitis in SSc is typically managed with acid suppression and sucralfate for symptomatic relief. Esophageal strictures are rarely observed in jSSc; if present, as in adults, mechanical dilatation via endoscopy may be required to allow for swallowing.[119]

Esophageal dysmotility is common and typically presents as dysphagia or a feeling of food getting stuck in the throat or chest area. A trial of prokinetic therapy is typically warranted. In jSSc, erythromycin or cyproheptadine are the preferred agents to begin (see **Table 2**). Low-dose erythromycin 2 to 3 times a day lowers esophageal pressure and increases gastric contractions to move food through the esophagus, whereas cyproheptadine assists in gut motility, gastric accommodation, and appetite stimulation, commonly used in pediatrics for different failure to thrive conditions. Metoclopramide is a useful prokinetic agent that increases esophageal sphincter pressure, improving peristalsis and gastric emptying, but has a more involved side-effect profile including tardive dyskinesia and prolonged QTc. Gastroparesis causes a feeling of early satiety and is treated with the same promotility agent strategy, best if taken before meals 3 times daily and at bedtime.[120–122]

Diarrhea and bloating are often caused by small intestinal bacterial overgrowth and treated by limited 7- to 10-day courses of antibiotics.[123–125] Antibiotic choice is empiric and includes rifaximin, amoxicillin with clavulanate, gentamicin, and fluoroquinolones. In refractory cases, metronidazole can be added for 5 to 7 days. Vitamins B12, vitamin D3, and iron for malabsorption and probiotics to improve bloating may be prescribed.[126] Acute intestinal pseudoobstruction can be treated with bowel rest and hydration. Once true mechanical obstruction is ruled out, promotility agents may be used similar to gastroparesis.[127] In addition, the somatostatin agonist octreotide may improve motility.[128]

Constipation due to colonic sclerosis is best treated with hydration and dietary fiber. Polyethylene glycol is commonly used, but osmotic laxatives should be avoided, as they can cause uncomfortable bloating. Fecal incontinence can be treated by biofeedback, pelvic floor exercises, or sacral nerve stimulation.[129]

A growing child or adolescent with SSc is especially vulnerable to malnutrition and associated growth delay. The cause can be involvement of any part of the GI tract, from malabsorption or from poor oral intake secondary to mechanical limitations from finger joint contractures or poor mouth opening or depression associated with chronic disease. In a patient with a BMI Z score less than or equal to 2.5, referral to a gastroenterologist, nutritionist, speech pathologist, dentist, and/or mental health provider should be considered.[130] Nasogastric or jejunostomy tube feeding and/or total parenteral nutrition may be recommended for severe malnutrition.

SUMMARY OF JUVENILE-ONSET SYSTEMIC SCLEROSIS TREATMENT

Similarities between pediatric and adult SSc allow for extrapolation of treatment approaches to some extent. However, there are important differences, necessitating studies of treatments in children. For example, the low rate of renal crisis may allow for increased use of GC to quickly halt the inflammatory stage of disease in children, even though GC should be avoided in adults. Although randomized control trials are challenging given the rarity of jSSc, other methods such as observational longitudinal studies and comparative effectiveness studies of consensus-driven treatment plans may provide data regarding treatment effectiveness.[131] Finally, treatment of specific organ dysfunction in jSSc could be assessed as part of studies in which multiple diseases are enrolled, such as clinical trials evaluating treatments for ILD, which may include enrollment of both idiopathic and connective-tissue disease–related ILD. Potentially curative treatment approaches such as ASCT would be especially amenable to this approach. The hope is that for a child with SSc, early diagnosis and comprehensive treatment may allow for disease reprogramming, inducing potential remodeling and regeneration of lung, skin, and GI tissue. Research will be imperative for improving future outcomes.

CLINICS CARE POINTS

- Supportive care and lifestyle modifications are equally important in treating jSSc, including physical therapy, avoidance of Raynaud triggers, and GERD precautions.
- There are now 2 FDA-approved therapies for SSc-related ILD in adults that can be extrapolated to children: tocilizumab and nintedanib.
- MMF has overtaken cyclophosphamide as first-line therapy for SSc-ILD. Tocilizumab has not been directly compared with either but is now also considered a first-line agent.
- Skin disease alone in jSSc should be treated with MMF or MTX.

- MSK involvement is more common in jSSc and should be treated similarly to juvenile idiopathic arthritis and juvenile dermatomyositis.
- Higher doses of GC can be given in jSSc than in adults but close monitoring is required for SRC.
- Calcium channel blockers remain first-line treatment of RP.
- Endothelin receptor agonists and phosphodiesterase inhibitors are effective and recommended in patients with recurrent DU.
- Prostanoids are the treatment of choice for acute digital ischemia, in addition to hospitalization with supportive care.
- GERD and esophageal dysmotility must be aggressively managed with pharmaceutical and supportive care to avoid significant weight loss, failure to thrive, and ILD progression.
- ASCT should be considered in patients with moderate-to-severe skin and lung disease at specialized centers with significant expertise and a multidisciplinary team.

DISCLOSURE

The author has received funding from the National Institutes of Health, Scleroderma Foundation, Scleroderma Research Foundation, and Nancy Taylor Foundation for Chronic Diseases Inc.

The author has no commercial or financial conflicts of interest and nothing to disclose.

ACKNOWLEDGMENTS

V. Sood, Pediatric Gastroenterology, Motility Disorders Clinic, Pediatric Scleroderma Center, UPMC.

F. Rosser, MD, Pediatric Pulmonologist, Pediatric Scleroderma Center, UPMC.

L. Farver, PT, DPT, Pulmonary Physical Therapist, Pediatric Scleroderma Center, UPMC.

K. Schollaert-Fitch, MS, Clinical Research Coordinator, Pediatric Scleroderma Center, UPMC.

REFERENCES

1. Herrick AL, Ennis H, Bhushan M, et al. Incidence of childhood linear scleroderma and systemic sclerosis in the UK and Ireland. Arthritis Care Res (Hoboken) 2010;62(2):213–8.
2. Beukelman T, Xie FL, Foeldvari I. Assessing the prevalence of juvenile systemic sclerosis in childhood using administrative claims data from teh United States. J Scleroderma Relat Disord 2018;3(2):189–90.
3. Pelkonen PM, Jalanko HJ, Lantto RK, et al. Incidence of systemic connective tissue diseases in children: a nationwide prospective study in Finland. Multicenter Study Research Support, Non-U.S. Gov't. J Rheumatol 1994;21(11):2143–6.
4. Scalapino K, Arkachaisri T, Lucas M, et al. Childhood onset systemic sclerosis: classification, clinical and serologic features, and survival in comparison with adult onset disease. Comparative Study Research Support, N.I.H., Extramural Research Support, Non-U.S. Gov't. J Rheumatol 2006;33(5):1004–13.
5. Martini G, Foeldvari I, Russo R, et al. Systemic sclerosis in childhood: clinical and immunologic features of 153 patients in an international database. Arthritis Rheum 2006;54(12):3971–8. https://doi.org/10.1002/art.22207.

6. Foeldvari I, Klotsche J, Kasapcopur O, et al. Differences sustained between diffuse and limited forms of juvenile systemic sclerosis in expanded international cohort. www.juvenile-scleroderma.com. Arthritis Care Res (Hoboken) 2021. https://doi.org/10.1002/acr.24609.

7. Stevens BE, Torok KS, Li SC, et al. Clinical characteristics and factors associated with disability and impaired quality of life in children with juvenile systemic sclerosis: results from the childhood arthritis and rheumatology research alliance legacy registry. Arthritis Care Res (Hoboken) 2018;70(12):1806–13.

8. Hawley DP, Baildam EM, Amin TS, et al. Access to care for children and young people diagnosed with localized scleroderma or juvenile SSc in the UK. Comparative Study. Rheumatology (Oxford) 2012;51(7):1235–9.

9. Foeldvari I, Klotsche J, Torok KS, et al. Are diffuse and limited juvenile systemic sclerosis different in clinical presentation? Clinical characteristics of a juvenile systemic sclerosis cohort. J Scleroderma Relat Disord 2018;4(1):49–61.

10. Foeldvari I, Torok KS. Review for best practice in clinical rheumatology juvenile systemic sclerosis - Updates and practice points. Best Pract Res Clin Rheumatol. 2021 Apr 22;101688. https://doi.org/10.1016/j.berh.2021.101688.

11. Foeldvari I, Culpo R, Sperotto F, et al. Consensus-based recommendations for the management of juvenile systemic sclerosis. Rheumatology (Oxford) 2021; 60(4):1651–8.

12. Showalter K, Hoffmann A, Rouleau G, et al. Performance of forced vital capacity and lung diffusion cutpoints for associated radiographic interstitial lung disease in systemic sclerosis. J Rheumatol 2018;45(11):1572–6.

13. Foeldvari I, Klotsche J, Hinrichs B, et al. Under detection of interstitial lung disease in juvenile systemic sclerosis (jSSc). Arthritis Care Res (Hoboken) 2020. https://doi.org/10.1002/acr.24499.

14. Ambartsumyan L, Zheng HB, Iyer RS, et al. Relationship between esophageal abnormalities on fluoroscopic esophagram and pulmonary function testing in juvenile systemic sclerosis. Arthritis Care Res (Hoboken) 2018. https://doi.org/10. 1002/acr.23778.

15. Kowal-Bielecka O, Fransen J, Avouac J, et al. Update of EULAR recommendations for the treatment of systemic sclerosis. Ann Rheum Dis 2017;76(8): 1327–39.

16. Fernandez-Codina A, Walker KM, Pope JE, et al. Treatment algorithms for systemic sclerosis according to experts. Arthritis Rheumatol 2018;70(11):1820–8.

17. Khanna D, Furst DE, Clements PJ, et al. Standardization of the modified Rodnan skin score for use in clinical trials of systemic sclerosis. J Scleroderma Relat Disord 2017;2(1):11–8.

18. Clements P, Lachenbruch P, Siebold J, et al. Inter and intraobserver variability of total skin thickness score (modified Rodnan TSS) in systemic sclerosis. Research Support, Non-U.S. Gov't Research Support, U.S. Gov't, P.H.S. J Rheumatol 1995;22(7):1281–5.

19. Domsic RT, Rodriguez-Reyna T, Lucas M, et al. Skin thickness progression rate: a predictor of mortality and early internal organ involvement in diffuse scleroderma. Ann Rheum Dis 2011;70(1):104–9.

20. Steen VD, Medsger TA Jr. Improvement in skin thickening in systemic sclerosis associated with improved survival. Arthritis Rheum 2001;44(12):2828–35.

21. van den Hoogen FH, Boerbooms AM, Swaak AJ, et al. Comparison of methotrexate with placebo in the treatment of systemic sclerosis: a 24 week randomized double-blind trial, followed by a 24 week observational trial. Br J Rheumatol 1996;35(4):364–72.

22. Pope JE, Bellamy N, Seibold JR, et al. A randomized, controlled trial of metho-trexate versus placebo in early diffuse scleroderma. Arthritis Rheum 2001;44(6): 1351–8.

23. Kowal-Bielecka O, Landewe R, Avouac J, et al. EULAR recommendations for the treatment of systemic sclerosis: a report from the EULAR Scleroderma Trials and Research group (EUSTAR). Consensus Development Conference Research Support, Non-U.S. Gov't. Ann Rheum Dis 2009;68(5):620–8.

24. Hinchcliff M, Huang CC, Wood TA, et al. Molecular signatures in skin associated with clinical improvement during mycophenolate treatment in systemic scle-rosis. J Invest Dermatol 2013;133(8):1979–89.

25. Hinchcliff M, Toledo DM, Taroni JN, et al. Mycophenolate mofetil treatment of systemic sclerosis reduces myeloid cell numbers and attenuates the inflamma-tory gene signature in skin. J Invest Dermatol 2018;138(6):1301–10.

26. Derk CT, Grace E, Shenin M, et al. A prospective open-label study of mycophe-nolate mofetil for the treatment of diffuse systemic sclerosis. Rheumatology (Ox-ford) 2009;48(12):1595–9.

27. Le EN, Wigley FM, Shah AA, et al. Long-term experience of mycophenolate mo-fetil for treatment of diffuse cutaneous systemic sclerosis. Ann Rheum Dis 2011; 70(6):1104–7.

28. Mendoza FA, Nagle SJ, Lee JB, et al. A prospective observational study of my-cophenolate mofetil treatment in progressive diffuse cutaneous systemic scle-rosis of recent onset. J Rheumatol 2012;39(6):1241–7.

29. Namas R, Tashkin DP, Furst DE, et al. Efficacy of mycophenolate mofetil and oral cyclophosphamide on skin thickness: post hoc analyses from two randomized placebo-controlled trials. Arthritis Care Res (Hoboken) 2018;70(3):439–44.

30. Tashkin DP, Elashoff R, Clements PJ, et al. Cyclophosphamide versus placebo in scleroderma lung disease. N Engl J Med 2006;354(25):2655–66.

31. Khanna D, Lin CJF, Furst DE, et al. Tocilizumab in systemic sclerosis: a rando-mised, double-blind, placebo-controlled, phase 3 trial. Lancet Respir Med 2020;8(10):963–74.

32. Khanna D, Spino C, Johnson S, et al. Abatacept in early diffuse cutaneous sys-temic sclerosis: results of a phase ii investigator-initiated, multicenter, double-blind, randomized, placebo-controlled trial. Arthritis Rheumatol 2020;72(1): 125–36.

33. Poelman CL, Hummers LK, Wigley FM, et al. Intravenous immunoglobulin may be an effective therapy for refractory, active diffuse cutaneous systemic scle-rosis. J Rheumatol 2015;42(2):236–42.

34. Jordan S, Distler JH, Maurer B, et al. Effects and safety of rituximab in systemic sclerosis: an analysis from the European Scleroderma Trial and Research (EU-STAR) group. Ann Rheum Dis 2015;74(6):1188–94.

35. Wang W, Bhattacharyya S, Marangoni RG, et al. The JAK/STAT pathway is acti-vated in systemic sclerosis and is effectively targeted by tofacitinib. J Sclero-derma Relat Disord 2019;5(1). p.40-50.

36. Avouac J, Clements PJ, Khanna D, et al. Articular involvement in systemic scle-rosis. Rheumatology (Oxford) 2012;51(8):1347–56.

37. Elhai M, Meunier M, Matucci-Cerinic M, et al. Outcomes of patients with sys-temic sclerosis-associated polyarthritis and myopathy treated with tocilizumab or abatacept: a EUSTAR observational study. Ann Rheum Dis 2013;72(7): 1217–20.

38. Omair MA, Phumethum V, Johnson SR. Long-term safety and effectiveness of tumour necrosis factor inhibitors in systemic sclerosis patients with inflammatory arthritis. Clin Exp Rheumatol 2012;30(2 Suppl 71):S55–9.

39. Lam GK, Hummers LK, Woods A, et al. Efficacy and safety of etanercept in the treatment of scleroderma-associated joint disease. J Rheumatol 2007;34(7):1636–7.

40. Steen VD, Medsger TA Jr. Case-control study of corticosteroids and other drugs that either precipitate or protect from the development of scleroderma renal crisis. Research Support, Non-U.S. Gov't. Arthritis Rheum 1998;41(9):1613–9.

41. Steen VD, Medsger TA Jr, Osial TA Jr, et al. Factors predicting development of renal involvement in progressive systemic sclerosis. Am J Med 1984;76(5):779–86.

42. Steen VD, Costantino JP, Shapiro AP, et al. Outcome of renal crisis in systemic sclerosis: relation to availability of angiotensin converting enzyme (ACE) inhibitors. Ann Intern Med 1990;113(5):352–7.

43. Steen VD, Medsger TA Jr. Long-term outcomes of scleroderma renal crisis. Ann Intern Med 2000;133(8):600–3.

44. Beckett VL, Donadio JV Jr, Brennan LA Jr, et al. Use of captopril as early therapy for renal scleroderma: a prospective study. Mayo Clin Proc 1985;60(11):763–71.

45. Foeldvari I, Nihtyanova SI, Wierk A, et al. Characteristics of patients with juvenile onset systemic sclerosis in an adult single-center cohort. J Rheumatol 2010;37(11):2422–6.

46. Foeldvari I, Tyndall A, Zulian F, et al. Juvenile and young adult-onset systemic sclerosis share the same organ involvement in adulthood: data from the EU-STAR database. Rheumatology (Oxford) 2012;51(10):1832–7.

47. Maricq HR. Wide-field capillary microscopy. Research Support, Non-U.S. Gov't. Arthritis Rheum 1981;24(9):1159–65.

48. Herrick AL. Evidence-based management of Raynaud's phenomenon. Ther Adv Musculoskelet Dis 2017;9(12):317–29.

49. Goldman W, Seltzer R, Reuman P. Association between treatment with central nervous system stimulants and Raynaud's syndrome in children: a retrospective case-control study of rheumatology patients. Arthritis Rheum 2008;58(2):563–6.

50. Thompson AE, Shea B, Welch V, et al. Calcium-channel blockers for Raynaud's phenomenon in systemic sclerosis. Arthritis Rheum 2001;44(8):1841–7.

51. Rademaker M, Cooke ED, Almond NE, et al. Comparison of intravenous infusions of iloprost and oral nifedipine in treatment of Raynaud's phenomenon in patients with systemic sclerosis: a double blind randomised study. BMJ 1989;298(6673):561–4.

52. Rodeheffer RJ, Rommer JA, Wigley F, et al. Controlled double-blind trial of nifedipine in the treatment of Raynaud's phenomenon. N Engl J Med 1983;308(15):880–3.

53. Lee EY, Park JK, Lee W, et al. Head-to-head comparison of udenafil vs amlodipine in the treatment of secondary Raynaud's phenomenon: a double-blind, randomized, cross-over study. Rheumatology (Oxford) 2014;53(4):658–64.

54. Phatak S, Ajmani S, Agarwal V, et al. Phosphodiesterase-5 inhibitors: Raynaud's and beyond. Indian J Rheumatol 2017;12(Suppl S1):227–31. Available at: http://www.indianjrheumatol.com/text.asp?2017/12/6/227/219076.

55. Roustit M, Blaise S, Allanore Y, et al. Phosphodiesterase-5 inhibitors for the treatment of secondary Raynaud's phenomenon: systematic review and meta-analysis of randomised trials. Ann Rheum Dis 2013;72(10):1696–9.

56. Stewart M, Morling JR. Oral vasodilators for primary Raynaud's phenomenon. Cochrane Database Syst Rev 2012;(7):CD006687.
57. Dziadzio M, Denton CP, Smith R, et al. Losartan therapy for Raynaud's phenomenon and scleroderma: clinical and biochemical findings in a fifteen-week, randomized, parallel-group, controlled trial. Arthritis Rheum 1999;42(12):2646–55.
58. Coleiro B, Marshall SE, Denton CP, et al. Treatment of Raynaud's phenomenon with the selective serotonin reuptake inhibitor fluoxetine. Rheumatology (Oxford) 2001;40(9):1038–43.
59. Curtiss P, Schwager Z, Cobos G, et al. A systematic review and meta-analysis of the effects of topical nitrates in the treatment of primary and secondary Raynaud's phenomenon. J Am Acad Dermatol 2018;78(6):1110–1118 e3.
60. Kuwana M, Okazaki Y, Kaburaki J. Long-term beneficial effects of statins on vascular manifestations in patients with systemic sclerosis. Mod Rheumatol 2009;19(5):530–5.
61. Neirotti M, Longo F, Molaschi M, et al. Functional vascular disorders: treatment with pentoxifylline. Angiology 1987;38(8):575–80.
62. Pope J, Fenlon D, Thompson A, et al. Iloprost and cisaprost for Raynaud's phenomenon in progressive systemic sclerosis. Cochrane Database Syst Rev 2000; 2:CD000953.
63. Rademaker M, Thomas RH, Provost G, et al. Prolonged increase in digital blood flow following iloprost infusion in patients with systemic sclerosis. Postgrad Med J 1987;63(742):617–20.
64. Tingey T, Shu J, Smuczek J, et al. Meta-analysis of healing and prevention of digital ulcers in systemic sclerosis. Arthritis Care Res (Hoboken) 2013;65(9): 1460–71.
65. Shenoy PD, Kumar S, Jha LK, et al. Efficacy of tadalafil in secondary Raynaud's phenomenon resistant to vasodilator therapy: a double-blind randomized crossover trial. Rheumatology (Oxford) 2010;49(12):2420–8.
66. Hachulla E, Hatron PY, Carpentier P, et al. Efficacy of sildenafil on ischaemic digital ulcer healing in systemic sclerosis: the placebo-controlled SEDUCE study. Ann Rheum Dis 2016;75(6):1009–15.
67. Abraham S, Steen V. Optimal management of digital ulcers in systemic sclerosis. Ther Clin Risk Manag 2015;11:939–47.
68. Wigley FM, Wise RA, Seibold JR, et al. Intravenous iloprost infusion in patients with Raynaud phenomenon secondary to systemic sclerosis. A multicenter, placebo-controlled, double-blind study. Ann Intern Med 1994;120(3):199–206.
69. Bettoni L, Geri A, Airo P, et al. Systemic sclerosis therapy with iloprost: a prospective observational study of 30 patients treated for a median of 3 years. Clin Rheumatol 2002;21(3):244–50.
70. Belch JJ, Newman P, Drury JK, et al. Intermittent epoprostenol (prostacyclin) infusion in patients with Raynaud's syndrome. A double-blind controlled trial. Lancet 1983;1(8320):313–5.
71. Trombetta AC, Pizzorni C, Ruaro B, et al. Effects of longterm treatment with bosentan and iloprost on nailfold absolute capillary number, fingertip blood perfusion, and clinical status in systemic sclerosis. J Rheumatol 2016;43(11): 2033–41.
72. Tomaino MM, Goitz RJ, Medsger TA. Surgery for ischemic pain and Raynaud's phenomenon in scleroderma: a description of treatment protocol and evaluation of results. Microsurgery 2001;21(3):75–9.
73. Drake DB, Kesler RW, Morgan RF. Digital sympathectomy for refractory Raynaud's phenomenon in an adolescent. J Rheumatol 1992;19(8):1286–8.

74. Uppal L, Dhaliwal K, Butler PE. A prospective study of the use of botulinum toxin injections in the treatment of Raynaud's syndrome associated with scleroderma. J Hand Surg Eur Vol 2014;39(8):876–80.

75. Momeni A, Sorice SC, Valenzuela A, et al. Surgical treatment of systemic sclerosis–is it justified to offer peripheral sympathectomy earlier in the disease process? Microsurgery 2015;35(6):441–6.

76. Del Papa N, Di Luca G, Andracco R, et al. Regional grafting of autologous adipose tissue is effective in inducing prompt healing of indolent digital ulcers in patients with systemic sclerosis: results of a monocentric randomized controlled study. Arthritis Res Ther 2019;21(1):7.

77. Galie N, Humbert M, Vachiery JL, et al. 2015 ESC/ERS guidelines for the diagnosis and treatment of pulmonary hypertension: The Joint Task Force for the Diagnosis and Treatment of Pulmonary Hypertension of the European Society of Cardiology (ESC) and the European Respiratory Society (ERS): endorsed by: association for European Paediatric and Congenital Cardiology (AEPC), International Society for Heart and Lung Transplantation (ISHLT). Eur Heart J 2016;37(1):67–119.

78. Galie N, Manes A, Farahani KV, et al. Pulmonary arterial hypertension associated to connective tissue diseases. Lupus 2005;14(9):713–7.

79. Solomon JJ, Olson AL, Fischer A, et al. Scleroderma lung disease. Eur Respir Rev 2013;22(127):6–19.

80. Roofeh D, Lin CJF, Goldin J, et al. Tocilizumab prevents progression of early systemic sclerosis associated interstitial lung disease. Arthritis Rheumatol 2021. https://doi.org/10.1002/art.41668.

81. Seibold JR, Maher TM, Highland KB, et al. Safety and tolerability of nintedanib in patients with systemic sclerosis-associated interstitial lung disease: data from the SENSCIS trial. Ann Rheum Dis 2020;79(11):1478–84.

82. Martini G, Vittadello F, Kasapcopur O, et al. Factors affecting survival in juvenile systemic sclerosis. Rheumatology (Oxford) 2009;48(2):119–22.

83. Tashkin DP, Elashoff R, Clements PJ, et al. Effects of 1-year treatment with cyclophosphamide on outcomes at 2 years in scleroderma lung disease. Am J Respir Crit Care Med 2007;176(10):1026–34.

84. Goldin J, Elashoff R, Kim HJ, et al. Treatment of scleroderma-interstitial lung disease with cyclophosphamide is associated with less progressive fibrosis on serial thoracic high-resolution CT scan than placebo: findings from the scleroderma lung study. Chest 2009;136(5):1333–40.

85. Roth MD, Tseng CH, Clements PJ, et al. Predicting treatment outcomes and responder subsets in scleroderma-related interstitial lung disease. Arthritis Rheum 2011;63(9):2797–808.

86. Tashkin DP, Roth MD, Clements PJ, et al. Mycophenolate mofetil versus oral cyclophosphamide in scleroderma-related interstitial lung disease (SLS II): a randomised controlled, double-blind, parallel group trial. Lancet Respir Med 2016;4(9):708–19.

87. Panopoulos ST, Bournia VK, Trakada G, et al. Mycophenolate versus cyclophosphamide for progressive interstitial lung disease associated with systemic sclerosis: a 2-year case control study. Lung 2013;191(5):483–9.

88. Shenoy PD, Bavaliya M, Sashidharan S, et al. Cyclophosphamide versus mycophenolate mofetil in scleroderma interstitial lung disease (SSc-ILD) as induction therapy: a single-centre, retrospective analysis. Arthritis Res Ther 2016; 18(1):123.

89. Yilmaz N, Can M, Kocakaya D, et al. Two-year experience with mycophenolate mofetil in patients with scleroderma lung disease: a case series. Int J Rheum Dis 2014;17(8):923–8.

90. Berezne A, Ranque B, Valeyre D, et al. Therapeutic strategy combining intravenous cyclophosphamide followed by oral azathioprine to treat worsening interstitial lung disease associated with systemic sclerosis: a retrospective multicenter open-label study. J Rheumatol 2008;35(6):1064–72.

91. Richeldi L, du Bois RM, Raghu G, et al. Efficacy and safety of nintedanib in idiopathic pulmonary fibrosis. N Engl J Med 2014;370(22):2071–82.

92. Distler O, Highland KB, Gahlemann M, et al. Nintedanib for systemic sclerosis-associated interstitial lung disease. N Engl J Med 2019;380(26):2518–28.

93. Khanna D, Albera C, Fischer A, et al. An open-label, Phase II study of the safety and tolerability of pirfenidone in patients with scleroderma-associated interstitial lung disease: the LOTUSS trial. J Rheumatol 2016;43(9):1672–9.

94. Keir GJ, Maher TM, Hansell DM, et al. Severe interstitial lung disease in connective tissue disease: rituximab as rescue therapy. Eur Respir J 2012;40(3):641–8.

95. Zulian F, Dal Pozzolo R, Meneghel A, et al. Rituximab for rapidly progressive juvenile systemic sclerosis. Rheumatology (Oxford) 2020;59(12):3793–7.

96. Lafyatis R, Kissin E, York M, et al. B cell depletion with rituximab in patients with diffuse cutaneous systemic sclerosis. Arthritis Rheum 2009;60(2):578–83.

97. Daoussis D, Liossis SN, Tsamandas AC, et al. Experience with rituximab in scleroderma: results from a 1-year, proof-of-principle study. Rheumatology (Oxford) 2010;49(2):271–80.

98. Sircar G, Goswami RP, Sircar D, et al. Intravenous cyclophosphamide vs rituximab for the treatment of early diffuse scleroderma lung disease: open label, randomized, controlled trial. Rheumatology (Oxford) 2018;57(12):2106–13.

99. Daoussis D, Melissaropoulos K, Sakellaropoulos G, et al. A multicenter, open-label, comparative study of B-cell depletion therapy with Rituximab for systemic sclerosis-associated interstitial lung disease. Semin Arthritis Rheum 2017;46(5):625–31.

100. Fraticelli P, Fischetti C, Salaffi F, et al. Combination therapy with rituximab and mycophenolate mofetil in systemic sclerosis. A single-centre case series study. Clin Exp Rheumatol 2018;36(Suppl 113):142–5.

101. Elhai M, Boubaya M, Distler O, et al. Outcomes of patients with systemic sclerosis treated with rituximab in contemporary practice: a prospective cohort study. Ann Rheum Dis 2019;78(7):979–87.

102. van Laar JM, Farge D, Sont JK, et al. Autologous hematopoietic stem cell transplantation vs intravenous pulse cyclophosphamide in diffuse cutaneous systemic sclerosis: a randomized clinical trial. JAMA 2014;311(24):2490–8.

103. Burt RK, Shah SJ, Dill K, et al. Autologous non-myeloablative haemopoietic stem-cell transplantation compared with pulse cyclophosphamide once per month for systemic sclerosis (ASSIST): an open-label, randomised phase 2 trial. Lancet 2011;378(9790):498–506.

104. Sullivan KM, Goldmuntz EA, Furst DE. Autologous Stem-Cell Transplantation for Severe Scleroderma. N Engl J Med 2018;378(11):1066–7.

105. Bernstein EJ, Peterson ER, Sell JL, et al. Survival of adults with systemic sclerosis following lung transplantation: a nationwide cohort study. Arthritis Rheumatol 2015;67(5):1314–22.

106. Schachna L, Medsger TA Jr, Dauber JH, et al. Lung transplantation in scleroderma compared with idiopathic pulmonary fibrosis and idiopathic pulmonary arterial hypertension. Arthritis Rheum 2006;54(12):3954–61.

107. Crespo MM, Bermudez CA, Dew MA, et al. Lung transplant in patients with scleroderma compared with pulmonary fibrosis. short- and long-term outcomes. Ann Am Thorac Soc 2016;13(6):784–92.

108. Martini A, Maccario R, Ravelli A, et al. Marked and sustained improvement two years after autologous stem cell transplantation in a girl with systemic sclerosis. Case Reports Research Support, Non-U.S. Gov't. Arthritis Rheum 1999;42(4):807–11.

109. Wulffraat NM, Sanders LA, Kuis W. Autologous hemopoietic stem-cell transplantation for children with refractory autoimmune disease. Curr Rheumatol Rep 2000;2(4):316–23.

110. Martini A, Maccario R, Ravelli A, et al. Efficacy and safety of autologous peripheral stem cell transplantation in three children with systemic sclerosis and progressive pulmonary involvement. Arthritis Rheum 2000;43(Suppl 9):1538.

111. Sullivan KM, Goldmuntz EA, Keyes-Elstein L, et al. Myeloablative autologous stem-cell transplantation for severe scleroderma. N Engl J Med 2018;378(1):35–47.

112. van Laar JM, Farge D, Tyndall A. Cardiac assessment before stem cell transplantation for systemic sclerosis–reply. JAMA 2014;312(17):1803–4.

113. Casale M, Sabatino L, Moffa A, et al. Breathing training on lower esophageal sphincter as a complementary treatment of gastroesophageal reflux disease (GERD): a systematic review. Eur Rev Med Pharmacol Sci 2016;20(21):4547–52.

114. Spruit MA, Singh SJ, Garvey C, et al. An official American Thoracic Society/European Respiratory Society statement: key concepts and advances in pulmonary rehabilitation. Am J Respir Crit Care Med 2013;188(8):e13–64.

115. Yuen HK, Weng Y, Bandyopadhyay D, et al. Effect of a multi-faceted intervention on gingival health among adults with systemic sclerosis. Clin Exp Rheumatol 2011;29(2 Suppl 65):S26–32.

116. Poole J, Conte C, Brewer C, et al. Oral hygiene in scleroderma: the effectiveness of a multi-disciplinary intervention program. Disabil Rehabil 2010;32(5):379–84.

117. Nagaraja V, McMahan ZH, Getzug T, et al. Management of gastrointestinal involvement in scleroderma. Curr Treatm Opt Rheumatol 2015;1(1):82–105.

118. Pakozdi A, Wilson H, Black CM, et al. Does long term therapy with lansoprazole slow progression of oesophageal involvement in systemic sclerosis? Randomized Controlled Trial Research Support, Non-U.S. Gov't. Clin Exp Rheumatol 2009;27(3 Suppl 54):5–8.

119. Lew RJ, Kochman ML. A review of endoscopic methods of esophageal dilation. J Clin Gastroenterol 2002;35(2):117–26.

120. Ramirez-Mata M, Ibanez G, Alarcon-Segovia D. Stimulatory effect of metoclopramide on the esophagus and lower esophageal sphincter of patients of patients with PSS. Arthritis Rheum 1977;20(1):30–4.

121. Mercado U, Arroyo de Anda R, Avendano L, et al. Metoclopramide response in patients with early diffuse systemic sclerosis. Effects on esophageal motility abnormalities. Clin Exp Rheumatol 2005;23(5):685–8.

122. Johnson DA, Drane WE, Curran J, et al. Metoclopramide response in patients with progressive systemic sclerosis. Effect on esophageal and gastric motility abnormalities. Arch Intern Med 1987;147(9):1597–601.

123. Parodi A, Sessarego M, Greco A, et al. Small intestinal bacterial overgrowth in patients suffering from scleroderma: clinical effectiveness of its eradication. Am J Gastroenterol 2008;103(5):1257–62.

124. Marie I, Ducrotte P, Denis P, et al. Small intestinal bacterial overgrowth in systemic sclerosis. Rheumatology (Oxford) 2009;48(10):1314–9.
125. Shah SC, Day LW, Somsouk M, et al. Meta-analysis: antibiotic therapy for small intestinal bacterial overgrowth. Aliment Pharmacol Ther 2013;38(8):925–34.
126. Frech TM, Khanna D, Maranian P, et al. Probiotics for the treatment of systemic sclerosis-associated gastrointestinal bloating/distention. Clin Exp Rheumatol 2011;29(2 Suppl 65):S22–5.
127. Folwaczny C, Laritz M, Meurer M, et al. [Effects of various prokinetic drugs on gastrointestinal transit times in patients with progressive systemic scleroderma]. Z Gastroenterol 1997;35(10):905–12. Einfluss verschiedener Prokinetika auf gastrointestinale Transitzeiten bei Patienten mit progressiv-systemischer Sklerodermie.
128. Nikou GC, Toumpanakis C, Katsiari C, et al. Treatment of small intestinal disease in systemic sclerosis with octreotide: a prospective study in seven patients. J Clin Rheumatol 2007;13(3):119–23.
129. Kenefick NJ, Vaizey CJ, Nicholls RJ, et al. Sacral nerve stimulation for faecal incontinence due to systemic sclerosis. Gut 2002;51(6):881–3.
130. Baron M, Bernier P, Cote LF, et al. Screening and therapy for malnutrition and related gastro-intestinal disorders in systemic sclerosis: recommendations of a North American expert panel. Clin Exp Rheumatol 2010;28(2 Suppl 58):S42–6.
131. Ringold S, Nigrovic PA, Feldman BM, et al. The childhood arthritis and rheumatology research alliance consensus treatment plans: toward comparative effectiveness in the pediatric rheumatic diseases. Arthritis Rheumatol 2018;70(5): 669–78.

Recent Advances in Pediatric Vasculitis

Laura Cannon, MD[a], Eveline Y. Wu, MD, MSCR[b,c],*

KEYWORDS

- Vasculitis • Vasculitides • Pediatric • Childhood • Systemic

KEY POINTS

- Childhood vasculitides are rare, and clinical manifestations are highly variable, making diagnosis challenging. Early recognition and timely treatment, however, are critical to improving outcomes and preventing organ damage.
- Recent work has advanced understanding of the pathogenesis of pediatric systemic vasculitides. In particular, identification of monogenic disease forms has characterized important disease pathways further and suggested more targeted treatments.
- Consensus-based guidelines are emerging for treatment of pediatric vasculitis, but pediatric-specific clinical trials are needed to fully determine the efficacy and safety of treatment options in children.

INTRODUCTION

Primary systemic vasculitides of childhood are a rare and heterogenous group of disorders characterized by inflammation of blood vessels. Classification of vasculitis is based on vessel size and other clinicopathologic features (**Fig. 1**).[1] The distribution of blood vessel involvement falls into 3 major categories: (1) large vessels, including the aorta and its major branches and the analogous veins; (2) medium vessels, including the main visceral arteries and veins and their initial branches; and (3) small vessels, including intraparenchymal arteries, arterioles, capillaries, venules, and veins.[1] Although classification reflects the predominant vessel size involved, it is important to emphasize that all 3 major categories can affect any size blood vessel.

Primary vasculitides are less common in children than adults, with an overall estimated incidence of 50 cases per 100,000 children per year.[2] The exceptions are immunoglobulin A (IgA) vasculitis and Kawasaki disease (KD), which occur predominantly in childhood.[2] Despite disease rarity, large registries, and international

[a] Division of Pediatric Rheumatology, Department of Pediatrics, Duke University, 2301 Erwin Road, DUMC Box 3212, Durham, NC 27710, USA; [b] Division of Pediatric Rheumatology, Department of Pediatrics, The University of North Carolina Chapel Hill, 030 MacNider Hall, CB #7231, Chapel Hill, NC 27599, USA; [c] Division of Allergy/Immunology, Department of Pediatrics, The University of North Carolina Chapel Hill, Chapel Hill, NC
* Corresponding author. Department of Pediatrics, The University of North Carolina Chapel Hill, 030 MacNider Hall, CB #7231, Chapel Hill, NC 27599
E-mail address: eveline.wu@unc.edu

Rheum Dis Clin N Am 47 (2021) 781–796
https://doi.org/10.1016/j.rdc.2021.07.007
0889-857X/21/© 2021 Elsevier Inc. All rights reserved.

rheumatic.theclinics.com

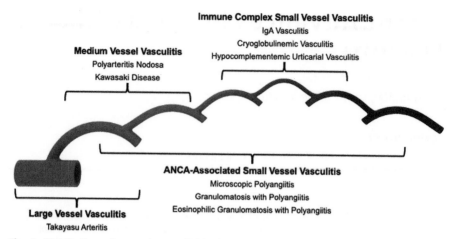

Fig. 1. Distribution of systemic vasculitides by vessel involvement. (*Adapted from* Jennette JC, Falk RJ, Bacon PA, et al. 2012 revised International Chapel Hill Consensus Conference Nomenclature of Vasculitides. *Arthritis Rheum.* 2013;65(1):1-11.) (*Courtesy of* Arthur Y. Wu.).

collaborations have produced significant advancements in the field of pediatric vasculitis research. This article aims to provide an overview of recent updates in the classification, pathogenesis, evaluation, and management of childhood vasculitides.

LARGE VESSEL VASCULITIS: TAKAYASU ARTERITIS

Takayasu arteritis (TA) is a chronic large vessel vasculitis affecting predominantly the aorta and its main branches. TA is characterized by a granulomatous panarteritis, and the inflammatory process eventually can lead to blood vessel stenosis, dilatation, or aneurysm.[3] Childhood TA (c-TA) typically involves the aorta and the renal, subclavian, and carotid arteries.[4] Although adult TA is reported worldwide, with the highest incidence in East Asia, the incidence in children remains unknown.[5,6] Median age of onset is 12 years to 14 years, although c-TA has been reported in infancy.[7–9] c-TA occurs more commonly in girls, with a 3:1 ratio of girls to boys.[4]

Early diagnosis of c-TA is challenging due to nonspecific presenting symptoms.[7] Large vessel biopsies often are not feasible, so diagnosis relies on clinical symptoms and confirmatory imaging. Frequent symptoms at diagnosis are nonspecific, including malaise, weight loss, and headache.[10] Arthritis and arthralgia are seen more frequently in c-TA than in adult TA.[3] Hypertension is a common finding, and a discrepancy between 4-extremity blood pressure measurements often is indicative of c-TA.[4,10] Up to half of children with c-TA present with a bruit.[7,10] Claudication and diminished or absent pulses often are observed distal to the affected vasculature, underscoring the importance of assessing 4-extremity pulses.

There is no specific laboratory finding diagnostic of c-TA, although erythrocyte sedimentation rate (ESR) commonly is elevated at diagnosis and can be a useful disease activity marker.[10] Imaging typically confirms c-TA diagnosis. Angiography is the gold standard, but it is invasive and does not detect thickened vessel walls, which may be an early sign of inflammation. Computed tomography (CT) and magnetic resonance angiograms (MRAs) are less invasive alternatives that detect luminal diameter changes and vessel wall thickening (**Fig. 2A–C**). Angiographic abnormalities of the aorta or its main branches and pulmonary arteries are mandatory criteria of the

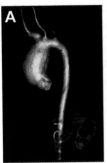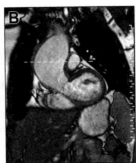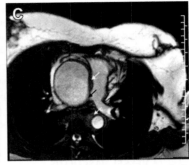

Fig. 2. TA. (*A*) Three-dimensional reconstruction of MRA shows severe dilation of the ascending aorta. (*B*) Coronal cine image of the ascending aortic aneurysm. (*C*) Axial cross-section of (*B*) (*yellow line*) demonstrating compression of the right pulmonary artery by the ascending aortic aneurysm (*black arrow*) and vessel wall thickness (*white arrows*) of the ascending and descending aorta. (*Courtesy* of M. Jay Campbell.)

validated classification criteria for c-TA proposed by the European League Against Rheumatism (EULAR), Paediatric Rheumatology European Society (PRES), and Paediatric Rheumatology International Trials Organisation (PRINTO) (**Table 1**).[11,12]

The goal of treatment in c-TA is control of vessel inflammation and prevention of irreversible vascular and organ damage. Treatment recommendations largely are extrapolated from adult observational cohort studies. Corticosteroids are first-line therapy; however, half of children need an additional immunosuppressant.[10] Treatment of c-TA with conventional synthetic disease-modifying anti-rheumatic drugs (csDMARD) and biologic DMARD (bDMARD) includes cyclophosphamide, azathioprine,

Table 1
European League Against Rheumatism//Paediatric Rheumatology International Trials Organisation/Paediatric Rheumatology European Society classification criteria for childhood Takayasu arteritis

Criterion	Glossary
Angiographic abnormality (mandatory criterion) plus 1 of the following:	Angiography of the aorta or its main branches and pulmonary arteries showing aneurysm/dilatation, narrowing, occlusion or thickened arterial wall
1. Pulse deficit or claudication	Lost/decreased/unequal peripheral artery pulse(s) Claudication: focal muscle pain induced by physical activity
2. Blood pressure discrepancy	Discrepancy of 4 limb systolic blood pressure >10 mm Hg difference in any limb
3. Bruits	Audible murmurs or palpable thrills over large arteries
4. Hypertension	Systolic or diastolic blood pressure >95th percentile for height
5. Elevated acute phase reactants	ESR >20 mm/h or CRP any value above normal

Data from Ozen S, Pistorio A, Iusan SM, et al. EULAR/PRINTO/PRES criteria for Henoch-Schönlein purpura, childhood polyarteritis nodosa, childhood Wegener granulomatosis and childhood Takayasu arteritis: Ankara 2008. Part II: Final classification criteria. *Ann Rheum Dis.* 2010;69(5):798-806.

methotrexate, mycophenolate mofetil (MMF), infliximab, and tocilizumab.[6,13-15] Recent studies suggest that tumor necrosis factor-α (TNF-α) inhibitors and interleukin (IL)-6 inhibition with tocilizumab may be promising options for refractory disease.[6,10] In 1 of the largest cohort studies of c-TA, the 2-year flare-free survival was significantly greater with bDMARD (80%) versus csDMARD (43%) therapies.[10] Children receiving bDMARD also were more likely to achieve inactive disease at last follow-up compared with children treated with nonbiologic agents.[10] Biologic DMARD increasingly are used in c-TA based on this favorable real-world evidence and anecdotal experience, but pediatric-specific trials are needed to inform evidence-based guidelines.

MEDIUM VESSEL VASCULITIS
Kawasaki Disease

KD is a medium vessel vasculitis and one of the most common childhood vasculitides. The cause of KD remains unknown, but seasonal variation in incidence suggests a possible viral trigger.[16] The epidemiology of KD varies geographically. Japan has the highest incidence of KD at 330 cases/100,000 children per year, which has increased over time.[17,18] Incidence has been relatively stable in the United States, at 20 cases per 100,000 hospitalized children less than 5 years old.[19] More than 75% of affected children are under 5 years old, with an average age of diagnosis of 3 years old.[19] Boys are affected more commonly than girls.[20]

Untreated KD is a triphasic disease.[20] The first phase is characterized by high fever in conjunction with other clinical features, including bilateral limbic-sparing, nonexudative bulbar conjunctivitis, involvement of the oropharyngeal mucous membranes, rash, unilateral anterior cervical lymphadenopathy, and peripheral extremity changes (**Fig. 3**A–D). During the subacute phase (2–4 weeks after diagnosis), desquamation of the hands and feet may be the only clinically evident feature (see **Fig. 3**E). Coronary artery aneurysms (CAAs) also develop during this phase (see **Fig. 3**F). The final or convalescent phase typically is asymptomatic.

Children with KD usually show evidence of inflammation with elevated ESR and C-reactive protein (CRP) and leukocytosis. Platelet counts may be normal at disease-onset but usually are significantly elevated by week 2 of illness. Sterile pyuria may be present but is of urethral origin, so a catheterized urine sample may be normal. If KD is suspected, timely evaluation for cardiovascular abnormalities should be performed with an echocardiogram. Although these findings are supportive, a diagnosis of KD depends on clinical criteria (**Box 1**).[21]

Intravenous immunoglobulin (IVIG), 2 g/kg, and aspirin are first-line therapies for KD. CAAs are a major morbidity of KD and are the leading cause of pediatric acquired heart disease in western countries.[20] IVIG treatment reduces CAA development by 5-fold and ideally should be administered within 10 days of fever onset.[21] Up to 20% of children fail to respond to initial IVIG therapy, and IVIG typically is redosed.[22] Due to ongoing inflammation, these patients are at higher risk of cardiac sequelae.

Determining a patient's risk of IVIG resistance and development of CAA is important in the context of initial treatment decisions, including consideration of adjunctive corticosteroid or TNF-α inhibitor therapy use with IVIG. Predictive tools developed in the Japanese population to determine risk of IVIG resistance and CAA are not generalizable to North American KD cohorts.[23] A recent risk model developed for prediction of CAA in North American KD cohorts included baseline z score of the left anterior descending or right coronary artery greater than or equal to 2.0, age less than 6 months, Asian race, and CRP greater than or equal to 13 mg/dL.[24] Prospective study is needed to determine the model's predictive utility in informing the early use of

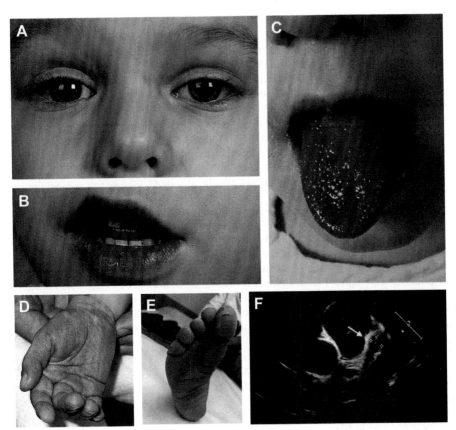

Fig. 3. KD. (*A*) Bilateral bulbar conjunctivitis. (*B*) Red, cracked lips. (*C*) Strawberry tongue. (*D*) Palmar erythema and edema. (*E*) Desquamation of the toes. (*F*) Echocardiogram demonstrating large aneurysm of the left anterior descending coronary artery (*arrow*). ([A], [B], [D] from Scuccimarri R. Kawasaki disease. *Pediatr Clin North Am.* 2012;59(2):425; with permission. [C] from Yoskovitch A, Tewfik TL, Duffy CM, et al. Head and neck manifestations of Kawasaki disease. *Int J Pediatr Otorhinolaryngol.* 2000;52(2):125; with permission.)

Box 1
European League Against Rheumatism//Paediatric Rheumatology European Society classification criteria for Kawasaki disease

Fever persisting for at least 5 days (mandatory criterion) plus 4 of the following:
1. Changes in peripheral extremities or perineal area
2. Polymorphous exanthema
3. Bilateral conjunctival injection
4. Changes of lips and oral cavity: injection of oral and pharyngeal mucosa
5. Cervical lymphadenopathy

In presence of coronary artery involvement and fever, fewer than 4 of the remaining 5 criteria are sufficient.

Data from Ozen S, Ruperto N, Dillon MJ, et al. EULAR/PRES endorsed consensus criteria for the classification of childhood vasculitides. *Ann Rheum Dis.* 2006;65(7):936-941.

adjunctive corticosteroids and/or other immunomodulatory medications, such as TNF-α inhibitors in KD.

In an effort to facilitate uniformity of care, the Single Hub and Access Point for Paediatric Rheumatology in Europe (SHARE) initiative has published evidence-based and consensus-based recommendations for diagnosis and treatment of pediatric vasculitides like KD.[25] The SHARE initiative recommends use of corticosteroids in children who are IVIG-resistant and proposes dosing regimens.[25] Less clear is whether there is any benefit in earlier corticosteroid treatment. A 2017 Cochrane review in KD found that the addition of corticosteroids to treatment regimens reduced occurrence of CAA, fever duration, time for ESR and CRP normalization, and length of hospital stay. Subgroup analysis showed the greatest benefit from corticosteroids in patients of Asian race, those with higher risk scores, and patients who received a longer corticosteroid course rather than a 1-time dose.[22] In the prospective, open-label RAISE study from Japan, significantly fewer children with KD randomized to receive IVIG and corticosteroids developed CAA compared with those treated with IVIG alone.[26] These results have not yet been replicated in non-Japanese populations. Although determining an optimal regimen for corticosteroids requires further study, corticosteroids are indicated for treatment-refractory KD and possibly as early adjunctive therapy to IVIG for patients with higher risk of treatment resistance and/or CAA.

There also has been interest in TNF-α inhibitor therapy for treatment-resistant KD. In a double-blind, randomized, placebo-controlled trial (RCT), the addition of infliximab to primary therapy resulted in faster resolution of fever and greater improvement in inflammatory markers. Early adjunctive infliximab therapy, however, did not reduce treatment resistance or coronary outcomes at 5-week follow-up.[27] In a small study of refractory KD, there were no differences in coronary outcomes between children receiving a second dose of IVIG versus infliximab.[28] As with corticosteroids, further studies are needed to determine the role of TNF-α inhibitors in the treatment of refractory KD.[29] Currently, there is no robust evidence that TNF-α inhibitors alter coronary artery outcomes in KD.

Polyarteritis Nodosa

Polyarteritis nodosa (PAN) is characterized by necrotizing inflammation of small and medium-sized arteries.[1] The disease spectrum ranges from self-limited cutaneous disease to the potentially life-threatening systemic form with widespread organ involvement.[30] Systemic PAN accounts for 3% of childhood vasculitides in the United States.[31] PAN occurs most frequently in elementary school-aged children and there is no gender predilection.[32,33]

The etiology of classic PAN is unclear. Recently, PAN-like necrotizing vasculitis was described in association with monogenic disorders. In deficiency of adenosine deaminase 2 (DADA2) due to loss-of-function mutations in CERC1, a PAN-like vasculopathy occurs. Young children present with intermittent fevers, lacunar strokes, livedoid rash, hepatosplenomegaly, and mild immune abnormalities.[34,35] An association between familial Mediterranean fever (FMF) and PAN also increasingly is appreciated. Children with both FMF and PAN typically have younger age at onset, more frequent hematomas, and an overall better prognosis than those with PAN alone.[36] Stimulator of interferon response genes–associated vasculopathy of infancy (SAVI) is an autoinflammatory disease characterized by severe vasculopathy and interstitial pulmonary disease.[37] Discovery of monogenic forms of PAN-like vasculitis may provide insight into critical pathways involved in the pathogenesis of classic PAN.

In the largest cohort of childhood PAN, the most common clinical features at presentation were fever, myalgia, and skin manifestations.[33] Cutaneous involvement has a variety of appearances, with livedo reticularis the most common.[32,33] Fixed, tender subcutaneous nodules can occur over affected vasculature,[33] and skin infarctions and autoamputation may be present during the disease course (**Fig. 4**A,B).[32]

Imaging in PAN reveals aneurysms, stenosis, or occlusion, which are reflective of the necrotizing vasculitis characteristic of the disease (see **Fig. 4**C). Conventional angiography remains the gold standard, but MRA and CTA are less invasive imaging modalities that are increasingly used. Angiographic changes are part of the childhood PAN EULAR/PRINTO/PRES classification criteria (**Table 2**).[11,38] Although nonspecific, inflammatory markers typically are elevated, antinuclear antibody (ANA) and antineutrophil cytoplasmic antibody (ANCA) usually are negative.[33]

As with other childhood vasculitides, PAN treatment largely is based on adult data and clinical experience. Corticosteroids are a mainstay of therapy. Cyclophosphamide may be considered for remission-induction.[32,33] Using a bayesian adaptive design, a recent open-label RCT was performed comparing MMF to cyclophosphamide for remission-induction in childhood PAN and found that remission rates were similar.[39] Biologic DMARD, such as TNF-α inhibitors and rituximab, reportedly are efficacious, including in treatment of refractory disease.[40,41] For monogenic PAN-like vasculitis, TNF-α inhibitors are recommended for DADA2 and Janus kinase (JAK) inhibitors have proved effective for SAVI.[34,37]

SMALL VESSEL VASCULITIS
Immunoglobulin A Vasculitis

IgA vasculitis (IgAV), formerly called Henoch-Schönlein purpura [HSP], is a leukocytoclastic vasculitis affecting predominantly small vessels. IgAV is the most common pediatric vasculitis,[42] accounting for approximately half of childhood systemic vasculitis cases in the United States.[43] IgAV affects mostly young children less than 10 years old.[44] There are reports of IgAV in infants, who usually have a milder course.[45] IgAV is more common in boys than girls.[44,46] IgAV occurs throughout the year, but seasonal variation has been observed,[47] with the highest number of cases occurring during the winter,[48] typically following a respiratory infection.[44]

IgAV is a clinical tetrad of palpable purpura, arthritis, abdominal pain, and glomerulonephritis. Non-thrombocytopenic petechiae and purpura on weight-bearing areas, such as the buttocks and legs, are characteristic. The EULAR/PRINTO/PRES criteria

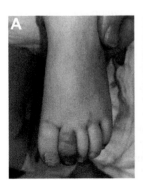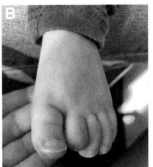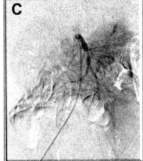

Fig. 4. Infant with PAN. (*A*) Progressive gangrene of the left second toe. (*B*) Autoamputation of the distal left second toe. (*C*) Arteriogram with aneurysmal dilatation of the proximal superior mesenteric artery (SMA) with mild stenosis proximal and distal to the aneurysm. Multiple microaneurysms in the distal branches of the SMA.

Table 2
European League Against Rheumatism//Paediatric Rheumatology International Trials Organisation/Paediatric Rheumatology European Society classification criteria for childhood polyarteritis nodosa

Criterion	Glossary
Histopathology	Evidence of necrotizing vasculitis in medium-sized or small arteries
Angiographic abnormality	Angiography showing aneurysm, stenosis, or occlusion of medium-sized or small arteries
Histopathology or angiographic abnormality (mandatory criterion) plus 1 of the following:	
1. Skin involvement	Livedo reticularis, skin nodules, or superficial or deep skin infarctions
2. Myalgia or muscle tenderness	Muscle pain or tenderness
3. Hypertension	Systolic or diastolic blood pressure >95th percentile for height
4. Peripheral neuropathy	Sensory peripheral neuropathy or motor mononeuritis multiplex
5. Renal involvement	Proteinuria >0.3 g/24 h or >30 mmol/mg of urine albumin/creatinine ratio on a spot morning sample

Data from Ozen S, Pistorio A, Iusan SM, et al. EULAR/PRINTO/PRES criteria for Henoch-Schönlein purpura, childhood polyarteritis nodosa, childhood Wegener granulomatosis and childhood Takayasu arteritis: Ankara 2008. Part II: Final classification criteria. Ann Rheum Dis. 2010;69(5):798-806.

for HSP (now called IgAV) requires the presence of lower limb–predominant palpable purpura in addition to one other feature (**Table 3**).[11] If characteristic rash is present, the diagnosis is straightforward. If the purpura is present in an atypical distribution, then consistent biopsy findings are required for diagnosis.[11] Gastrointestinal symptoms and arthritis/arthralgia may precede cutaneous findings by up to 2 weeks, making diagnosis more challenging.[44] Gastrointestinal symptoms range from colicky abdominal pain to overt bowel perforation. A rare but serious gastrointestinal complication is intussusception.[49] Renal involvement occurs in approximately one-third of IgAV patients, typically within 6 months of onset, and 2% of children develop end-stage renal disease.[43,50]

Although there are no diagnostic laboratory findings, platelets are normal or increased, distinguishing IgAV from purpura caused by thrombocytopenia. Serum IgA is increased in the acute phase of illness in approximately half of patients.[51] If diagnosis is uncertain, skin biopsy demonstrating leukocytoclastic vasculitis with IgA deposition can be helpful.

There is ongoing debate about the role of corticosteroids in IgAV treatment. In patients with more severe symptoms, prednisone reduces the intensity of abdominal and joint pain compared with placebo.[52] In severe IgAV cases requiring hospitalization, corticosteroids also are associated with improved gastrointestinal outcomes.[53] A meta-analysis of patients treated with corticosteroids versus supportive care found that corticosteroids resulted in a 5-fold increase in the odds of abdominal pain resolution within 24 hours.[43]

Renal disease is a relatively rare but potentially severe complication of IgAV; however, currently available data do not support universal administration of corticosteroids to

Table 3
European League Against Rheumatism//Paediatric Rheumatology International Trials Organisation/Paediatric Rheumatology European Society classification criteria for Henoch-Schönlein purpura

Criterion	Glossary
Purpura (mandatory criterion) and at least 1 of the following:	Purpura or petechiae, with lower limb predominance (not related to thrombocytopenia)
1. Abdominal pain	Diffuse abdominal colicky pain with acute onset assessed by history and physical examination. May include intussusception and gastrointestinal bleeding
2. Histopathology	Typically, leukocytoclastic vasculitis with predominant IgA deposit or proliferative glomerulonephritis with predominant IgA deposit
3. Arthritis or arthralgias	Arthritis of acute onset defined as joint swelling or joint pain with limitation on motion Arthralgia of acute onset defined as joint pain without joint swelling or limitation on motion
4. Renal involvement	Proteinuria >0.3 g/24 h or >30 mmol/mg on spot urine albumin/creatinine ratio

Data from Ozen S, Pistorio A, Iusan SM, et al. EULAR/PRINTO/PRES criteria for Henoch-Schönlein purpura, childhood polyarteritis nodosa, childhood Wegener granulomatosis and childhood Takayasu arteritis: Ankara 2008. Part II: Final classification criteria. *Ann Rheum Dis.* 2010;69(5):798-806.

prevent kidney disease. A recent double-blind RCT did not detect a difference in the prevalence of proteinuria at 12 months in IgAV patients treated with corticosteroids versus placebo.[54] This was consistent with a systematic review of other RCTs in IgAV renal disease that demonstrated corticosteroids did not change renal outcomes.[55] Children require close monitoring for renal involvement after diagnosis, particularly in the first months when risk is highest. Patients who develop renal involvement should be treated with corticosteroids as first-line therapy, either oral or pulse intravenous (IV), depending on nephritis severity. As with other systemic small vessel vasculitides, the SHARE initiative recommends pulse IV methylprednisolone and IV cyclophosphamide for severe IgAV nephritis.[56] Plasmapheresis may be indicated for rapidly progressive glomerulonephritis (RPGN).[55,57] Azathioprine, cyclosporine, MMF, and cyclophosphamide may be considered for induction in moderate IgAV nephritis or for maintenance therapy.[55–57]

Antineutrophil Cytoplasmic Antibody–associated Vasculitis

In ANCA-associated vasculitis (AAV), there is ANCA production and small to medium-sized vessel inflammation and necrosis.[1] ANCAs typically are directed toward proteinase 3 (PR3-ANCA) or myeloperoxidase (MPO-ANCA). Clinical phenotypes include granulomatosis with polyangiitis (GPA), microscopic polyangiitis (MPA), eosinophilic GPA (EGPA), and renal-limited AAV.[1] Although AAV is rare in children, epidemiologic data suggest an increase in cases over the last 10 to 25 years, likely due to improved clinical recognition, ANCA testing, and disease classification. Estimated incidence rates of pediatric AAV currently are 0.4 per million per year to 6.39 per million per year.[58,59] The median age at diagnosis is 10 years to 14 years, and, in contrast to adults, childhood-onset AAV is more common in girls.[58,60,61]

AAV pathogenesis involves genetic susceptibility factors, environmental exposures, and abnormalities in innate and adaptive immunity. Genome-wide association studies have identified both major histocompatibility complex (MHC) and non-MHC associations in AAV and suggest associations more strongly align with ANCA specificity rather than clinical phenotype. The strongest genetic associations include *HLA-DP*, *SERPINA1* (encoding α_1-antitrypsin), and *PRTN3* (encoding PR3) with PR3-ANCA and *HLA-DQ* with MPO-ANCA.[62] Environmental triggers include infections (e.g., *Staphylococcus aureus*), drugs (e.g., hydralazine, propylthiouracil, levamisole-adulterated cocaine, and others), and air pollutants (e.g., silica).[63] AAV immunopathogenesis is complex and not fully elucidated, but neutrophils are a central effector cell. T-cell dysregulation and B-cell dysregulation with pathogenic ANCA production are additional key contributors.[63] There also is increasing appreciation that complement activation plays a role in AAV pathogenesis.[64] EGPA classically is considered a type 2 helper T cell–driven hyperinflammatory response directed by cytokines IL-4, IL-5, and IL-13, and eosinophils are a predominant cell type.[65]

AAV clinical phenotypes have overlapping features. Like other systemic vasculitides of childhood, nonspecific symptoms of fever, malaise, and weight loss are common, occurring in more than 80% of children with AAV.[61] A triad of ear, nose, and throat disease; lower respiratory tract involvement; and renal disease presenting as pauci-immune crescentic glomerulonephritis often characterizes GPA, but cutaneous, gastrointestinal, and musculoskeletal manifestations also occur (**Fig. 5A–C**).[61] Renal disease is common in MPA and often presents as an RPGN.[58] EGPA characteristically develops in 3 sequential phases: (1) prodromal allergic with asthma, allergic rhinitis, and sinusitis; (2) eosinophilic with peripheral eosinophilia and eosinophilic tissue infiltration; and (3) vasculitic with peripheral neuropathy, palpable purpura, and pauci-immune necrotizing glomerulonephritis.[65]

Diagnosis can be challenging, especially because ANCA positivity is not universal. In a large pediatric AAV cohort, 26% of MPA patients and 5% of GPA patients were ANCA negative.[61] Elevations in CRP and ESR and anemia are common laboratory findings.[61] Although adult classification algorithms have been applied to children, the only pediatric-specific classification criteria are those proposed by EULAR/ PRINTO/PRES for GPA (**Table 4**).[11] In a pediatric AAV cohort, the EULAR/

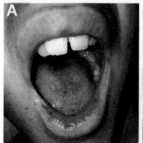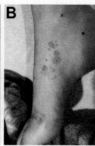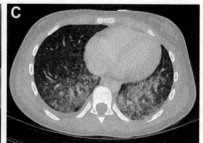

Fig. 5. GPA. (*A*) Oral ulcers, focal erythema, and petechiae. (*B*) Cutaneous small vessel vasculitis. (*C*) Axial image from chest CT with bilateral ground-glass alveolar opacities due to diffuse alveolar hemorrhage.

Table 4
European League Against Rheumatism//Paediatric Rheumatology International Trials Organisation/Paediatric Rheumatology European Society classification criteria for childhood granulomatosis with polyangiitis

Criterion	Glossary
1. Histopathology	Granulomatous inflammation within the wall of an artery or in the perivascular or extravascular area
2. Upper airway involvement	Chronic purulent or blood nasal discharge or recurrent epistaxis/crusts/granulomata Nasal septum perforation or saddle nose deformity Chronic or recurrent sinus inflammation
3. Laryngotracheobronchial involvement	Subglottic, tracheal, or bronchial stenosis
4. Pulmonary involvement	Chest radiograph or CT showing presence of nodules, cavities, or fixed infiltrates
5. ANCA	ANCA positivity by immunofluorescence or by ELISA
6. Renal involvement	Proteinuria >0.3 g/24 h or >30 mmol/mg of urine albumin/creatinine ratio on a spot morning sample

Data from Ozen S, Pistorio A, Iusan SM, et al. EULAR/PRINTO/PRES criteria for Henoch-Schönlein purpura, childhood polyarteritis nodosa, childhood Wegener granulomatosis and childhood Takayasu arteritis: Ankara 2008. Part II: Final classification criteria. *Ann Rheum Dis.* 2010;69(5):798-806.

PRINTO/PRES criteria were more sensitive than those of the American College of Rheumatology but less sensitive than the European Medicines Agency criteria in classifying pediatric GPA.[66] Even still, many children with AAV are unclassifiable using adult criteria, emphasizing the need to validate pediatric-specific classification criteria for all AAV subtypes. The poor sensitivity of adult criteria in classifying pediatric AAV also may highlight clinical differences. Compared with adult counterparts, children with AAV experience kidney and multiorgan involvement, nasal deformities, and subglottic stenosis more frequently.[67] More than one-half of children with AAV have organ damage present early in the disease course.[68] Childhood-onset AAV also is associated with more frequent disease relapse and longer exposure to toxic therapies.

Efforts to create validated outcome measures for disease assessment of pediatric AAV are progressing. The Paediatric Vasculitis Activity Score is adapted from the Birmingham Vasculitis Activity Score and has been validated.[69] A pediatric Vasculitis Damage Index was proposed, and the PRES and Childhood Arthritis and Rheumatology Research Alliance (CARRA) vasculitis workgroups are working toward validation of the pediatric modification.[68]

AAV treatment includes induction and maintenance phases and is based on disease severity, although corticosteroids continue to be the cornerstone of therapy. The CARRA vasculitis workgroup recently published consensus treatment plans for new-onset, severe AAV, suggesting either cyclophosphamide IV or rituximab in conjunction with corticosteroids for remission-induction. Options for remission-maintenance include rituximab, methotrexate, and azathioprine.[70] Recent reviews of landmark trials for adult AAV are published, but pediatric-specific therapeutic trials are lacking.[71]

SUMMARY

Recent research has resulted in substantial advances in the understanding and care of childhood vasculitides. Identification of monogenic disorders associated with systemic vasculitis has characterized disease pathways further and revealed new treatment targets. Multicenter and international collaborations have led to the development of classification criteria and consensus-based treatment recommendations for several pediatric vasculitides. There remain, however, critical areas of unmet need. Disease rarity poses a significant barrier making collaboration the key to accelerating progress in the field. International collaborations facilitate the establishment of adequate diagnostic criteria and shared biobanks may expedite the discovery of additional genetic susceptibility factors and more reliable disease biomarkers. Harmonized international registries and databases can improve understanding of the natural history of the rare vasculitides, and multicenter studies are needed to perform high-quality clinical trials to inform tailored treatment approaches. Working collaboratively is critical to improving the care and outcomes of these rare vasculitides in children.

CLINICS CARE POINTS

- Key challenges remain in early recognition and timely diagnosis of childhood vasculitides.
- Despite published recommendations for the diagnosis and classification of several pediatric vasculitides, these guidelines are limited by a paucity of pediatric-specific evidence, underscoring the need for more research.
- Further research is necessary to better define the genetic susceptibility and pathogenesis of pediatric vasculitides as well as identify reliable disease biomarkers.
- For many pediatric systemic vasculitides, treatment recommendations largely are extrapolated from adult data. Consensus-based guidelines like those from the SHARE initiative and CARRA help harmonize management and reduce variability in the treatment of pediatric vasculitis.
- Patients and providers urgently need therapeutic trials in pediatric vasculitis to refine treatment regimens that safely reduce corticosteroid exposure, incorporate newer approaches involving biologic agents, and outline duration of induction and maintenance therapy.

DISCLOSURE

Dr Cannon's work was supported by an Arthritis Foundation 2020 Fellowship Grant. Dr Wu's work was supported by the National Center for Advancing Translational Sciences; National Institutes of Health, through Grant KL2TR002490; and through generous donations from the Kioti Tractor Company, the Kim family, and the Smith family. The content is solely the responsibility of the authors and does not necessarily represent the official views of the NIH. Dr Wu receives consulting and Advisory Board fees from Pharming Healthcare, Inc., and research funding from AstraZeneca and Bristol-Myers Squibb.

ACKNOWLEDGMENTS

The authors are grateful to Arthur Y. Wu and Dr M. Jay Campbell for providing figures for this article.

REFERENCES

1. Jennette JC, Falk RJ, Bacon PA, et al. 2012 revised International Chapel Hill Consensus Conference Nomenclature of Vasculitides. Arthritis Rheum 2013; 65(1):1–11.

2. Sag E, Batu ED, Ozen S. Childhood systemic vasculitis. Best Pract Res Clin Rheumatol 2017;31(4):558–75.

3. Brunner J, Feldman BM, Tyrrell PN, et al. Takayasu arteritis in children and adolescents. Rheumatology 2010;49(10):1806–14.

4. Cakar N, Yalcinkaya F, Duzova A, et al. Takayasu arteritis in children. J Rheumatol 2008;35(5):913–9.

5. de Souza AW, de Carvalho JF. Diagnostic and classification criteria of Takayasu arteritis. J Autoimmun 2014;48-49:79–83.

6. Batu ED, Sonmez HE, Hazirolan T, et al. Tocilizumab treatment in childhood Takayasu arteritis: case series of four patients and systematic review of the literature. Semin Arthritis Rheum 2017;46(4):529–35.

7. Sahin S, Hopurcuoglu D, Bektas S, et al. Childhood-onset Takayasu arteritis: a 15-year experience from a tertiary referral center. Int J Rheum Dis 2019;22(1):132–9.

8. Fan L, Zhang H, Cai J, et al. Clinical course and prognostic factors of childhood Takayasu's arteritis: over 15-year comprehensive analysis of 101 patients. Arthritis Res Ther 2019;21(1):31.

9. Singh N, Hughes M, Sebire N, et al. Takayasu arteritis in infancy. Rheumatology 2013;52(11):2093–5.

10. Aeschlimann FA, Eng SWM, Sheikh S, et al. Childhood Takayasu arteritis: disease course and response to therapy. Arthritis Res Ther 2017;19(1):255.

11. Ozen S, Pistorio A, Iusan SM, et al. EULAR/PRINTO/PRES criteria for Henoch-Schönlein purpura, childhood polyarteritis nodosa, childhood Wegener granulomatosis and childhood Takayasu arteritis: Ankara 2008. Part II: Final classification criteria. Ann Rheum Dis 2010;69(5):798–806.

12. Ruperto N, Ozen S, Pistorio A, et al. EULAR/PRINTO/PRES criteria for Henoch-Schönlein purpura, childhood polyarteritis nodosa, childhood Wegener granulomatosis and childhood Takayasu arteritis: Ankara 2008. Part I: overall methodology and clinical characterisation. Ann Rheum Dis 2010;69(5):790–7.

13. Ozen S, Duzova A, Bakkaloglu A, et al. Takayasu arteritis in children: preliminary experience with cyclophosphamide induction and corticosteroids followed by methotrexate. J Pediatr 2007;150(1):72–6.

14. Szugye HS, Zeft AS, Spalding SJ. Takayasu Arteritis in the pediatric population: a contemporary United States-based single center cohort. Pediatr Rheumatol Online J 2014;12:21.

15. Stern S, Clemente G, Reiff A, et al. Treatment of pediatric Takayasu arteritis with infliximab and cyclophosphamide: experience from an American-Brazilian cohort study. J Clin Rheumatol 2014;20(4):183–8.

16. Rowley AH, Shulman ST. The epidemiology and pathogenesis of Kawasaki disease. Front Pediatr 2018;6:374.

17. Makino N, Nakamura Y, Yashiro M, et al. Descriptive epidemiology of Kawasaki disease in Japan, 2011-2012: from the results of the 22nd nationwide survey. J Epidemiol 2015;25(3):239–45.

18. Rife E, Gedalia A. Kawasaki disease: an update. Curr Rheumatol Rep 2020; 22(10):75.

19. Holman RC, Belay ED, Christensen KY, et al. Hospitalizations for Kawasaki syndrome among children in the United States, 1997-2007. Pediatr Infect Dis J 2010;29(6):483–8.

20. Sundel RP. Kawasaki disease. Rheum Dis Clin North Am 2015;41(1):63–73, viii.

21. McCrindle BW, Rowley AH, Newburger JW, et al. Diagnosis, treatment, and long-term management of Kawasaki disease: a scientific statement for health professionals from the American Heart Association. Circulation 2017;135(17):e927–99.

22. Wardle AJ, Connolly GM, Seager MJ, et al. Corticosteroids for the treatment of Kawasaki disease in children. Cochrane Database Syst Rev 2017;1(1): Cd011188.

23. Son MBF, Gauvreau K, Kim S, et al. Predicting coronary artery aneurysms in Kawasaki disease at a North American Center: an assessment of baseline z scores. J Am Heart Assoc 2017;6(6).

24. Son MBF, Gauvreau K, Tremoulet AH, et al. Risk model development and validation for prediction of coronary artery aneurysms in Kawasaki disease in a North American population. J Am Heart Assoc 2019;8(11):e011319.

25. de Graeff N, Groot N, Ozen S, et al. European consensus-based recommendations for the diagnosis and treatment of Kawasaki disease - the SHARE initiative. Rheumatology 2019;58(4):672–82.

26. Kobayashi T, Saji T, Otani T, et al. Efficacy of immunoglobulin plus prednisolone for prevention of coronary artery abnormalities in severe Kawasaki disease (RAISE study): a randomised, open-label, blinded-endpoints trial. Lancet 2012; 379(9826):1613–20.

27. Tremoulet AH, Jain S, Jaggi P, et al. Infliximab for intensification of primary therapy for Kawasaki disease: a phase 3 randomised, double-blind, placebo-controlled trial. Lancet 2014;383(9930):1731–8.

28. Burns JC, Best BM, Mejias A, et al. Infliximab treatment of intravenous immunoglobulin-resistant Kawasaki disease. J Pediatr 2008;153(6):833–8.

29. Yamaji N, da Silva Lopes K, Shoda T, et al. TNF-α blockers for the treatment of Kawasaki disease in children. Cochrane Database Syst Rev 2019;8(8): Cd012448.

30. Dillon MJ, Eleftheriou D, Brogan PA. Medium-size-vessel vasculitis. Pediatr Nephrol 2010;25(9):1641–52.

31. Bowyer S, Roettcher P. Pediatric rheumatology clinic populations in the United States: results of a 3 year survey. Pediatric Rheumatology Database Research Group. J Rheumatol 1996;23(11):1968–74.

32. Ozen S, Anton J, Arisoy N, et al. Juvenile polyarteritis: results of a multicenter survey of 110 children. J Pediatr 2004;145(4):517–22.

33. Eleftheriou D, Dillon MJ, Tullus K, et al. Systemic polyarteritis nodosa in the young: a single-center experience over thirty-two years. Arthritis Rheum 2013; 65(9):2476–85.

34. Caorsi R, Penco F, Grossi A, et al. ADA2 deficiency (DADA2) as an unrecognised cause of early onset polyarteritis nodosa and stroke: a multicentre national study. Ann Rheum Dis 2017;76(10):1648–56.

35. Navon Elkan P, Pierce SB, Segel R, et al. Mutant adenosine deaminase 2 in a polyarteritis nodosa vasculopathy. N Engl J Med 2014;370(10):921–31.

36. Ozen S, Ben-Chetrit E, Bakkaloglu A, et al. Polyarteritis nodosa in patients with Familial Mediterranean Fever (FMF): a concomitant disease or a feature of FMF? Semin Arthritis Rheum 2001;30(4):281–7.

37. Liu Y, Jesus AA, Marrero B, et al. Activated STING in a vascular and pulmonary syndrome. N Engl J Med 2014;371(6):507–18.

38. Ozen S, Ruperto N, Dillon MJ, et al. EULAR/PReS endorsed consensus criteria for the classification of childhood vasculitides. Ann Rheum Dis 2006;65(7):936–41.
39. Brogan PA, Arch B, Hickey H, et al. Mycophenolate mofetil versus cyclophosphamide for remission induction in childhood polyarteritis nodosa: an open label, randomised, Bayesian, non-inferiority trial. Arthritis Rheumatol March 24, 2021. https://doi.org/10.1002/art.41730.
40. Ginsberg S, Rosner I, Slobodin G, et al. Infliximab for the treatment of refractory polyarteritis nodosa. Clin Rheumatol 2019;38(10):2825–33.
41. Eleftheriou D, Melo M, Marks SD, et al. Biologic therapy in primary systemic vasculitis of the young. Rheumatology 2009;48(8):978–86.
42. Gardner-Medwin JM, Dolezalova P, Cummins C, et al. Incidence of Henoch-Schönlein purpura, Kawasaki disease, and rare vasculitides in children of different ethnic origins. Lancet 2002;360(9341):1197–202.
43. Weiss PF, Feinstein JA, Luan X, et al. Effects of corticosteroid on Henoch-Schönlein purpura: a systematic review. Pediatrics 2007;120(5):1079–87.
44. Saulsbury FT. Henoch-Schönlein purpura in children. Report of 100 patients and review of the literature. Medicine 1999;78(6):395–409.
45. Al-Sheyyab M, El-Shanti H, Ajlouni S, et al. The clinical spectrum of Henoch-Schönlein purpura in infants and young children. Eur J Pediatr 1995;154(12): 969–72.
46. Calviño MC, Llorca J, García-Porrúa C, et al. Henoch-Schönlein purpura in children from northwestern Spain: a 20-year epidemiologic and clinical study. Medicine 2001;80(5):279–90.
47. Weiss PF, Klink AJ, Luan X, et al. Temporal association of Streptococcus, Staphylococcus, and parainfluenza pediatric hospitalizations and hospitalized cases of Henoch-Schönlein purpura. J Rheumatol 2010;37(12):2587–94.
48. Farley TA, Gillespie S, Rasoulpour M, et al. Epidemiology of a cluster of Henoch-Schönlein purpura. Am J Dis Child 1989;143(7):798–803.
49. Huber AM, King J, McLaine P, et al. A randomized, placebo-controlled trial of prednisone in early Henoch Schönlein Purpura [ISRCTN85109383]. BMC Med 2004;2:7.
50. Narchi H. Risk of long term renal impairment and duration of follow up recommended for Henoch-Schonlein purpura with normal or minimal urinary findings: a systematic review. Arch Dis Child 2005;90(9):916–20.
51. Trygstad CW, Stiehm ER. Elevated serum IgA globulin in anaphylactoid purpura. Pediatrics 1971;47(6):1023–8.
52. Ronkainen J, Koskimies O, Ala-Houhala M, et al. Early prednisone therapy in Henoch-Schönlein purpura: a randomized, double-blind, placebo-controlled trial. J Pediatr 2006;149(2):241–7.
53. Weiss PF, Klink AJ, Localio R, et al. Corticosteroids may improve clinical outcomes during hospitalization for Henoch-Schönlein purpura. Pediatrics 2010; 126(4):674–81.
54. Dudley J, Smith G, Llewelyn-Edwards A, et al. Randomised, double-blind, placebo-controlled trial to determine whether steroids reduce the incidence and severity of nephropathy in Henoch-Schonlein Purpura (HSP). Arch Dis Child 2013;98(10):756–63.
55. Chartapisak W, Opastiraku S, Willis NS, et al. Prevention and treatment of renal disease in Henoch-Schönlein purpura: a systematic review. Arch Dis Child 2009;94(2):132–7.

56. Ozen S, Marks SD, Brogan P, et al. European consensus-based recommendations for diagnosis and treatment of immunoglobulin A vasculitis-the SHARE initiative. Rheumatology 2019;58(9):1607–16.

57. Saulsbury FT. Henoch-Schönlein purpura. Curr Opin Rheumatol 2010;22(5): 598–602.

58. Sacri AS, Chambaraud T, Ranchin B, et al. Clinical characteristics and outcomes of childhood-onset ANCA-associated vasculitis: a French nationwide study. Nephrol Dial Transpl 2015;30(Suppl 1):i104–12.

59. Jariwala MP, Laxer RM. Primary vasculitis in childhood: GPA and MPA in childhood. Front Pediatr 2018;6:226.

60. Hirano D, Ishikawa T, Inaba A, et al. Epidemiology and clinical features of childhood-onset anti-neutrophil cytoplasmic antibody-associated vasculitis: a clinicopathological analysis. Pediatr Nephrol 2019;34(8):1425–33.

61. Cabral DA, Canter DL, Muscal E, et al. Comparing presenting clinical features in 48 children with microscopic polyangiitis to 183 children who have granulomatosis with polyangiitis (Wegener's): An ARChiVe cohort study. Arthritis Rheumatol 2016;68(10):2514–26.

62. Lyons PA, Rayner TF, Trivedi S, et al. Genetically distinct subsets within ANCA-associated vasculitis. N Engl J Med 2012;367(3):214–23.

63. Jennette JC, Falk RJ. Pathogenesis of antineutrophil cytoplasmic autoantibody-mediated disease. Nat Rev Rheumatol 2014;10(8):463–73.

64. Wu EY, McInnis EA, Boyer-Suavet S, et al. Measuring circulating complement activation products in myeloperoxidase- and proteinase 3-antineutrophil cytoplasmic antibody-associated vasculitis. Arthritis Rheumatol 2019;71(11): 1894–903.

65. Wu EY, Hernandez ML, Jennette JC, et al. Eosinophilic granulomatosis with polyangiitis: clinical pathology conference and review. J Allergy Clin Immunol Pract 2018;6(5):1496–504.

66. Uribe AG, Huber AM, Kim S, et al. Increased sensitivity of the European medicines agency algorithm for classification of childhood granulomatosis with polyangiitis. J Rheumatol 2012;39(8):1687–97.

67. Iudici M, Pagnoux C, Quartier P, et al. Childhood- versus adult-onset ANCA-associated vasculitides: a nested, matched case-control study from the French Vasculitis Study Group Registry. Autoimmun Rev 2018;17(2):108–14.

68. Morishita KA, Moorthy LN, Lubieniecka JM, et al. Early outcomes in children with antineutrophil cytoplasmic antibody-associated vasculitis. Arthritis Rheumatol 2017;69(7):1470–9.

69. Dolezalova P, Price-Kuehne FE, Özen S, et al. Disease activity assessment in childhood vasculitis: development and preliminary validation of the Paediatric Vasculitis Activity Score (PVAS). Ann Rheum Dis 2013;72(10):1628–33.

70. Morishita KA, Wagner-Weiner L, Yen EY, et al. Consensus treatment plans for severe pediatric antineutrophil cytoplasmic antibody-associated vasculitis. Arthritis Care Res March 6, 2021. https://doi.org/10.1002/acr.24590.

71. Lee JJY, Alsaleem A, Chiang GPK, et al. Hallmark trials in ANCA-associated vasculitis (AAV) for the pediatric rheumatologist. Pediatr Rheumatol Online J 2019;17(1):31.

COVID-19 in Pediatrics

Siobhan Mary Case, MD, MHS[a,b],*, Mary Beth Son, MD[a]

KEYWORDS

- COVID-19 • Coronavirus • Multisystem inflammatory syndrome in children
(MIS-C) • Pediatric inflammatory multisystem syndrome temporally
related to SARS CoV-2 (PIMS-TS)

KEY POINTS

- Coronavirus disease 2019 in children is typically milder than adults; symptoms commonly include headache, fever, and cough.
- Severe coronavirus disease 2019 has been reported in the pediatric population, typically in children with underlying conditions.
- Multisystem inflammatory syndrome in children is a postinfectious sequela of severe acute respiratory syndrome coronavirus 2 infection that has prominent cardiovascular and gastrointestinal symptomatology.
- There are patients with features of both severe acute coronavirus disease 2019 and multisystem inflammatory syndrome in children, suggesting that further work is needed to characterize this overlap and refine disease definitions.

CORONAVIRUS DISEASE 2019 IN CHILDREN AND ADOLESCENTS

In 2019, a novel coronavirus emerged called severe acute respiratory syndrome coronavirus 2 (SARS-CoV-2), which causes coronavirus disease 2019 (COVID-19). Initially identified in Wuhan, China, COVID-19 spread internationally and became a global pandemic. Most pediatric COVID-19 cases were milder than in adults, but in the early spring of 2020, a new inflammatory syndrome emerged in children who had evidence of prior SARS CoV-2 infection, called multisystem inflammatory syndrome in children (MIS-C). This article describes the features, diagnosis, and treatment of pediatric COVID-19 and MIS-C based on the data available at the time of publication.

Incidence and Mortality Rates

As of March 2021, there were approximately 2,592,619 cases of COVID-19 in people under 18 in the United States and 300 deaths.[1] Of all American cases, 2.1% were in

[a] Division of Immunology, Boston Children's Hospital, 300 Longwood Avenue, Fegan, 6th Floor, Boston, Massachusetts 02115, USA; [b] Division of Rheumatology, Inflammation and Immunity, Brigham and Women's Hospital, 60 Fenwood Road, 3rd Floor, Boston, MA 02115, USA
* Corresponding author.
E-mail address: siobhan.case@childrens.harvard.edu
Twitter: @sio322 (S.M.C.)

Rheum Dis Clin N Am 47 (2021) 797–811
https://doi.org/10.1016/j.rdc.2021.07.006
0889-857X/21/© 2021 Elsevier Inc. All rights reserved.

rheumatic.theclinics.com

children aged 0 to 4 years old, and another 10.2% were in those aged 5 to 17.[1] Prevalence varies by age, with estimates ranging from 17% for children under 2 years old to 25% of children ages 6 to 10 years old, and 23% in 10 to 14 years old.[2]

The severity of the disease is generally lower for children, with only 1% to 5% of pediatric cases qualifying as severe versus to 10% to 20% in adults.[3] This finding is thought to reflect the lower levels of angiotensin-converting enzyme 2 expression in alveolar cells, which is the mechanism by which SARS-CoV-2 enters cells.[3] Likewise, mortality rates are estimated at 0.3% (95% confidence interval, 0.1–0.4) in patients under 21 years of age,[2] in comparison with 5.8% for American adults.[4] Being older than 12 years and having a high initial C-reactive protein (CRP) are risk factors for admission to a pediatric intensive care unit, and high CRP, leukocytosis, and thrombocytopenia are risk factors for organ dysfunction.[5] Viral load and young age, specifically children under 1 year of age, are other risk factors for more severe disease.[6]

Clinical Features

Presenting symptoms in pediatric COVID-19 cases are variable (**Table 1**).[2] Estimates of asymptomatic infection range from 13% to 50% of pediatric cases.[2] The median time from exposure to onset of symptoms is 7 days.[7] Of symptomatic cases, headache occurs in approximately two-thirds and fever and cough in about one-half.[2] Gastrointestinal symptoms, sore throat, and rhinorrhea are rare,[2] although patients with more severe COVID-19 experience gastrointestinal and upper respiratory symptoms.[8]

The definition of severe COVID-19 in children varies, but includes requiring inpatient care and having at least 1 severe organ system manifestation and a positive reverse transcriptase polymerase chain reaction test for SARS CoV-2 infection.[8] Among severe cases described in the United States Overcoming COVID-19 network, the majority (71%) had severe respiratory disease, whereas less than 3% had severe cardiovascular involvement and 9% had severe cardiorespiratory involvement. Of these patients, one-half required some form of respiratory support, including 15% on mechanical ventilation and 1.4% on extracorporeal membrane oxygenation.[8] Neurologic manifestations were noted in 20% of patients in the same cohort.[9] When considering both patients with severe COVID-19 and MIS-C with neurologic manifestations, 12% had potentially life-threatening complications, including encephalopathy, stroke, cerebral edema, demyelination, and Guillain–Barré syndrome.[9]

Comorbidities

Previously healthy children are susceptible to a severe COVID-19 course, including death.[10] However, the majority of severe and/or hospitalized cases had comorbidities, such as asthma, immunosuppression, and neurologic disease.[10–12] A history of prematurity, asthma, or diabetes; an immunocompromised state; and gastrointestinal disease are associated with an increased odds of admission.[13] Furthermore, those with asthma and gastrointestinal disease are more likely to require respiratory support.[13] Obesity is associated with a higher risk of severe COVID-19.[12] Patients with chronic conditions may have a concomitant worsening of their underlying disease, including diabetic ketoacidosis and acute chest syndrome.[5]

Coinfection with other viruses and bacteria is an important consideration. A meta-analysis found that 5.6% of pediatric patients had a coinfection; within this group, 58% had *Mycoplasma pneumoniae*, 11.1% had influenza A or B, 9.7% had respiratory syncytial virus; the remainder had other common types of viral and bacterial infections.[11]

Table 1
Symptoms in pediatric COVID-19 and MIS-C

Symptom	Pediatric COVID-19	MIS-C
Asymptomatic	13%[2]	0% by definition
Fever	55%[2]	100% by definition
Respiratory	Cough in 45%, dyspnea in 19%[2]	14%[2]
Cardiovascular	N/A[a]	71%[2] Shock in 35%, cardiac dysfunction in 40%, hypotension in 50%[41]
Gastrointestinal	6%[2]	87%[2] Abdominal pain, vomiting, and diarrhea
Mucocutaneous	N/A[b]	73%[2] Rash in 53%, conjunctivitis in 48%, mucocutaneous lesions in 35%[41]
Neurologic	Headache in 67%[2]	22%[2]

Abbreviation: N/A, not applicable.
[a] In severe cases, 2.9%.[8]
[b] In severe cases, 10.2%.[8]

Thrombotic complications from COVID-19 such as deep vein thrombosis and pulmonary embolism were seen in 2.1% of pediatric cases in a multicenter retrospective cohort study in the United States, sometimes despite thromboprophylaxis.[14]

Laboratory evaluations

In a meta-analysis of pediatric cases, the most common laboratory findings were high ferritin and procalcitonin in approximately 25% and high CRP in approximately 20% of patients.[2] The mean CRP among pediatric cases of COVID-19 is estimated at 9.4 mg/L.[11] In contrast with adult cases, the leukocyte count was normal in around 70% of cases, with 15% each having leukopenia or leukocytosis.[15] D-Dimer, IL-6, and creatinine kinase may also be elevated.[11]

Imaging

In reported pediatric cases, the chest radiographs were normal in roughly one-third, and another one-third showed focal consolidations; the remainder demonstrated ground glass opacities.[2,11] A systematic review of chest computed tomography (CT) scans in pediatric cases found that 61.5% showed either consolidations or ground glass opacities; 26.5% were normal.[16]

Treatment

Patients with mild or moderate symptoms of COVID-19 often do well with supportive care alone. However, therapies such as monoclonal antibodies, antiviral therapy, glucocorticoids (GC), and immunosuppression may be indicated.

Monoclonal antibodies, such as bamlanivimab–etesevimab and casirivimab–imdevimab, have emergency use authorization through the US Food and Drug Administration in pediatric patients who present with mild to moderate disease and who are at high risk for progression to severe disease.[17,18] High-risk conditions include obesity, chronic respiratory disease, chronic kidney disease, and immunocompromised states, such as those with rheumatologic disease who are on immunosuppressive therapy.

Antiviral therapy with remdesivir should be considered for patients with a positive SARS-CoV-2 polymerase chain reaction test and severe or critical manifestations of either COVID-19.

GC may be an option for pediatric patients who require respiratory support, but data are lacking.[19] GC may also be considered for patients with concurrent acute respiratory distress syndrome, septic shock, or adrenal insufficiency.

Convalescent plasma has an emergency use authorization from the US Food and Drug Administration for adult patients who are critically ill with COVID-19,[20] but its use has not been well-studied in pediatric patients with COVID-19.[21] If considered, it should be administered early in the course of illness, especially if there is no improvement after remdesivir and GC, and for those patients with impaired humoral immunity.

Finally, antiplatelet and anticoagulation therapy should be considered to prevent thrombotic complications. Experts have recommended prophylactic low molecular weight heparin in children hospitalized for COVID-19 or MIS-C who are at higher risk for thrombosis, including elevated D-dimer, risk factors for severe SARS-CoV-2–related disease, or risk factors for venous thromboembolism, such as a family history, obesity, and chronic inflammatory conditions.[22]

Treatment resistance and complications
A subset of adult patients develop high levels of inflammation around the second week of COVID-19, termed COVID-19–associated hyperinflammatory syndrome.[23] Frequent manifestations include fever, high ferritin, liver injury, hematologic abnormalities, coagulopathy, and high levels of inflammatory cytokines, specifically CRP and IL-6. There have been several adult trials for COVID-19–associated hyperinflammatory syndrome, primarily with tocilizumab, with conflicting results.[24,25] The use of tocilizumab in pediatric patients with COVID-19 has not been studied formally. The American College of Rheumatology (ACR) has issued guidelines for pediatric patients with COVID-19 who develop hyperinflammation; recommendations include anakinra and consideration of other therapies with less evidence, including GC and tociliuzumab.[26]

Outcomes and Long-Term Recommendations

Data are still emerging on the long-term outcomes after COVID-19 in children. In a small case series from China, a repeat CT scan approximately 30 days after discharge showed that one-half of pediatric patients had imaging abnormalities, but dyspnea scores were all mild and improving, and no patients required oxygen.[27]

In adults, long COVID has been described with symptoms of headache, fatigue, dyspnea, and anosmia lasting for weeks to months after infection.[28] The full spectrum of long COVID, or postacute sequelae of SARS-CoV-2 infection, has not yet been fully characterized in children, but efforts are underway.

Currently, messenger RNA vaccines against SARS-CoV-2 have been approved for patients age 12 and older; large pediatric trials are assembled with results expected by summer 2021. Vaccination is recommended for eligible people who have had COVID-19, but delaying vaccination for 90 days after the acute illness is recommended.

COVID-19 in Pediatric Rheumatic Diseases

The ACR has issued guidance regarding medication management in children with rheumatologic disease in the setting of the SARS-CoV-2 pandemic.[29] Pediatric patients with chronic rheumatologic disease do not uniformly seem to be at a higher risk of COVID-19. In adults, there is a higher odds of death in those with moderate to high rheumatologic disease activity and certain medications, including GC, rituximab, and sulfasalazine.[30] Similar data have not been reported in pediatric rheumatic diseases, but are being collected. To date, specific guidance has not been issued regarding SARS-CoV-2 vaccination in pediatric rheumatology patients, but the ACR has recommended holding certain immunosuppressives for adults with rheumatic disease around vaccination.[31]

MULTISYSTEM INFLAMMATORY SYNDROME IN CHILDREN

MIS-C is a potentially life-threatening condition that can have acute, severe cardiovascular symptoms. It is presumably a post infectious phenomenon following SARS-CoV-2 infection and[32,33] is considered on the spectrum of postacute sequelae of SARS-CoV-2 infection manifestations. This syndrome was first described with a cluster of children presenting with hyperinflammatory shock in London in mid-April of 2020.[34] Soon thereafter, cases rose globally, prompting the Centers for Disease Control and Prevention (CDC) to define MIS-C in May.[35] The case definition for MIS-C from the CDC, the World Health Organization (WHO),[36] and Royal College of Pediatrics and Child Health[37] are outlined in **Table 2**.

The timing of symptom onset is typically 3 to 6 weeks after exposure to SARS-CoV-2 (**Fig. 1**).[38] The majority of patients with MIS-C did not have significant illness at the time of the inciting SARS-CoV-2 infection. Of note, this time frame is longer than that seen for hyperinflammatory states from COVID-19.

Incidence and Mortality Rates

As of early April 2021, there were 3185 cases of MIS-C in the United States and 36 deaths reported to the CDC.[35] The incidence is low, with an estimated 2 in 200,000 people under 21 years of age.[39] In a systematic review of global cases including 665 patients, 11 patients (1.7%) died.[40]

MIS-C is more commonly seen in males (59%) than females.[38] The median age is between 7.3 and 10.0 years,[40,41] and a similar illness can rarely be seen in adults.[42] Patients with MIS-C aged 6 to 12 and 13 to 20 years were more likely than those aged 0 to 5 years to require intensive care.[43] There is a greater incidence among patients identifying as racial or ethnic minorities, especially people with African, Afro-Caribbean, and Hispanic ancestries.[26,40] In a meta-analysis, between 31% and 62% of patients identified as Black or Afro-Caribbean, and 36% to 39% as Hispanic.[38] Intensive care unit admission is also more common among patients identifying as non-Hispanic Black, compared with non-Hispanic White.[43] It is not clear whether these race-based differences are due to genetics, inequities in social determinants of health impacting exposure to SARS-CoV-2, or both.[38,41] Obesity is common in patients with MIS-C, with roughly one-half of patients qualifying as overweight or obese based on body mass index.[44]

Clinical Features

Patients with MIS-C have fever and involvement of at least 2 organ systems. The most common symptoms are gastrointestinal, mucocutaneous, and cardiovascular (see **Table 1**).[38] The mucocutaneous features and rash in MIS-C have invoked comparisons to Kawasaki disease.[45] The rash is variable, and mucocutaneous symptoms occur quickly, within a mean of 2.7 days after start of fever.[46] Roughly one-quarter to one-half of patients with MIS-C also met the criteria for Kawasaki disease, most commonly the incomplete presentation.[26,40] Nearly one-quarter of patients have myocarditis, making hypotension and shock common presenting symptoms.[40] Other

Table 2
Definitions of MIS-C and PIMS-TS

Organization	Centers for Disease Control and Prevention	World Health Organization	Royal College of Pediatrics and Child Health
Population	Individuals aged <21 y	Individuals aged <20 y	Children
Clinical symptoms	Fever: >38.0 °C for ≥24 h, or report of subjective fever lasting ≥24 h AND both of the following: Evidence of clinically severe illness requiring hospitalization Multisystem (>2) organ involvement: cardiac, renal, respiratory, hematologic, gastrointestinal, dermatologic or neurologic	Fever: >3 d AND two of the following: Rash or bilateral nonpurulent conjunctivitis or mucocutaneous inflammation signs (oral, hands or feet) Hypotension or shock Features of myocardial dysfunction, pericarditis, valvulitis, or coronary abnormalities (including echocardiographic findings or elevated troponin/N-terminal pro B-type natriuretic protein) Evidence of coagulopathy (by prothrombin time, partial thromboplastin time, elevated D-dimers) Acute gastrointestinal problems (diarrhea, vomiting, or abdominal pain)	Fever: >38.5 °C and persistent AND evidence of single or multiorgan dysfunction: Shock Cardiac disorder Respiratory disorder Renal disorder Gastrointestinal disorder Neurologic disorder
Laboratory evidence of inflammation	AND one or more of the following: Elevated CRP Elevated ESR Elevated fibrinogen Elevated ferritin Elevated LDH Elevated IL-6	AND elevated markers of inflammation such as: ESR CRP Procalcitonin	AND inflammation: Neutrophilia Elevated CRP Lymphopenia

Elevated neutrophils
Low lymphocytes
Low albumin

SARS-CoV-2 testing	AND one of the following: Positive for current or recent SARS-CoV-2 infection by RT-PCR, serology, or antigen test COVID-19 exposure within the 4 wk before the onset of symptoms	AND one of the following: Evidence of COVID-19: RT-PCR, antigen test or serology positive Likely contact with patients with COVID-19	AND: Positive or negative SARS-CoV-2 PCR testing
Evaluation of other diagnoses	AND: No alternative plausible diagnoses	AND: No other obvious microbial cause of inflammation, including bacterial sepsis, staphylococcal or streptococcal shock syndromes	AND: Exclusion of any other microbial cause, including bacterial sepsis, staphylococcal or streptococcal shock syndromes, infections associated with myocarditis such as enterovirus (waiting for results of these investigations should not delay seeking expert advice) This may include children fulfilling full or partial criteria for Kawasaki disease

Abbreviations: ESR, erythrocyte sedimentation rate; RT-PCR, reverse transcriptase polymerase chain reaction test.

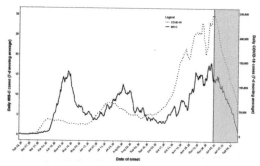

Fig. 1. CDC daily MIS-C cases and COVID-19 cases (7-day moving average). The graph shows the 7-day average number of MIS-C and COVID-19 cases with MIS-C date of onset between February 19, 2020, and February 21, 2021. The grayed-out area on the right side represents the most recent 6 weeks of data, for which reporting of MIS-C cases is still incomplete. (From Centers for Disease C. Daily MIS-C Cases and COVID-19 Cases (Seven-Day Moving Average). https://www.cdc.gov/mis-c/cases/index.html Published 2021. Accessed March 1, 2021.)

cardiac complications include arrhythmia, left ventricular (LV) dysfunction, and coronary artery ectasia or aneurysms.[6] Neurologic symptoms occur in 22%, including headache, altered mental status, and aseptic meningitis.[9,40] In contrast with patients with acute COVID-19, rhinorrhea and cough are only seen in 13% and 7% of patients, respectively.[44]

The ACR has issued guidelines for a tiered diagnostic evaluation of MIS-C (**Table 3**).[26] Hospitalization is recommended for patients with potential MIS-C, because patients are at risk for rapid evolution to severe illness. Hypotension, driven by either decreased LV function and/or vasodilatory shock, can require urgent intervention.[8,32]

Differential diagnosis

A broad differential, including infection and malignancy, should be entertained when considering MIS-C, because many features are nonspecific and overlap with sepsis.[26] Patients with MIS-C may have superimposed bacterial infections and should be covered empirically with antibiotics when indicated clinically.[6]

The presentation of MIS-C has similarities to other inflammatory conditions including Kawasaki disease, toxic shock syndrome, and macrophage activation syndrome. Among patients with Kawasaki-like features, 26% experienced shock, which is much higher than the 5% typically seen in US patients who present with Kawasaki disease shock syndrome.[47] A British study compared pediatric patients with MIS-C with patients with Kawasaki disease with or without shock, and toxic shock syndrome.[48] Patients with MIS-C were older (median age, 9.0 years vs 2.7 years), had more hematologic abnormalities, and higher elevations in CRP, troponin, and fibrinogen compared with those with Kawasaki disease. Compared with patients with toxic shock syndrome, patients with MIS-C were older with more profound anemia and higher CRP and alanine aminotransferase levels. Both patients with macrophage activation syndrome and MIS-C have cytopenias, hyperferritinemia, coagulopathy, and high soluble IL-2 receptor.[49] However, increases in ferritin, high soluble IL-2 receptor, IL-18, and CXCL9 are less marked in MIS-C as compared with macrophage activation syndrome.[49]

Laboratory features

Inflammatory markers are elevated, including the erythrocyte sedimentation rate, CRP, and ferritin.[40] The median initial CRP is higher among patients requiring pediatric intensive care unit admission and in those who develop organ dysfunction.[5]

Table 3
ACR guidelines for diagnostic evaluation of MIS-C

Patient Population	Testing
Patients presenting with: 1. Fever 2. An epidemiologic link to SARS-CoV-2 3. AND clinical features of MIS-C: gastrointestinal symptoms, neurologic symptoms, and features of Kawasaki disease And without shock	Tier 1: Complete blood cell count Complete metabolic panel ESR CRP SARS CoV-2 PCR and antibodies
Patients with concerning features on tier 1 testing: Elevated inflammatory markers (ESR ≥40 mm/h or CRP ≥5 mg/dL) AND one other suggestive laboratory feature (absolute lymphocyte count <1000/μL, neutrophilia, platelet count <150,000/μL, sodium <135 mmol/L, hypoalbuminemia)	Tier 2: B-type natriuretic peptide Troponin T Procalcitonin Ferritin Prothrombin Partial thromboplastin time D-Dimer Fibrinogen Lactate dehydrogenase Urinalysis Cytokine panel Triglycerides SARS-CoV-2 serologies (if not sent in tier 1) Electrocardiogram Echocardiogram

Abbreviation: ESR, erythrocyte sedimentation rate.
 Data from Henderson LA, Canna SW, Friedman KG, et al. American College of Rheumatology Clinical Guidance for Pediatric Patients with Multisystem Inflammatory Syndrome in Children (MIS-C) Associated with SARS-CoV-2 and Hyperinflammation in COVID-19. Version 2. Arthritis Rheumatol. 2020.

Lymphopenia is common (58%), and approximately 20% have neutrophilia, anemia, or thrombocytopenia.[40] A higher median initial white blood cell count and lower median initial platelet count were seen in patients who develop organ dysfunction.[5] As for cardiac markers, around 40% have elevated B-type natriuretic peptide and more than 30% have high troponin.[40] High B-type natriuretic peptide and troponin, and low platelets and lymphocytes are associated with need for intensive care.[43] Coagulation studies commonly show elevations in D-dimer and fibrinogen. Cytokine levels are typically elevated for IL-6, IL-10, soluble IL-2 receptor, and tumor necrosis factor.[26,49,50]

 After the initial evaluation, the erythrocyte sedimentation rate, CRP, B-type natriuretic peptide, and troponin T levels should be trended closely to monitor for development of sometimes rapidly progressive cardiac involvement and ongoing inflammation.[26]

 Approximately 75% to 100% of patients have positive SARS-CoV-2 antibodies (IgG or IgM), whereas reverse transcriptase polymerase chain reaction testing is more variable, ranging from 13% to 69%.[26,38] In 1 study, 7% had positive antibodies and reverse transcriptase polymerase chain reaction test, whereas another 15% had negative testing but had been exposed to family members who were positive.[40]

Imaging

Reports of lung imaging abnormalities have varied, with a meta-analysis demonstrating that 13.7% of patients with MIS-C had findings on radiographs or CT scans,[40] which is less than in acute COVID-19. A recent study comparing severe acute COVID-19 versus MIS-C in a single large cohort (n = 1116) revealed similarities in rates of infiltrates on chest radiography, with 37% of acute severe COVID-19 versus 38% of patients with MIS-C having the finding.[8]

Echocardiography can reveal a decreased LV ejection fraction and coronary artery ectasia or aneurysm. Arrythmias have been reported, usually during the acute illness,[51] and ACR guidelines recommend obtaining electrocardiograms every 48 hours during hospitalization and at follow-up visits, with escalation to telemetry and possible outpatient Holter monitoring for those with conduction abnormalities.[26] Echocardiograms are likewise recommended at diagnosis and during subsequent follow-up, including 1 to 2 weeks and 4 to 6 weeks after presentation at a minimum.[26] A cardiac CT scan may be needed to identify distal coronary artery aneurysms not seen on an echocardiogram. Cardiac MRI may be indicated for those with significant or persistent LV dysfunction.[26]

Treatment

The ACR guidelines for treatment of MIS-C recommend[26] intravenous immunoglobulin (IVIG, 2 g/kg per ideal body weight), which may need to be administered slowly for those with abnormal cardiac function and/or volume overload. For those with moderate to severe symptoms, IVIG with GC is the first tier of therapy.[26] GC can also be given for refractory disease at low-to-moderate doses of 1 to 2 mg/kg/d, with a taper over 2 to 3 weeks. For patients refractory to first-line therapy, pulse doses of methylprednisolone (10–30 mg/kg/dose) and/or anakinra can be considered. Observational studies have suggested that giving IVIG and GC together was superior to IVIG alone in regard to the resolution of fever within 2 days, need for second-line therapy or hemodynamic support, acute LV dysfunction after the initial therapy, duration of intensive care unit stay,[52] and time to improvement of cardiac function.[53]

Antiplatelet therapy and anticoagulation may be indicated for patients with MIS-C.[26] The ACR recommends low-dose aspirin of 3 to 5 mg/kg/d up to a maximum dose of 81 mg in those with features of Kawasaki disease, coronary artery aneurysm, or thrombocytosis. Anticoagulation should be started for patients with coronary artery aneurysm with a z-score of more than 10, and considered for those with LV ejection fraction of less than 35%. If vasopressor agents are required, epinephrine followed by norepinephrine is recommended; dobutamine may also be effective for those with severe myocardial dysfunction.[6]

Short-term outcomes and complications

The median hospital stay for patients with MIS-C is 7.9 ± 0.6 days.[44] A study early in the pandemic noted that 80% of patients required intensive care unit admission.[33] In a systematic review of 505 cases, more than one-half of patients (57%) required vasopressor agents, 26% required mechanical ventilation, and 5% required extracorporeal membrane oxygenation.[54] Nearly 12% had acute kidney injury. Thromboses were rare, in only 3.5% of patients, but this finding was in the setting of more than one-half of patients receiving anticoagulation.

The cardiovascular burden in MIS-C is significant. In a European cohort study, the most common findings in MIS-C included shock, arrhythmias, pericardial effusion, and coronary artery aneurysm.[32] More than one-half of the patients had a depressed

LV ejection fraction and the majority had high troponin. A recent CDC report found that elevated CRP, ferritin, d-Dimer, and markers of cardiac injury (troponin, B-type natriuretic peptide, and pro B-type natriuretic peptide) were associated with decreased cardiac function in a cohort of more than 1000 children with MIS-C.[43] Rates of coronary artery abnormalities have ranged from 13%[8] to almost 19%.[41] The majority of aneurysms reported to date have been small with z scores of 2.5 to 5.0 or greater,[8,32,33] with very few giant aneurysms reported.[48] First-degree atrioventricular block has also been noted in approximately 20% of patients with MIS-C in several small retrospective cohort studies,[51,55] and can progress to second- or third-degree atrioventricular block.[51] Short-term follow-up has not been studied extensively yet, but Feldstein and colleagues[8] reported that decreased LV systolic function resolved in 91% (156 of 172 patients), as did the coronary artery aneurysms in 79% (45 of 57 patients) at 30 days of follow-up. An example of cardiac dysfunction on echocardiogram and first degree atrioventricular block on electrocardiogram are shown in **Fig. 2**.

There are reports of venous thromboembolism in 6.5% of patients with MIS-C, compared with 2.1% with symptomatic and 0.7% of asymptomatic COVID-19 cases.[14] This finding is thought to be related to abnormalities in the coagulation

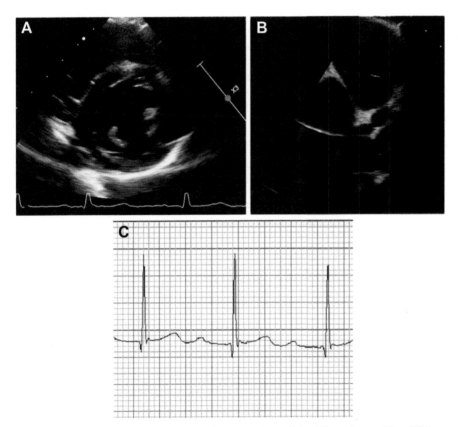

Fig. 2. Cardiac dysfunction in MIS-C. (*A*) Short axis view of the bilateral ventricles. (*B*) Parasternal short axis showing the aortic valve and coronary aneurysms of the left main coronary artery and proximal left anterior descending artery. (*C*) Electrocardiogram with first-degree atrioventricular block and a PR interval of 280 ms. (Courtesy of Audrey Dionne)

cascade. Risk factors include age greater than 12 years, cancer, and central venous catheters.[14]

Outcomes and Long-Term Recommendations

Studies are needed on the long-term outcomes and recommendations for monitoring for patients with a history of MIS-C. Patients should be followed by rheumatology, infectious disease, cardiology, hematology, and other subspecialties as needed based on disease manifestations.

FUTURE DIRECTIONS

In May of 2020, the CDC definition of MIS-C was made deliberately broad to capture all cases of a newly emergent syndrome as well as the spectrum of illness in MIS-C. However, the definition likely needs to be refined and narrowed. Increasing seroprevalence to SARS CoV-2 owing to natural infection in addition to vaccination will also complicate the ability to make the diagnosis going forward. Last, the cause of the disproportionate burden of MIS-C in Black and Hispanic children and adolescents requires further investigation.

SUMMARY AND DISCUSSION

The manifestations of COVID-19 are typically milder in children than adults, although severe cases can occur in otherwise healthy children and more commonly in those with underlying conditions. MIS-C is a postinfectious hyperinflammatory syndrome occurring weeks after SARS-CoV-2 exposure that has distinct clinical features including gastrointestinal, mucocutaneous, and cardiac symptoms, and is characterized by high levels of inflammation. More data is needed to define optimal treatments of both pediatric COVID-19 and MIS-C, as well as long-term outcomes.

CLINICS CARE POINTS

- COVID-19 infection in children can be mild or asymptomatic. Patients at a greater risk for severe disease or complications include children under 1 year of age, as well as those with obesity, other chronic conditions and Black or Hispanic race/ethnicity.
- Consider MIS-C in patients with previous COVID-19 or exposure who present with fever, high levels of inflammation, and gastrointestinal, mucocutaneous, and cardiovascular symptoms.
- The criteria for MIS-C are broad. Alternative and comorbid diagnoses should be considered, including hyperinflammatory response to acute COVID-19, toxic shock syndrome and other bacterial infections, autoimmune disease, and malignancy.

DISCLOSURE

The authors have nothing to disclose.

REFERENCES

1. Centers for Disease Control. Demographic trends of COVID-19 cases and deaths in the US reported to CDC 2021. Available at: https://covid.cdc.gov/covid-data-tracker/?CDC_AA_refVal=https%3A%2F%2Fwww.cdc.gov%2Fcoronavirus%2F2019-ncov%2Fcases-updates%2Fcases-in-us.html#demographics. Accessed April 7, 2021.

2. Badal S, Thapa Bajgain K, Badal S, et al. Prevalence, clinical characteristics, and outcomes of pediatric COVID-19: a systematic review and meta-analysis. J Clin Virol 2020;135:104715.
3. Kabeerdoss J, Pilania RK, Karkhele R, et al. Severe COVID-19, multisystem inflammatory syndrome in children, and Kawasaki disease: immunological mechanisms, clinical manifestations and management. Rheumatol Int 2021;41(1):19–32.
4. Loomba RS, Aggarwal G, Aggarwal S, et al. Disparities in case frequency and mortality of coronavirus disease 2019 (COVID-19) among various states in the United States. Ann Med 2021;53(1):151–9.
5. Fisler G, Izard SM, Shah S, et al. Characteristics and risk factors associated with critical illness in pediatric COVID-19. Ann Intensive Care 2020;10(1):171.
6. Jiang L, Tang K, Levin M, et al. COVID-19 and multisystem inflammatory syndrome in children and adolescents. Lancet Infect Dis 2020;20(11):e276–88.
7. Patel NA. Pediatric COVID-19: systematic review of the literature. Am J Otolaryngol 2020;41(5):102573.
8. Feldstein LR, Tenforde MW, Friedman KG, et al. Characteristics and outcomes of US children and adolescents with multisystem inflammatory syndrome in children (MIS-C) compared with severe acute COVID-19. JAMA 2021;325(11):1074–87.
9. LaRovere KL, Riggs BJ, Poussaint TY, et al. Neurologic involvement in children and adolescents hospitalized in the United States for COVID-19 or multisystem inflammatory syndrome. JAMA Neurol 2021;78(5):536–47.
10. Oualha M, Bendavid M, Berteloot L, et al. Severe and fatal forms of COVID-19 in children. Arch Pediatr 2020;27(5):235–8.
11. Hoang A, Chorath K, Moreira A, et al. COVID-19 in 7780 pediatric patients: a systematic review. EClinicalMedicine 2020;24:100433.
12. Tsankov BK, Allaire JM, Irvine MA, et al. Severe COVID-19 infection and pediatric comorbidities: a systematic review and meta-analysis. Int J Infect Dis 2021;103:246–56.
13. Graff K, Smith C, Silveira L, et al. Risk factors for severe COVID-19 in children. Pediatr Infect Dis J 2021;40(4):e137–45.
14. Whitworth HB, Sartain SE, Kumar R, et al. Rate of thrombosis in children and adolescents hospitalized with COVID-19 or MIS-C. Blood 2021;138(2):190–8.
15. Henry BM, Lippi G, Plebani M. Laboratory abnormalities in children with novel coronavirus disease 2019. Clin Chem Lab Med 2020;58(7):1135–8.
16. Katal S, Johnston SK, Johnston JH, et al. Imaging findings of SARS-CoV-2 infection in pediatrics: a systematic review of coronavirus disease 2019 (COVID-19) in 850 patients. Acad Radiol 2020;27(11):1608–21.
17. Federal Drug Administration: Silver Spring, Maryland, USA. Fact sheet for health care providers emergency use authorization (EUA) of bamlanivimab [press release] 2020.
18. Federal Drug Administration: Silver Spring, Maryland, USA. Fact sheet for health care providers emergency use authorization (EUA) of casirivimab and imdevimab [press release] 2020.
19. WHO. Rapid evidence appraisal for COVID-19 Therapies Working Group, Sterne JAC, Murthy S, Diaz JV, et al. Association between administration of systemic corticosteroids and mortality among critically Ill patients with COVID-19: a meta-analysis. JAMA 2020;324(13):1330–41.
20. Fact sheet for healthcare providers: emergency use authorization (EUA) of COVID-19 convalescent plasma for treatment of hospitalized patients with COVID-19 [press release]; Silver Spring, Maryland, USA:Federal Drug Administration.

21. Diorio C, Anderson EM, McNerney KO, et al. Convalescent plasma for pediatric patients with SARS-CoV-2-associated acute respiratory distress syndrome. Pediatr Blood Cancer 2020;67(11):e28693.

22. Goldenberg NA, Sochet A, Albisetti M, et al. Consensus-based clinical recommendations and research priorities for anticoagulant thromboprophylaxis in children hospitalized for COVID-19-related illness. J Thromb Haemost 2020;18(11):3099–105.

23. Webb BJ, Peltan ID, Jensen P, et al. Clinical criteria for COVID-19-associated hyperinflammatory syndrome: a cohort study. Lancet Rheumatol 2020;2(12):e754–63.

24. Tocilizumab reduces deaths in patients hospitalised with COVID-19 [press release]; Oxford, United Kingdom: Nuffield Department of Population Health.

25. Okoh AK, Bishburg E, Grinberg S, et al. Tocilizumab use in COVID-19-associated pneumonia. J Med Virol 2021;93(2):1023–8.

26. Henderson LA, Canna SW, Friedman KG, et al. American College of Rheumatology clinical guidance for pediatric patients with multisystem inflammatory syndrome in children (MIS-C) associated with SARS-CoV-2 and hyperinflammation in COVID-19. Version 2. Arthritis Rheumatol 2020;2(11):1791–805.

27. Zhang C, Huang L, Tang X, et al. Pulmonary sequelae of pediatric patients after discharge for COVID-19: an observational study. Pediatr Pulmonol 2021.

28. Nalbandian A, Sehgal K, Gupta A, et al. Post-acute COVID-19 syndrome. Nat Med 2021;27(4):601–15.

29. Wahezi DM, Lo MS, Rubinstein TB, et al. American College of Rheumatology guidance for the management of pediatric rheumatic disease during the COVID-19 pandemic: version 1. Arthritis Rheumatol 2020;72(11):1809–19.

30. Strangfeld A, Schafer M, Gianfrancesco MA, et al. Factors associated with COVID-19-related death in people with rheumatic diseases: results from the COVID-19 Global Rheumatology Alliance physician-reported registry. Ann Rheum Dis 2021;80(7):930–42.

31. Rheumatology ACo:Atlanta, Georgia, USA. COVID-19 vaccine clinical guidance summary for patients with rheumatic and Musculoskeletal diseases 2021.

32. Valverde I, Singh Y, Sanchez-de-Toledo J, et al. Acute cardiovascular manifestations in 286 children with multisystem inflammatory syndrome associated with COVID-19 infection in Europe. Circulation 2021;143(1):21–32.

33. Feldstein LR, Rose EB, Horwitz SM, et al. Multisystem inflammatory syndrome in U.S. children and adolescents. N Engl J Med 2020;383(4):334–46.

34. Riphagen S, Gomez X, Gonzalez-Martinez C, et al. Hyperinflammatory shock in children during COVID-19 pandemic. Lancet 2020;395(10237):1607–8.

35. Health department-reported cases of multisystem inflammatory syndrome in children (MIS-C) in the United States. Centers for Disease Control. 2021. Available at: https://www.cdc.gov/mis-c/cases/index.html. Accessed April 4, 2021.

36. World Health Organization. Multisystem inflammatory syndrome in children and adolescents with COVID-19. 2021. Available at: https://www.who.int/publications/i/item/multisystem-inflammatory-syndrome-in-children-and-adolescents-with-covid-19. Accessed April 4th, 2021.

37. Royal College of Paediatrics and Child Health. Guidance: paediatric multisystem inflammatory syndrome temporally associated with COVID-19. 2020. Available at: https://www.rcpch.ac.uk/resources/paediatric-multisystem-inflammatory-syndrome-temporally-associated-covid-19-pims-guidance. Accessed April 4th, 2021.

38. Abrams JY, Godfred-Cato SE, Oster ME, et al. Multisystem inflammatory syndrome in children associated with severe acute respiratory syndrome coronavirus 2: a systematic review. J Pediatr 2020;226:45–54.
39. Dufort EM, Koumans EH, Chow EJ, et al. Multisystem inflammatory syndrome in children in New York State. N Engl J Med 2020;383(4):347–58.
40. Kaushik A, Gupta S, Sood M, et al. A systematic review of multisystem inflammatory syndrome in children associated with SARS-CoV-2 infection. Pediatr Infect Dis J 2020;39(11):e340–6.
41. Godfred-Cato S, Bryant B, Leung J, et al. COVID-19-associated multisystem inflammatory syndrome in children - United States, March-July 2020. MMWR Morb Mortal Wkly Rep 2020;69(32):1074–80.
42. Morris SB, Schwartz NG, Patel P, et al. Case series of multisystem inflammatory syndrome in adults associated with SARS-CoV-2 infection - United Kingdom and United States, March-August 2020. MMWR Morb Mortal Wkly Rep 2020;69(40):1450–6.
43. Abrams JY, Oster ME, Godfred-Cato SE, et al. Factors linked to severe outcomes in multisystem inflammatory syndrome in children (MIS-C) in the USA: a retrospective surveillance study. Lancet Child Adolesc Health 2021;5(5):323–31.
44. Ahmed M, Advani S, Moreira A, et al. Multisystem inflammatory syndrome in children: a systematic review. EClinicalMedicine 2020;26:100527.
45. Verdoni L, Mazza A, Gervasoni A, et al. An outbreak of severe Kawasaki-like disease at the Italian epicentre of the SARS-CoV-2 epidemic: an observational cohort study. Lancet 2020;395(10239):1771–8.
46. Young TK, Shaw KS, Shah JK, et al. Mucocutaneous manifestations of multisystem inflammatory syndrome in children during the COVID-19 pandemic. JAMA Dermatol 2020;157(2):207–12.
47. McCrindle BW, Rowley AH, Newburger JW, et al. Diagnosis, treatment, and long-term management of Kawasaki disease: a scientific statement for health professionals from the American Heart Association. Circulation 2017;135(17):e927–99.
48. Whittaker E, Bamford A, Kenny J, et al. Clinical characteristics of 58 children with a pediatric inflammatory multisystem syndrome temporally associated with SARS-CoV-2. JAMA 2020;324(3):259–69.
49. Lee PY, Day-Lewis M, Henderson LA, et al. Distinct clinical and immunological features of SARS-CoV-2-induced multisystem inflammatory syndrome in children. J Clin Invest 2020;130(11):5942–50.
50. Diorio C, Henrickson SE, Vella LA, et al. Multisystem inflammatory syndrome in children and COVID-19 are distinct presentations of SARS-CoV-2. J Clin Invest 2020;130(11):5967–75.
51. Dionne A, Mah DY, Son MBF, et al. Atrioventricular block in children with multisystem inflammatory syndrome. Pediatrics 2020;146(5). e2020009704.
52. Ouldali N, Toubiana J, Antona D, et al. Association of intravenous immunoglobulins plus methylprednisolone vs immunoglobulins alone with course of fever in multisystem inflammatory syndrome in children. JAMA 2021;325(9):855–64.
53. Belhadjer Z, Auriau J, Meot M, et al. Addition of corticosteroids to immunoglobulins is associated with recovery of cardiac function in multi-inflammatory syndrome in children. Circulation 2020;142(23):2282–4.
54. Aronoff SC, Hall A, Del Vecchio MT. The natural history of SARS-Cov-2 related multisystem inflammatory syndrome in children (MIS-C): a systematic review. J Pediatr Infect Dis Soc 2020;9(6):746–51.
55. Choi NH, Fremed M, Starc T, et al. MIS-C and cardiac conduction abnormalities. Pediatrics 2020;146(6). e2020009738.

UNITED STATES POSTAL SERVICE®

Statement of Ownership, Management, and Circulation
(All Periodicals Publications Except Requester Publications)

1. Publication Title: RHEUMATIC DISEASE CLINICS OF NORTH AMERICA

2. Publication Number: 006 – 272

3. Filing Date: 9/18/2021

4. Issue Frequency: FEB, MAY, AUG, NOV

5. Number of Issues Published Annually: 4

6. Annual Subscription Price: $362.00

7. Complete Mailing Address of Known Office of Publication *(Not printer)* *(Street, city, county, state, and ZIP+4®)*
ELSEVIER INC.
230 Park Avenue, Suite 800
New York, NY 10169

Contact Person: Malathi Samayan
Telephone *(Include area code)*: 91-44-4299-4507

8. Complete Mailing Address of Headquarters or General Business Office of Publisher *(Not printer)*
ELSEVIER INC.
230 Park Avenue, Suite 800
New York, NY 10169

9. Full Names and Complete Mailing Addresses of Publisher, Editor, and Managing Editor *(Do not leave blank)*

Publisher *(Name and complete mailing address)*
Dolores Meloni, ELSEVIER INC.
1600 JOHN F KENNEDY BLVD. SUITE 1800
PHILADELPHIA, PA 19103-2899

Editor *(Name and complete mailing address)*
LAUREN BOYLE, ELSEVIER INC.
1600 JOHN F KENNEDY BLVD. SUITE 1800
PHILADELPHIA, PA 19103-2899

Managing Editor *(Name and complete mailing address)*
PATRICK MANLEY, ELSEVIER INC.
1600 JOHN F KENNEDY BLVD. SUITE 1800
PHILADELPHIA, PA 19103-2899

10. Owner *(Do not leave blank. If the publication is owned by a corporation, give the name and address of the corporation immediately followed by the names and addresses of all stockholders owning or holding 1 percent or more of the total amount of stock. If not owned by a corporation, give the names and addresses of the individual owners. If owned by a partnership or other unincorporated firm, give its name and address as well as those of each individual owner. If the publication is published by a nonprofit organization, give its name and address.)*

Full Name	Complete Mailing Address
WHOLLY OWNED SUBSIDIARY OF REED/ELSEVIER, US HOLDINGS	1600 JOHN F KENNEDY BLVD, SUITE 1800 PHILADELPHIA, PA 19103-2899

11. Known Bondholders, Mortgagees, and Other Security Holders Owning or Holding 1 Percent or More of Total Amount of Bonds, Mortgages, or Other Securities. If none, check box ► ☐ None

Full Name	Complete Mailing Address
N/A	

12. Tax Status *(For completion by nonprofit organizations authorized to mail at nonprofit rates)* *(Check one)*
The purpose, function, and nonprofit status of this organization and the exempt status for federal income tax purposes:
☒ Has Not Changed During Preceding 12 Months
☐ Has Changed During Preceding 12 Months *(Publisher must submit explanation of change with this statement)*

PS Form **3526**, July 2014 *[Page 1 of 4 (see instructions page 4)]* PSN: 7530-01-000-9931 PRIVACY NOTICE: See our privacy policy on www.usps.com.

---

13. Publication Title: RHEUMATIC DISEASE CLINICS OF NORTH AMERICA

14. Issue Date for Circulation Data Below: MAY 2021

15. Extent and Nature of Circulation

			Average No. Copies Each Issue During Preceding 12 Months	No. Copies of Single Issue Published Nearest to Filing Date
a. Total Number of Copies *(Net press run)*			179	165
b. Paid Circulation *(By Mail and Outside the Mail)*	(1)	Mailed Outside-County Paid Subscriptions Stated on PS Form 3541 *(Include paid distribution above nominal rate, advertiser's proof copies, and exchange copies)*	85	79
	(2)	Mailed In-County Paid Subscriptions Stated on PS Form 3541 *(Include paid distribution above nominal rate, advertiser's proof copies, and exchange copies)*	0	0
	(3)	Paid Distribution Outside the Mails Including Sales Through Dealers and Carriers, Street Vendors, Counter Sales, and Other Paid Distribution Outside USPS®	56	51
	(4)	Paid Distribution by Other Classes of Mail Through the USPS *(e.g., First-Class Mail®)*	0	0
c. Total Paid Distribution *(Sum of 15b (1), (2), (3), and (4))* ►			141	130
d. Free or Nominal Rate Distribution *(By Mail and Outside the Mail)*	(1)	Free or Nominal Rate Outside-County Copies included on PS Form 3541	24	21
	(2)	Free or Nominal Rate In-County Copies Included on PS Form 3541	0	0
	(3)	Free or Nominal Rate Copies Mailed at Other Classes Through the USPS *(e.g. First-Class Mail)*	0	0
	(4)	Free or Nominal Rate Distribution Outside the Mail *(Carriers or other means)*	0	0
e. Total Free or Nominal Rate Distribution *(Sum of 15d (1), (2), (3) and (4))* ►			24	21
f. Total Distribution *(Sum of 15c and 15e)* ►			165	151
g. Copies not Distributed *(See Instructions to Publishers #4 (page 3))* ►			14	14
h. Total *(Sum of 15f and g)* ►			179	165
i. Percent Paid *(15c divided by 15f times 100)* ►			85.45%	86.09%

* If you are claiming electronic copies, go to line 16 on page 3. If you are not claiming electronic copies, skip to line 17 on page 3.

16. Electronic Copy Circulation

	Average No. Copies Each Issue During Preceding 12 Months	No. Copies of Single Issue Published Nearest to Filing Date
a. Paid Electronic Copies ►		
b. Total Paid Print Copies (Line 15c) + Paid Electronic Copies (Line 16a) ►		
c. Total Print Distribution (Line 15f) + Paid Electronic Copies (Line 16a) ►		
d. Percent Paid (Both Print & Electronic Copies) (16b divided by 16c × 100) ►		

☒ I certify that 50% of all my distributed copies (electronic and print) are paid above a nominal price.

17. Publication of Statement of Ownership
☒ If the publication is a general publication, publication of this statement is required. Will be printed in the NOVEMBER 2021 issue of this publication. ☐ Publication not required.

18. Signature and Title of Editor, Publisher, Business Manager, or Owner

Malathi Samayan - Distribution Controller

Malathi Samayan

Date: 9/18/2021

I certify that all information furnished on this form is true and complete. I understand that anyone who furnishes false or misleading information on this form or who omits material or information requested on the form may be subject to criminal sanctions (including fines and imprisonment) and/or civil sanctions (including civil penalties).

PS Form **3526**, July 2014 (Page 3 of 4) PRIVACY NOTICE: See our privacy policy on www.usps.com.

Printed and bound by CPI Group (UK) Ltd, Croydon, CR0 4YY

08/05/2025

01864713-0004